CRC SERIES IN AGING

Editors-in-Chief

Richard C. Adelman, Ph.D.
Executive Director
Institute on Aging
Temple University
Philadelphia, Pennsylvania

George S. Roth, Ph.D.
Research Chemist
Gerontology Research Center
National Institute on Aging
Baltimore City Hospitals
Baltimore, Maryland

HANDBOOK OF BIOCHEMISTRY IN AGING
Editor
James Florini, Ph.D.
Department of Biology
Syracuse University
Syracuse, New York

HANDBOOK OF IMMUNOLOGY IN AGING
Editors
Marguerite M. B. Kay, M.D. and
Takashi Makinodan, Ph.D.
Geriatric Research Education and Clinical Center
V.A. Wadsworth Medical Center
Los Angeles, California

SENESCENCE IN PLANTS
Editor
Kenneth V. Thimann, Ph.D.
The Thimann Laboratories
University of California
Santa Cruz, California

HANDBOOK OF PHYSIOLOGY IN AGING
Editor
Edward J. Masoro, Ph.D.
Department of Physiology
University of Texas
Health Science Center
San Antonio, Texas

IMMUNOLOGICAL TECHNIQUES APPLIED TO AGING RESEARCH
Editors
William H. Adler, M.D. and
Albert A. Nordin, Ph.D.
Gerontology Research Center
National Institute on Aging
Baltimore City Hospitals
Baltimore, Maryland

CURRENT TRENDS IN MORPHOLOGICAL TECHNIQUES
Editor
John E. Johnson, Jr., Ph.D.
Gerontology Research Center
National Institute on Aging
Baltimore City Hospitals
Baltimore, Maryland

Additional topics to be covered in this series include Cell Biology of Aging, Microbiology of Aging, Pharmacology of Aging, Evolution and Genetics, Animal Models for Aging Research, Hormonal Regulatory Mechanisms, Detection of Altered Proteins, Insect Models, Lower Invertebrate Models, Testing the Theories of Aging, and Nutritional Approaches to Aging Research.

CRC Handbook of Biochemistry in Aging

Editor

James R. Florini, Ph.D.
Professor of Biochemistry
Biology Department
Syracuse University
Syracuse, New York

CRC Series in Aging

Editors-in-Chief

Richard C. Adelman, Ph.D.
Executive Director
Institute on Aging
Temple University
Philadelphia, Pennsylvania

George S. Roth, Ph.D.
Research Chemist
Gerontology Research Center
National Institute on Aging
Baltimore City Hospitals
Baltimore, Maryland

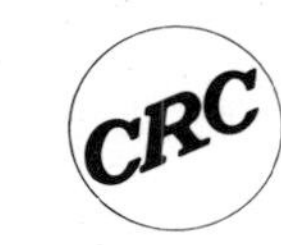

CRC Press, Inc.
Boca Raton, Florida

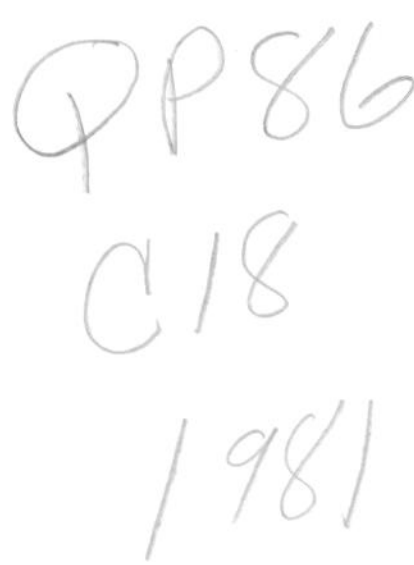

Library of Congress Cataloging in Publication Data

Main entry under title:

CRC handbook of biochemistry in aging.

(CRC series in aging)
Bibliography: p.
Includes index.
1. Aging. 2. Biological chemistry. I. Florini, James Ralph, 1931- II. Title: Handbook of biochemistry in aging. III. Series. DNLM: 1. Genetics, Biochemical. 2. Aging. 3. Hormones—Pharmacodynamics. 4. Cells—Physiology. WI104 C104]
P86.C18 599.03'72 80-23060
ISBN 0-8493-3141-2

This book represents information obtained from authentic and highly regarded sources. Reprinted material is quoted with permission, and sources are indicated. A wide variety of references are listed. Every reasonable effort has been made to give reliable data and information, but the author and the publisher cannot assume responsibility for the validity of all materials or for the consequences of their use.

Direct all inquiries to CRC Press, Inc., 2000 N.W. 24th Street, Boca Raton, Florida 33431.

International Standard Book Number 0-8493-3141-2

Library of Congress Card Number 80-23060
Printed in the United States

PREFACE

This handbook has been assembled by a group of experienced biochemical gerontologists to serve as a reference book for beginners in the field and for those working on other aspects of aging related to the ones covered here. Like all other branches of science, gerontology has been limited by the availability of appropriate subjects and reliable techniques for the desired experiments. For example, most gerontologists agree that studies done with animals of unknown pathology and disease history are of questionable significance, but it is not necessarily true that *all* measurements made with these animals are not valid. Thus it has been difficult for the reviewers to determine which studies to include in the tabulations presented here. In general, we have tried to be comprehensive rather than narrowly selective; in the long run, each investigator must decide for himself what data he considers reliable. Wherever possible, we have presented some criteria on which such decisions might be based.

The handbook is organized to present first a consideration of the components and processes involved in gene expression. This is followed by sections on organ and tissue composition and function. Next the control of biological processes (particularly by hormones) is considered, and the book ends with an evaluation of current theories on the biology of aging by a pioneer in biological gerontology. Although acutely aware of the unavoidable deficiencies in this handbook, the authors and I hope that it will be useful to the rapidly growing number of investigators who share our interest in the biochemical changes associated with aging.

James R. Florini

EDITORS-IN-CHIEF

Dr. Richard C. Adelman is currently Executive Director of the Temple University Institute on Aging, Philadelphia, Pa., as well as Professor of Biochemistry in the Fels Research Institute of the Temple University College of Medicine. An active gerontologist for more than 10 years, he has achieved international prominence as a researcher, educator, and administrator. These accomplishments span a broad spectrum of activities ranging from the traditional disciplinary interests of the research biologist to the advocacy, implementation, and administration of multidisciplinary issues of public policy of concern to elderly people.

Dr. Adelman pursued his pre- and postdoctoral research training under the guidance of two prominent biochemists, each of whom is a member of the National Academy of Sciences: Dr. Sidney Weinhouse as Director of the Fels Research Institute, Temple University, and Dr. Bernard L. Horecker as Chairman of the Department of Molecular Biology, Albert Einstein College of Medicine, Bronx, N.Y. His accomplishments as a researcher can be expressed in at least the following ways. He is the author and/or editor of more than 70 publications, including original research papers in referred journals, review chapters, and books. His research efforts have been supported by grants from the National Institutes of Health for the past 10 years, at a current annual level of approximately $300,000. He continues to serve as an invited speaker at seminar programs, symposiums, and workshops all over the world. He is the recipient of the IntraScience Research Foundation Medalist Award, an annual research prize awarded by peer evaluation for major advances in newly emerging areas of the life sciences. He is the recipient of an Established Investigatorship of the American Heart Association.

As an educator, Dr. Adelman is also involved in a broad variety of activities. His role in research training consists of responsibility for pre- and postdoctoral students who are assigned specific projects in his laboratory. He teaches an Advanced Graduate Course on the Biology of Aging, lectures on biomedical aspects of aging to medical students, and is responsible for the biological component of the basic course in aging sponsored by the School of Social Administration. Training activities outside the University include membership in the Faculty of the National Institute on Aging summer course on the Biology of Aging; programs on the biology of aging for AAA's throughout Pennsylvania and Ohio; and the implementation and teaching of Biology of Aging for the Nonbiologist locally, for the Gerontology Society of America and other national organizations, as well as for the International Association of Gerontology.

Dr. Adelman has achieved leadership positions across equally broad areas. Responsibilities of this position include the integration of multidisciplinary programs in research, consultation and education, and health service, as well as advocacy for the University on all matters dealing with aging. He coordinates a city-wide consortium of researchers from Temple University, the Wistar Institute, the Medical College of Pennsylvania, Drexel University, and the Philadelphia Geriatric Center, conducting collaborative research projects, training programs, and symposiums. He was a past President of the Philadelphia Biochemists Club. He serves on the editorial boards of the *Journal of Gerontology, Mechanisms of Ageing and Development, Experimental Aging Research*, and *Gerontological Abstracts*. He was a member of the Biomedical Research Panel of the National Advisory Council of the National Institute on Aging. He chairs a subcommittee of the National Academy of Sciences Committee on Animal Models for Aging Research. As an active Fellow of the Gerontological Society of America, he is a past Chairman of the Biological Sciences section; a past Chairman of the Society Public Policy Committee for which he prepared Congressional testimony and represented the Society on the Leadership Council of the Coalition of National Aging Organizations; and is Secretary-Treasurer of the North American Executive

Committee of the International Association of Gerontology. Finally, as the highest testimony of his leadership capabilities, he continues to serve on National Advisory Committee which impact on diverse key issues dealing with the elderly. These include a 4-year appointment as a member of the NIH Study Section on Pathobiological Chemistry; the Executive Committee of the Health Resources Administration Project on publication of the recent edition of *Working with Older People — A Guide to Practice;* a recent appointment as reviewer of AOA applications fo Career Preparation Programs in Gerontology; and a 4-year appointment on the Veterans Administration Long-Term Care Advisor Council responsible for evaluating their program on Geriatric Research, Education, and Clinical Centers (GRECC).

Dr. George S. Roth is a Research Chemist at the Gerontology Research Center of the National Institute on Aging, Baltimore, Md. Dr. Roth received his B.S. in Biology from Villanova University in 1968 and his Ph.D. in Microbiology from Temple University School of Medicine in 1971. He received postdoctoral training in Biochemistry at the Fels Research Institute in Philadelphia, Pa. Since coming to NIA in 1972, Dr. Roth has also been affiliated with the Graduate Schools of Georgetown University and George Washington University, Washington, D.C.

He is an officer of the Gerontological Society of America, a co-editor of the CRC series, *Methods of Aging Research*, an associate editor of *Neurobiology of Aging*, and a referee for numerous other journals. Dr. Roth has published extensively in the area of hormone action and aging and has lectured throughout the world on this subject.

THE EDITOR

Dr. James R. Florini is currently Professor of Biochemistry in the Biology Department at Syracuse University. He was born in Gillespie, Ill., in 1931 and received a B.A. degree in chemistry from Blackburn College (Carlinville, Ill.) in 1953 and a Ph.D. in biochemistry from the University of Illinois (Urbana) in 1956. Upon completion of his graduate training, he joined the research staff at the Lederle Laboratories division of American Cyanamid where he worked initially on the action and metabolism of glucocorticoids, and subsequently on the mechanisms and control of muscle protein synthesis. In 1966, he moved to his present location where his research has continued to emphasize the biochemical endocrinology of muscle growth and differentiation.

As a result of his participation in an NIH-sponsored course on tissue culture and aging at the W. Alton Jones Cell Science Center in 1971, his recent research has concentrated on the control of muscle cell growth and differentiation in culture. His concurrent research on aging has involved age-related changes in protein and nucleic acid synthesis as well as in the levels and actions of the somatomedins (the hormones his group has found most active in stimulating growth and differentiation of muscle in culture).

Dr. Florini is a member of the American Society of Biological Chemists, the American Society for Cell Biology, the Gerontological Society of America, the Endocrine Society, and the Tissue Culture Association. He has served as Program Committee Co-Chairman and is currently Chairman-elect of the Biological Sciences Section of the Gerontological Society of America, Chairman of the Education Committee of the Tissue Culture Association, and as a member of various other professional committees. He is currently a member of the Pathobiological Chemistry Study Section (NIH) and the Muscular Dystrophy Association's Postdoctoral Fellowship Review Subcommittee. He has chaired Gordon Research Conference on Hormone Action (1969) and Biology of Aging (1980).

Dr. Florini's outside interests center on aviation and music. He is a licensed commercial pilot and flight instructor and has served as president of both the Central New York Pilots Association and the Syracuse Flying Club. His interests in music involve choral singing and harpsichords building; his home is currently crowded by four harpsichords and one clavichord, and the office in which this volume was assembled contains a small fretted clavichord which was rather sadly neglected while work was being done on the CRC Handbook.

ADVISORY BOARD

CONTRIBUTORS

Charles H. Barrows, Jr.
Head, Section on Comparative Nutrition
Gerontology Research Center
Baltimore City Hospitals
Baltimore, Maryland

Kerry L. Dearfield
Research Associate
Laboratory of Environmental and Radiological Hazard Research
Department of Radiology and Pharmacology
George Washington University School of Medicine and Health Sciences
Washington, D.C.

Henry Donato, Jr.
Assistant Professor
Department of Chemistry
Southern Methodist University
Dallas, Texas

Richard G. Hansford
Research Chemist
Gerontology Research Center
National Institute on Aging
National Institutes of Health
Baltimore City Hospitals
Baltimore, Maryland

Gertrude C. Kokkonen
Research Biochemist
Gerontology Research Center
Baltimore City Hospitals
Baltimore, Maryland

Sharon W. Krauss
Senior Fellow of the American Cancer Society
Department of Biochemistry
University of California
Berkeley, Califofnia

Laura L. Mays
Gerontology Research Center
Baltimore City Hospitals
Baltimore, Maryland

Anna E. Miller
Research Associate
Department of Physiology
Michigan State University
East Lansing, Michigan

Mark F. Obenrader
Temple University Institute on Aging
School of Medicine
Philadelphia, Pennsylvania

Arlan Richardson
Professor
Department of Chemistry
Illinois State University
Normal, Illinois

Gail D. Riegle
Professor of Physiology and Animal Husbandry
Department of Physiology
Michigan State University
East Lansing, Michigan

Morton Rothstein
Professor
Cell and Molecular Biology
State University of New York
Buffalo, New York

James L. Sartin
Fels Research Institute
School of Medicine
Philadelphia, Pennsylvania

Edward L. Schneider
Associate Director for Biomedical Research and Clinical Medicine
National Institute on Aging
National Institutes of Health
Bethesda, Maryland

Sarah Seifert
Postdoctoral Fellow
Department of Biology
Syracuse University
Syracuse, New York

Nathan W. Shock
Scientist Emeritus
Gerontology Research Center
National Institute on Aging
Baltimore City Hospitals
Baltimore, Maryland

R. S. Sohal
Professor
Department of Biology
Southern Methodist University
Dallas, Texas

Marvin L. Tanzer
Professor
Department of Biochemistry
University of Connecticut Health Center
Farmington, Connecticut

J. Herbert Waite
Assistant Professor
Division of Orthopaedic Surgery
University of Connecticut Health Center
Farmington, Connecticut

Jerry R. Williams
Research Professor
Department of Radiology and Pharmacology
George Washington University
School of Medicine and Health Sciences
Washington, D.C.

Patricia D. Wilson
Research Fellow
Department of Cellular Pathology
Imperial Cancer Research Fund
London, England

TABLE OF CONTENTS

Gene Expression

Replication and Repair

DNA REPLICATION IN AGING

Sharon Wald Krauss

Genomic DNA is synthesized by DNA polymerases during the S phase of the cell cycle and during cellular repair processes. These enzymes synthesize DNA in the 5′ → 3′ direction in the presence of deoxynucleoside triphosphates, a divalent cation, and a DNA template-primer. Eukaryotic replicative synthesis probably is a discontinuous process (as in prokaryotes) in which short pieces of DNA are synthesized, processed, and ligated.

Currently, there are three generally accepted classes of eukaryotic DNA polymerases: α, β, and γ.[1-3] These are distinguished by their size, their ability to copy various synthetic template-primers, and their sensitivities to agents such as N-ethyl-maleimide, KCl, phosphate, 2′:3′ dideoxythymidine-5′-triphosphate, and aphidicolin. The α and β classes are heterogeneous in many systems, and γ has also been isolated in several forms. Mitochondria contain a polymerase activity which is closely related to or identical with the γ activity of the cytoplasm after aqueous extraction.[4] The properties previously associated with a unique mitochondrial polymerase appear to be attributable to mycoplasma present in the tissue culture samples. Thus, in studies of DNA polymerases from cultured cells, it is imperative to rigorously test for the presence of this common contaminant.

The precise roles of the α, β, and γ polymerases in DNA replication or repair have not been determined due to a lack of well-defined mutants. Instead, polymerase activities have been correlated with stimulation of rapid DNA synthesis, phases of the cell cycle in synchronized populations, or developmental stages. Such observations suggest that α polymerase participates directly in cellular DNA replication, and that β polymerase may have the major role in repair processes.[1-3,5] However, recent studies with the α inhibitor aphidicolin indicate that α polymerase also may be involved in some types of repair.[6] The only polymerase present in mitochondria, γ polymerase, presumably is responsible for mitochondrial DNA synthesis.

In addition to DNA polymerase, other enzymes and protein factors are necessary for replicative synthesis. Some of these (such as ligases, primases, unwinding proteins, and initiation activities) have been isolated and partially characterized. Recently, Brun and Weissbach[7] have reconstructed a system from HeLa nuclei components which in vitro can support several of the initial phases of the in vivo replicative process.

Research on changes in DNA replication during aging stems largely from three types of observations.

1. Untransformed cell cultures (such as WI-38, IMR-90, and MRC-5) show increased population doubling times and eventual cessation of cell division (phase III) with serial passaging.[8]
2. When cells from patient or animal explants are cultured, the population doublings remaining correlate inversely with the age of the donor.[8,9]
3. Changes in the kinetics of the cell cycle occur during aging.[10]

Data on age-associated changes in cell division times are summarized in Table 1. Information on age-associated changes in the induction of DNA synthesis is presented in Table 2. Note that it is sometimes unclear whether the DNA synthesis observed is due to replication and/or repair. Finally, experiments reporting age-associated effects on DNA polymerase function are listed in Table 3. Age-associated changes in the fidelity of DNA polymerases perhaps are more relevant to an understanding of cellular

Table 1
PERTURBATIONS OF CELL CYCLE DURING AGING

System employed	Observations and conclusions	Ref.
Mouse duodenal epithial cells and crypt cells	Length of cell cycle increased with age	16—18
Mouse colon epithial cells	Length of cell cycle increased with age	19
Mouse alveolar cells	Mean generation times increased with age	20
Mouse ear epithial cells	Mitotic index decreased with age	21
Rat liver regeneration	Time to reach peak of [^{14}C]thymine incorporation into DNA increased with age; prereplicative phase of cell cycle (G_0) increased with age	22
Rat salivary glands stimulated with isoproterenol	Prereplicative phase of cell cycle (G_0) increased with age	23
Human fetal lung fibroblasts	Senescent cultures have increased proportion of cells in G_1	24—26
	Interdivision time in late-passage cells is longer and more variable	27

Table 2
INDUCTION OF DNA SYNTHESIS DURING AGING

System employed	Observations and conclusions	Ref.
	Chemical Stimulation	
Human fetal lung fibroblasts	Cortisone and dihydrocortisone extend in vitro life span by about 20%	28—30
Rat salivary glands	Time course of isoproterenol-stimulated DNA synthesis varies with age; age-associated decrease in fraction of cells synthesizing DNA in response to isoproterenol	23
Human lymphocytes	Age-associated decrease in fraction of cells which divide after phytohemagglutinin stimulation	31
	Rate of thymidine incorporation after phytohemagglutinin is the same in young and old adults	32
Human fetal lung fibroblasts and human foreskin	Transformed cells isolated after prolonged cultivation following carcinogen exposure	33, 34
	Replication of DNA Viruses	
Human fetal lung fibroblasts	Polio, Herpes simplex, and VSV had no significant alteration in viral yield, heat stability, or mutant virus frequency when grown on late-passage cells	35
Human skin fibroblasts	VSV replication and yield on cells from old donors was not statistically different from cells of young donors	36

Table 2 (continued)
INDUCTION OF DNA SYNTHESIS DURING AGING

System employed	Observations and conclusions	Ref.
Cell Hybridizations or Fusions		
Human skin fibroblasts	Fusions between aged cells or young and senescent cells failed to produce viable hybrids; senescence is dominant	37
	DNA synthesis was inhibited in nuclei of low-passage cells when fused to postreplicative cells	12
Human fetal lung fibroblasts	In fusions between whole cells and enucleate cells, cytoplasmic factors did not appear to control in vitro cellular senescence	38, 39
Human skin fibroblasts	Doubling potential of hybrids between young and old cells is intermediate between that of the parents; regulation of life span is codominant	40
Human fetal lung fibroblasts	In fusions between karyoplasts and cytoplasts from old and young cells, a decreased number of cell divisions is observed with nuclei or cytoplasm from old cells; both nucleic and cytoplasmic factors from old cells can regulate young components	41
Human diploid fibroblasts	Reinitiation of DNA synthesis in senescent nuclei when fused to HeLa or SV40 transformed cells	42
Human skin fibroblasts	[^{3}H]thymidine incorporation in heterokaryons from fusions of postmitotic human diploid cells and a murine cell line; cells of unlimited proliferative capacity can stimulate DNA synthesis in senescent nuclei	43
Human fetal lung fibroblasts	Phase II, but not phase III nucleated or enucleated fibroblasts could reactivate chick erythrocyte nuclei; senescent cells lack factors necessary for reactivation	44

senescence than the age-associated decline of polymerase activity.[11] DNA polymerase activities which become "error-prone" could introduce changes in DNA base sequence both during replication of mitotic cell populations or in repair processes in mitotic and postmitotic cells. Such alterations, if expressed, may be deleterious to the cell.

The implication of a causal relationship between loss of cell division potential *in vitro* and cellular senescence is controversial for the following reasons:[8,10,12-14] first, subculturing may cause diploid cells to become refactory to further mitotic stimulation ("terminal differentiation" hypothesis); second, cell populations in vivo probably never reach the limit of their replicative potential; third, cells do not "die" in phase III and can be maintained in a viable nonproliferating state for prolonged periods; and fourth, nondividing ("fixed postmitotic") cells show age changes. Hayflick[15] has stressed that aging may be due to other functional decrements which occur prior to loss of ability to replicate, and that loss of cell division potential per se is a reflection of more universal genomic processes operating during senescence.

Table 3
DNA POLYMERIZATION DURING AGING

System employed	Observations and conclusions	Ref.
Human fetal lung fibroblasts	Length of grain tracks in DNA fiber autoradiography decreased at late passage; rate of DNA chain elongation is slower in senescent cells	45
Rat bone marrow cells	Analysis of BrdUrd-labeled cells indicated that populations from old rats replicate more slowly	46
Human lung fibroblasts	Fidelities in vitro of DNA polymerase activities from late-passage cells are decreased relative to those from early passage; amount of polymerase activity decreased with increasing passage	11
Human lymphocytes	α polymerases isolated after phytohemagglutinin stimulation of cells from young and old adults have similar fidelities; α polymerase from old adults was more thermolabile than that from young adults	32
Chick fibroblasts	α polymerases from senescent cells had altered heat lability, sensitivity to ribonucleoside triphosphates, KCl, NEM, and altered template-primer utilization; age-related alterations in enzymatic properties may reflect structural or conformational changes in α polymerases	47
Mouse liver	A low molecular weight DNA polymerase isolated from aged mice had decreased fidelity in vitro relative to enzyme from young adults	48

REFERENCES

1. **Bollum, F. J.**, Mammalian DNA polymerases, *Prog. Nucleic Acid Res. Mol. Biol.*, 15, 109, 1975.
2. **Weissbach, A.**, Eukaryotic DNA polymerases, in *Annu. Rev. Biochem.*, Vol. 46, Snell, E. S., Ed., Annual Reviews, Palo Alto, Calif., 1977, 25.
3. **Dube, D. K., Travaglini, E. C., and Loeb, L. A.**, Isolation and characterization of DNA polymerases from eukaryotic cells, in *Methods in Cell Biol. XIX*, Stein, G., Stein, J., and Kleinsmith, L. J., Eds., Academic Press, San Francisco, 1978, 27.
4. **Bolden, A., Pedrali-Noy, G., and Weissbach, A.**, DNA polymerase of mitochondria is a γ polymerase, *J. Biol. Chem.*, 252, 3351, 1977.
5. **Hübscher, U., Kuenzle, C., and Spardari, S.**, Functional roles of DNA polymerases β and γ, *Proc. Natl. Acad. Sci. U.S.A.*, 76, 2316, 1979.
6. **Hanaoka, F., Kata, H., Ikegami, S., Ohashi, M., and Yamada, M.**, Aphidicolin does inhibit repair replication, *Biochem. Biophys. Res. Commun.*, 87, 575, 1979.
7. **Brun, G. and Weissbach, A.**, Initiation of Hela cell DNA synthesis in a subnuclear system, *Proc. Natl. Acad. Sci. U.S.A.*, 75, 5931, 1978.
8. **Hayflick, L.**, The cellular basis for biological aging, in *Handbook of the Biology of Aging*, Finch, C. E. and Hayflick, L., Eds., Van Nostrand Reinhold, San Francisco, 1977, 159.
9. **Schneider, E. L. and Mitsui, Y.**, The relationship between *in vitro* cellular aging and *in vivo* human age, *Proc. Natl. Acad. Sci. U.S.A.*, 73, 3584, 1976.
10. **Baserga, R. L.**, Cell division and the cell cycle, in *Handbook of the Biology of Aging*, Finch, C. E. and Hayflick, L., Eds., Van Nostrand Reinhold, San Francisco, 1977, 101.
11. **Linn, S., Kairis, M., and Holliday, R.**, Decreased fidelity of DNA polymerase activity isolated from aging human fibroblasts, *Proc. Natl. Acad. Sci. U.S.A.*, 73, 2818, 1976.
12. **Martin, G. M., Sprague, C. A., Norwood, T. H., and Pendergrass, W. R.**, Clonal selection, attenuation, and differentiation in an *in vitro* model of hyperplasia, *Am. J. Pathol.*, 74, 137, 1974.
13. **Bell, E., Marek, L. F., Levinstone, D. S., Merrill, C., Sher, S., Young, I. T., and Eden, M.**, Loss of division potential *in vitro:* aging or differentiation?, *Science*, 202, 1158, 1978.
14. **Daniel, C.**, Cell longevity *in vivo*, in *Handbook of the Biology of Aging*, Finch, C. E. and Hayflick, L., Eds., Van Nostrand Reinhold, San Francisco, 1977, 122.
15. **Hayflick, L.**, Cell biology of aging, *Fed. Proc.*, 38, 1847, 1979.
16. **Lesher, S., Fry, R. J. M., and Kohn, H. I.**, Influence of age on the transit time of the mouse intestinal epithelium. I. Duodenum, *Lab. Invest.*, 10, 291, 1961.
17. **Lesher, S., Fry, R. J. M., and Kohn, H. I.**, Age and the generation time of the mouse duodenal cells, *Exp. Cell Res.*, 24, 334, 1961.
18. **Thrasher, J. D. and Greulich, R. C.**, The duodenal cell progenitor population. I. Age-related increase in the duration of the cryptal progenitor cycle, *J. Exp. Zool.*, 159, 39, 1965.
19. **Thrasher, J. D.**, Age and the cell cycle of the mouse colonic epithelium, *Anal. Rec.*, 157, 621, 1967.
20. **Simmet, J. D. and Hepplestone, A. G.**, Cell renewal in the mouse lung, *Lab. Invest.*, 15, 1793, 1966.
21. **Whiteley, H. T. and Horton, D. L.**, The effect of age on the mitotic activity of the ear epithelium in the CBA mouse, *J. Gerontol.*, 18, 335, 1963.
22. **Bucher, N. L. R.**, Regeneration of mammalian liver, *Int. Rev. Cytol.*, 15, 245, 1963.
23. **Adelman, R. C., Stein, G., Roth, G. S., and Englander, D.**, Age-dependent regulation of mammalian DNA synthesis and cell proliferation *in vivo*, *Mech. Aging Dev.*, 1, 49, 1972.
24. **Schneider, E. L. and Fowlkes, B. J.**, Measurement of DNA content and cell volume in senescent human fibroblasts utilizing flow multiparameter single cell analysis, *Exp. Cell Res.*, 98, 298, 1976.
25. **Yanishevsky, R. and Carrano, A. V.**, Prematurely condensed chromosomes of dividing and nondividing cells in aging human cell culture, *Exp. Cell Res.*, 90, 169, 1975.
26. **Yanishevsky, R., Mendelsohn, M. L., Mayall, B. H., and Cristofalo, V. J.**, Proliferative capacity and DNA content of aging human diploid cells in culture: a cytophotometric and autoradiographic analysis, *J. Cell. Physiol.*, 84, 165, 1974.
27. **Absher, R. M., Absher, R. G., and Barnes, W. D.**, Geneology of clones of diploid fibroblasts, *Exp. Cell Res.*, 88, 95, 1974.
28. **Macieira-Coelho, A.**, Action of cortisone on human fibroblasts *in vitro*, *Experientia*, 22, 390, 1966.
29. **Cristofalo, V. J.**, Metabolic aspects of aging in diploid human cells, in *Aging in Cell and Tissue Culture*, Holečková, E. and Cristofalo, V. J., Eds., Plenum Press, New York, 1970, 83.
30. **Bilgin, B. A. and Cristofalo, V. J.**, Effect of hydrocortisone on the transition probability of WI-38 cells during aging, *In Vitro*, 14, 359, 1978.
31. **Oh, Y. H. and Conard, R. A.**, Effect of aging on thymidine incorporation in nuclei of lymphocytes stimulated with phytohemmagglutinin, *Life Sci.*, 11, 677, 1972.

32. **Agarwal, S. S., Tuffner, M., and Loeb, L. A.,** DNA replication in human lymphocytes during aging, *J. Cell. Physiol.,* 96, 235, 1978.
33. **Milo, G. E. and Di Poalo, J. A.,** Neoplastic transition of human diploid cells *in vitro* after chemical carcinogen treatment, *Nature,* 275, 130, 1978.
34. **Kakunaga, T.,** Neoplastic transformation of human diploid fibroblast cells by chemical carcinogens, *Proc. Natl. Acad. Sci. U.S.A.,* 75, 1334, 1978.
35. **Holland, J. J., Koline, D., and Doyle, M. V.,** Analysis of viral replication in aging human fibroblasts, *Nature,* 245, 316, 1973.
36. **Danner, D. B., Schneider, E. L., and Pitha, J.,** Macromolecular synthesis in human diploid fibroblasts: a viral probe examining the effect of *in vivo* aging, *Exp. Cell Res.,* 114, 63, 1978.
37. **Littlefield, J. W.,** Attempted hybridization with senescent human fibroblasts, *J. Cell. Physiol.,* 82, 129, 1973.
38. **Wright, W. E. and Hayflick, L.,** Contribution of cytoplasmic factors to *in vitro* cellular senescence, *Fed. Proc.,* 34, 76, 1975.
39. **Wright, W. E. and Hayflick, L.,** Nuclear control of cellular aging demonstrated by hubridization of anuclear and whole cultured normal human fibroblasts, *Exp. Cell Res.,* 96, 113, 1975.
40. **Hoehn, H., Bryant, E. M., and Martin, G. M.,** The replicative life span of euploid hybrids derived from short-lived and long-lived human skin fibroblast cultures, *Cytogenet. Cell Genet.,* 21, 282, 1978.
41. **Muggleton-Harris, A. and Hayflick, L.,** Cellular aging studied by the reconstruction of replicating cells from nuclei and cytoplasms isolated from normal human diploid cells, *Exp. Cell Res.,* 103, 321, 1976.
42. **Norwood, T. H., Pendergrass, W. R., and Martin, G. M.,** Reinitiation of DNA synthesis in senescent human fibroblasts upon fusion with cells of unlimited growth potential, *J. Cell Biol.,* 64, 551, 1975.
43. **Norwood, T. H., Rabinovitch, P. S., and Zeigler, C. J.,** Complementation in heterokaryons derived from a thymidine kinase deficient cell line and senescent human diploid cells, *Fed. Proc.,* 38, 1868, 1979.
44. **Roa, M. V.,** Reactivation of chick erythrocyte nuclei in young and senescent WI-38 cells, *Exp. Cell Res.,* 102, 25, 1976.
45. **Petes, T. D., Farber, R. A., Tarrant, G. M., and Holliday, R.,** Altered rate of DNA replication in ageing human fibroblast cultures, *Nature,* 251, 434, 1974.
46. **Schneider, E. L.,** Cell replication and aging: *in vitro* and *in vivo* studies, *Fed. Proc.,* 38, 1857, 1979.
47. **Fry, M., and Weisman-Shomer, P.,** Altered nuclear deoxyribonucleic acid α polymerases in senescent cultured chick embryo fibroblasts, *Biochemistry,* 15, 4319, 1976.
48. **Barton, R. W., Waters, L. C., and Young, W. K.,** *In vitro* synthesis by low-molecular-weight DNA polymerases: increased infidelity associated with aging, *Fed. Proc.,* 34(Abstr. 1102), 1419, 1974.

CELLULAR EFFECTS OF AGE-RELATED CHANGES IN DNA REPLICATION

Edward L. Schneider

INTRODUCTION

This section will be divided into two major areas: studies of cellular replication in vitro (chiefly, human diploid cell cultures) and in vivo studies of laboratory rodent cell populations. It is hoped that information gained from these complementary systems will be applicable to human cellular aging in vivo.

Unfortunately, there is a dearth of substantial laboratory observations on the effect of aging on replicating cell populations in vivo. One of the most well-defined changes with aging in humans and other mammals is a decline in the function of the immunological system. This decline can be seen at the cellular level as the decreased ability of immune cells to mount an effective response to antigen challenge.[1-3] Diminished immune response can have several possible components: decreased recognition of the antigen, failure to stimulate cells to replicate, decline in the replication rate of the stimulated cells, and diminished functional ability of the replicated cell population. Although it is difficult to discriminate between all these components of in vivo immune response, Albright and Makinodan[4] found that a decline in cellular proliferation does appear to play a role in the decreased immune response found with aging.

It has been reported that red blood cell counts[5] and hematocrits[6] are diminished with aging. However, recent studies indicate that at least in the laboratory mouse, the ability to respond to anemic stress may not be seriously impaired as a function of aging.[7]

The dermal fibroblast is another proliferating cell which has been reported to decline in function with aging. Decreased dermal fibroblast replication may be responsible for the delay in wound healing that has been reported to occur with aging.[8] Unfortunately, there is little data to support this observation other than the general observations of surgeons. Recently, Grove and his co-workers[9] have developed quantitative dermatologic assays for measuring wound healing. Their preliminary findings suggest a significant decline in the kinetics of wound healing with human aging.

It is important to think in terms of alterations in cellular proliferation with aging instead of merely decreased replication. Although this section of the handbook will focus on evidence for decreased cellular replication in both in vivo and in vitro replicating cell populations, an increase in cellular replication may occur with aging in certain cell populations. Among the cell populations whose replication rate may increase with aging are the smooth muscle cells in arterial walls and prostatic cells.

Finally, it is well-known that aging is related to an increased incidence of altered cell replication manifested by a variety of malignancies. Although enormous energies have been expanded in delineating the mechanisms of malignant transformation, little attention has been given to the changes at the cellular level with aging which predispose to malignant alterations.

IN VITRO STUDIES

Total Replicative Capabilities — The Hayflick Phenomenon

Initial studies of the behavior of cells in tissue culture indicated that the constraints of mortality were removed in tissue culture.[10,11] Cell populations, once established in tissue culture, appeared able to be propagated indefinitely. Therefore, the reports by

Table 1
EFFECT OF SERIAL IN VITRO PASSAGE ON CELL REPLICATION PARAMETERS

Observation	Ref.
Decreased replicating cells in the cell population	16
Increased percent slowly replicating cells	17 18
Increased modal cell volumes	20 21
Increased frequency of G_1 cells	22 23 24
Increased heterogeneity of cell replication times	27 28
Diminished replicative potential of individual cells	29 31

Swim and Parker[12] and Hayflick and Moorhead[13] that human diploid cells had a finite in vitro life span were greeted with great skepticism. However, in a series of elegant experiments, Hayflick demonstrated that the limited proliferative capability of human fetal lung fibroblasts was not due to any trivial explanation. After a period of sustained rapid replication, human diploid cell replication slows, and then is arrested. Indeed, with only a few interesting exceptions, this onset of cell culture senescence and limited in vitro life span have been confirmed in a wide variety of human diploid cells in numerous laboratories through the world.

Metabolic vs. Calendar Time

What is the determinant of the limited proliferative ability of human diploid fibroblasts in tissue culture? Is it the total number of DNA replication cycles or the length of time in tissue culture? Hayflick demonstrated that when cell populations were frozen and preserved in liquid nitrogen at various levels of their in vitro life span and then returned to tissue culture, the total cumulative number of cell population replications remained unchanged.[14] More recently, Dell'Orco et al. have shown that when human diploid fibroblasts are maintained in a nondividing state with low serum concentrations and then returned to conditions favoring cell replication, their in vitro life span is dependent on the number of cell population doublings previously attained, rather than the total time in tissue culture.[15] Therefore, regulation of the total replicative capacity of human fibroblasts is independent of calendar time, and dependent on the previous numbers of DNA replications.

Cell Population Kinetics

In contrast to the relatively homogenous nature of cellular replication in established or permanent cell lines, individual cell replication is quite variable in human diploid cell cultures. This has been demonstrated by a variety of different approaches. The effect of serial in vitro passage on several cell replication parameters is summarized in Table 1.

Percent replicating cells — Utilizing tritiated thymidine labeling of cell cultures for 48 hr followed by autoradiography, Cristofalo and Sharf[16] demonstrated that the number of rapidly replicating cells in the cell population diminishes as a function of in vitro passage. This technique has been subssquently utilized to identify the passage level of certain human fetal lung fibroblast cell cultures. Initially, it was suggested that cells that did not replicate under these conditions were nonreplicating. However, when labeling periods were extended well past 48 hr, it was shown that most of the nonlabeled cells at 48 hr were slowly replicating cells.[17,18] Another approach to measuring the percent of rapidly replicating cells is by incubating cells with bromodeoxyuridine (BrdU) and determining the number of cell nuclei with depressed fluorescent labeling after staining with fluorescent DNA stains.[19]

Cell volume — With increasing in vitro serial passage, a substantial increase is observed in the cell volumes of human diploid cells.[20,21] This increase in cell volume appears to be closely related to the increased replication times of these cells. Thus, large cells comprise the slowly dividing or nondividing cells, while small cells are rapidly replicating cells. Flow microfluorometric analyses have demonstrated that slowly replicating cells in G1 as well as G2 are enlarged at late passage.[22]

Cell cycle — Flow microfluorometric[22] and microdensitometric[23,24] analyses have revealed that with increasing in vitro passage, an increasing proportion of the cell population accumulates in the G1 phase of the cell cycle, and a corresponding decrease is seen in the percent of cells in the G2 and S phases of the cell cycle.

Cell separation studies — Since large cells accumulate with in vitro passage and are slowly or nondividing cells, removal of these cells from a culture by physical means might be expected to affect the proliferative capacity of a cell culture. Cells from late passage cultures can be readily separated on the basis of volume by velocity sedimentation at 1 g. Cell fractions can be obtained from senescent cell populations that are comprised of approximately 99% small, rapidly replicating cells.[25] However, upon return of these cells to tissue culture, they rapidly return to the characteristics of an unfractionated cell population; they have no substantial increase in proliferative rate,[25] cloning capabilities, or in vitro life span.[26] Similarly, cell fractions enriched for large, nondividing or slow dividing cells quickly returned to the characteristics of the unfractionated cell population.

Microcinematographic analysis of in vitro proliferation — Microcinematographic analyses of cells at late in vitro passage reveal enormous heterogeneity of cell replication times[27,28] when compared to cell cultures at early passage. These investigations also demonstrated that large, apparently nonreplicating cells can quickly return to small cells and reinitiate replication.

Clonal Analysis of Cellular Replication

Most studies of fetal lung fibroblasts were conducted on cell populations. However, it is equally important to examine the behavior of individual cells. The most comprehensive work in this area has been conducted by Smith and Hayflick and Martin et al.[29-31] They observed that even in early passage cell cultures, individual cells had markedly different proliferative capabilities. While some cells possessed extensive proliferative capabilities, others had severely limited replicative abilities. With increasing passage, fewer cells have substantial remaining proliferative capabilities. In fact, the number of cells able to form colonies with 16 or more cells (4 doublings) is an excellent indicator of the remaining in vitro life span of a cell culture.[30]

Somatic Cell Genetic Analysis Of The Lost Proliferative Capacity Of Senescent Cells

The development of the field of somatic cell genetics has led to the creation of new techniques for examining the mechanisms of the decline in cellular proliferation that occurs as a function of the in vitro serial passage of human diploid cells. Several of these techniques have been applied to this problem.

Heterokaryon analysis — This technique involves the fusion of two cells, and the analysis of the product of the fusion — the heterokaryon. Measurement of DNA syn-

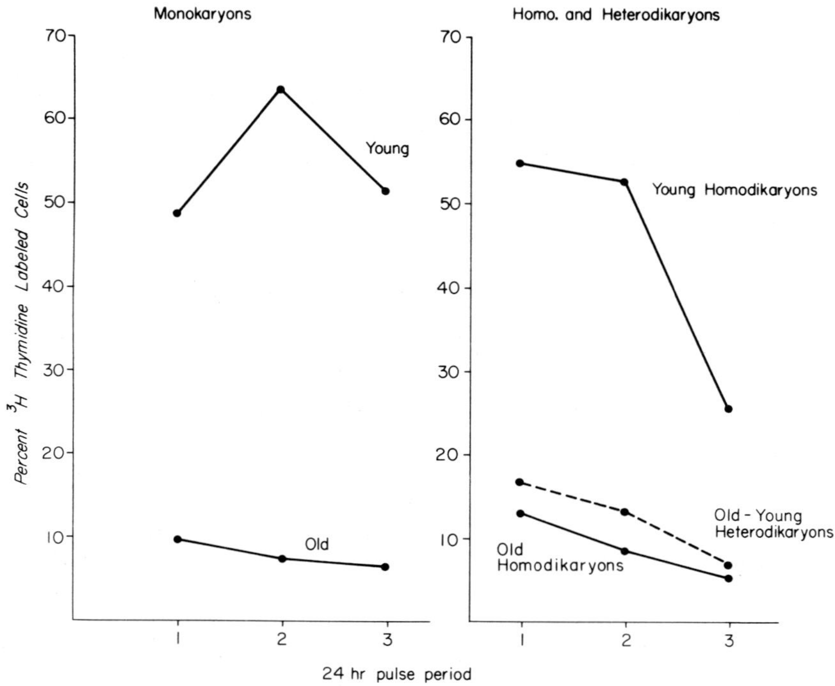

FIGURE 1. ^{3}H-TdR labeling indexes of human diploid cell mono-, homo-, and heterodikaryons following Sendai-virus-mediated cell fusion between senescent and low-passage, actively dividing human diploid cells of the same strain. The slightly higher labeling indexes of the old-young heterodikaryons in comparison with those of old homodikaryons are not significant. (From Martin, G. M., Sprague, C. A., Norwood, T. H., Pendergrass, W. R., Bornstein, P., Hoehn, H., and Arend, W. P., *Adv. Exp. Med. Biol.*, 53, 67, 1975. With permission.)

thesis in heterokaryons made from early passage and senescent human diploid fibroblasts revealed that the senescent nucleus inhibited DNA synthesis in the early passage cell nucleus (Figure 1).[31] The senescent nucleus did not appear to be stimulated by the presence of the early passage nucleus. Heterokaryons have also been prepared from senescent human diploid fibroblasts and aneuploid permanent cell lines.[32,33] However, these studies had different outcomes. Fusion of senescent human diploid cells with Hela cells resulted in stimulation of DNA synthesis in the senescent nucleus,[32] while fusion of senescent cells with T98G human glioblastoma cells resulted in failure to stimulate DNA synthesis in the senescent nucleus.[33] This apparent discordance may be due to differences between the two aneuploid permanent cell strains used in these studies.

Synkaryon analysis — Synkaryons are formed from the fusion of the two nuclei of the heterokaryon, and can lead to production of proliferating hybrid cells. Many attempts have been made to fuse senescent and early passage cells, and to examine the resultant hybrid. After exhaustive attempts, Littlefield was unable to produce a proliferative hybrid from these parental cell types.[34] Many other laboratories have tried, but also without success. This failure may reflect the dominant nature of the senescent phenotype indicated by the outcome of heterokaryon studies.

Enucleation studies — Another approach to the question of analyzing the senescent phenotype is through the enucleation of early passage and senescent cells. The resultant cytoplasts can then be fused with either whole cells or nucleoplasts (nuclei with residual cytoplasmic contaminants). Using these techniques, Wright and Hayflick[35] found the senescent phenotype to be determined by the cell nucleus rather than the cytoplasm. Utilizing a slightly different approach which involves micromanipulation, Muggleton-Harris and Hayflick[36] found that the cytoplasm may contribute to the senescent phenotype. Further studies are clearly necessary to discriminate between the contribution of the nucleus and cytoplasm to the inhibition of cellular replication that occurs as a function of in vitro passage.

Modulation of In Vitro Life Span (Total Proliferative Potential)

Several agents have been shown to be capable of modulating the in vitro life span of cultured cells. These agents include serum albumin,[37] corticosteroids,[38,39] and fetal bovine serum.[40] Although initial reports indicated that vitamin E could significantly lengthen in vitro life span,[41] subsequent reports indicate that the interaction of vitamin E and a particular serum lot were responsible for this effect.[42] In a study of the effect of in vivo human age on the in vitro life span of cultured human skin fibroblast cultures, Schneider et al. found that the batch of fetal bovine serum utilized played a crucial role in determining the length of the in vitro life span of these cell cultures.[40] Perhaps the most well-defined prolongation of life span is accomplished by hydrocortisone. However, this extension of life span may be limited to a specific cell type since hydrocortisone appears to severely inhibit acute and chronic cell replication in both adult and fetal skin fibroblast cultures.[43]

Relation of In Vitro Life Span to In Vivo Cellular Aging

Human Fibroblasts

Hayflick was the first to demonstrate that in vitro life span is related to the age of the cell culture donor. He demonstrated that lung fibroblast cultures derived from adult human lung tissues had significantly shorter in vitro life spans than fibroblast cultures derived from fetal lungs.[14] This relationship was further examined by Goldstein et al.[44] and Martin et al.[45] in skin fibroblast cultures derived from adult human donors of varying ages. These studies revealed a gradual decline in the in vitro life span of these cell cultures as a function of the age of the cell culture donor. This question has been further pursued, utilizing cell cultures derived from volunteer members of the Baltimore Longitudinal Study.[46] This group is comprised of relatively healthy male subjects, ages 20 to 95, who visit the Gerontology Research Center every 18 months for a comprehensive series of physiologic and psychologic studies. Therefore, this group of subjects is as close to an ideal population that can be currently obtained for studies of human biomedical aging. All cell cultures from these subjects were obtained from the same standardized site — the inner aspect of the left upper arm. This area was chosen because of its limited light exposure. All cell cultures were established and subcultured under identical protocols to minimize variations in tissue culture. In addition to measuring the total cumulative cell populations of each cell culture (in vitro life span), Schneider and Mitsui[46] also determined the number of cell populations that transpired between establishment of the culture and the onset of cell culture senescence. The results of these studies (summarized in Table 2) reveal that cell cultures derived from older human subjects had significantly earlier onsets of cell culture senescence and shorter in vitro life spans than parallel cultures obtained from young human subjects.[46]

Other Cell Systems

LeGuilly et al.[49] examined liver cell cultures (derived from post-mortem liver tissue) and found that those cultures derived from older subjects had significantly reduced in vitro life spans. Another cell type which has gained much recent attention is the cul-

Table 2
SUMMARY OF STUDIES OF CELLULAR REPLICATION CONDUCTED ON SKIN FIBROBLAST CULTURES DERIVED FROM YOUNG AND OLD HUMAN SUBJECTS[46]

Replication parameter	Young subjects (20—35 years)	Old subjects (65 + years)
Onset of senescent phase (PD)[a]	35.2 ± 2.1 (23)[b]	22.5 ± 1.7 (21)
In vitro life span (PD)	44.6 ± 2.5 (23)	33.6 ± 2.1 (21)
Cell population replication rate (hr)	20.8 ± 0.8 (18)	24.3 ± 0.9 (18)
Percent replicating cells[c]	87.7 ± 1.6 (7)	79.6 ± 2.5 (7)
Cell number at confluency (× 10^4 cells/cm^2)	7.31 ± 0.42 (18)	5.06 ± 0.52 (18)
Percent cells able to form colony > 16 cells[d]	69.0 ± 3.3 (9)	48.0 ± 4.4 (8)

[a] PD = population doublings.
[b] Numbers within parentheses indicate number of cell cultures examined. Values are mean ± standard error of the mean.
[c] Determined by incubating cells for 24 hr with tritiated thymidine and then measuring the frequency of labeled nuclei by autoradiography.
[d] Two weeks after plating at low cell densities.

tured human epidermal keratinocyte.[48] Although these investigators were not primarily concerned with the effect of aging, Rheinwald and Green found that cell cultures derived from newborns have considerably longer in vitro life spans than cultures derived from adults.[48]

Human Genetic Disorders Which Have Features Resembling Premature Aging

Cell cultures derived from patients with the two autosomal recessive human genetic disorders which have many features resembling premature aging — the Werner syndrome and progeria — had significantly reduced in vitro life spans.[45] In two more common disorders which have some features of premature aging — diabetes mellitus[44] and the Down syndrome[49] — significant decreases in in vitro life span were also observed. However, this author questions the importance of studies which show diminished in vitro life spans in conditions which have severe metabolic disturbances; emphasis should instead be placed on finding conditions which manifest increased in vitro life spans.

Acute Cell Replication and Aging

Human Skin Fibroblasts

In addition to examining the chronic replicative capacities of skin fibroblast cultures derived from members of the Baltimore Longitudinal Study, several determinations of acute replication have been performed.[46] These determinations were conducted at early in vitro passage on cells derived from young and old subjects well before the onset of cell culture senescence. The percent of rapidly replicating cells was determined by incubating cells with tritiated thymidine for 24 hr and then using autoradiography to enumerate the number of labeled nuclei (Table 2). Although the decline in percent of rapidly replicating cells with donor age is not of the magnitude observed as a function of in vitro serial passage ('' in vitro aging''), it is statistically significant.[46]

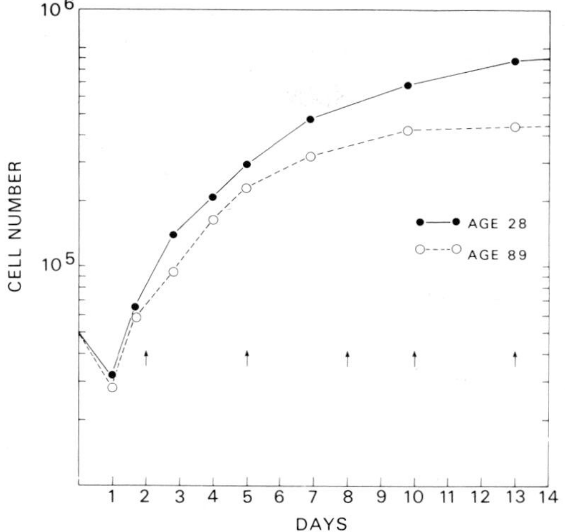

FIGURE 2. Cell population growth curves of skin fibroblast cultures derived from a young and an old donor. Arrows indicate change of medium. (From Grove, G., personal communication, 1979. With permission.)

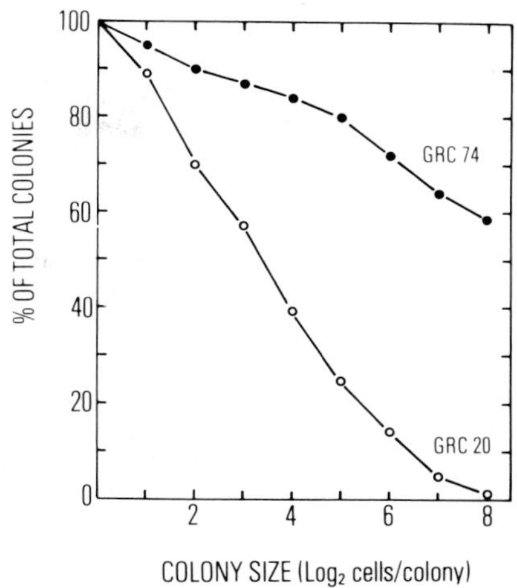

FIGURE 3. Percentage of colonies able to attain at least a specified size vs. colony size. Colony size is expressed as log of the number of cells per colony. Adult human skin cultures from a young (GRC74, age 33 years) and an old (GRC20, age 80 years) donor were cloned at the tenth PD in vitro. (From Hayflick, L., *Exp. Cell Res.*, 37, 614, 1965. With permission.)

Cell population replication rate and cell number at confluency were determined from young and old donor cell culture growth curves (Figure 2). The drop in cell number after transfer, sometimes referred to as the "plating efficiency", was similar in young and old donor cell cultures. Cell population doubling times were significantly longer in cell cultures derived from old human donors when compared to parallel cultures derived from young subjects (Table 2). The greatest difference between young and old donor cell cultures was in the cell number at confluency.[46] Cell cultures derived from young subjects had almost 50% higher cell numbers at confluency when compared to old subject cultures (Table 1).

Colony-size distributions of young and old donor subjects were also determined.[50] Typical colony-size distributions of cells derived from a young and old donor cell culture are seen in Figure 3. Note that while 60% of cloned young donor cells were able to form large colonies with over 256 cells (8 population doublings), only 2% of old donor cells have this replicative ability. When colony-size distributions from many young and old donor cell cultures were examined, a significantly greater number of cells from young donor cultures were able to reach a colony size of ≥16 cells (Table 2). Thus, under both mass culture conditions and as isolated colonies, cells derived from younger subjects had greater replicative abilities than cells from older subjects examined at the same early population doubling levels.

Human Lymphocytes

Although human peripheral lymphocytes do not normally replicate in tissue culture, they can be stimulated by several mitogens to commence DNA synthesis. It has been shown by several authors that lymphocyte cell cultures derived from older subjects have diminished replicative responses to stimulation by a T-cell mitogen — phytohemagglutinin (PHA) — when compared with cells derived from young subjects.[51-54] This decreased response is not due to a decline in T-cell number, but rather to intrinsic defects in the T cells of older subjects.[54,55]

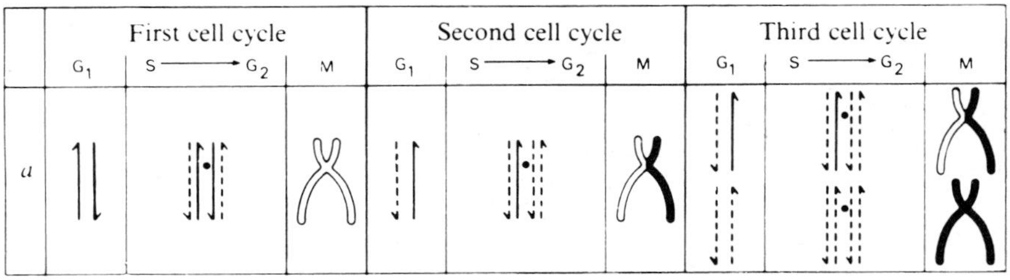

	First cell cycle			Second cell cycle			Third cell cycle		
	G_1	S ⟶ G_2	M	G_1	S ⟶ G_2	M	G_1	S ⟶ G_2	M
a									

FIGURE 4. Schema demonstrating the differential chromatid staining patterns of metaphase cells which have replicated in the presence of BrdU. Solid lines represent unsubstituted DNA while dashed lines represent BrdU-substituted DNA. White chromatid indicates bright fluorescent staining, while black chromatid indicates dull fluorescence.

The development of the BrdU differential chromatid staining techniques[56,57] permits the examination of cellular replication in vivo,[58] as well as in vitro.[59] This technique is based on the observation that BrdU containing DNA fluoresces less intensely than unsubstituted DNA. The schema presented in Figure 4 demonstrates how incubation of cells with BrdU permits the identification of cells which have replicated once, twice, or three or more times in the presence of this nucleotide analog. Typical first, second, and third replication cycle cells are seen in Figure 5.

Utilizing this technique, Tice et al.[60] were able to investigate whether the decline in PHA-stimulated cell replication with human aging was due to fewer old cells responding to PHA and/or to a diminished replication rate of the PHA responding cells. In Figure 6, the percent of lymphocyte metaphases in first, second, third, and subsequent cell cycles is shown as a function of time after PHA stimulation in four young and old donor lymphocyte cultures. Computer analysis of these data yields minimum cell cycle times of 10.6 hr in young cultures vs. 10.0 hr in old donor cell cultures; mean cell cycle durations of 12.3 hr in young donor cell cultures and 15.0 hr in old donor cell cultures; and maximum cell cycle durations of 15.6 hr in young donor cell cultures and 25.0 hr in old donor cell cultures[60] (Table 3). These results closely approximate what occurs in human fibroblasts as a function of in vitro passage (in vitro aging); minimum cell cycle times are not significantly altered, but mean and particularly maximum cell cycle times are significantly lengthened.

In addition to examining the cell cycle duration of cells stimulated by PHA, the BrdU differential staining techniques can be modified to examine percent of replicating cells in the cell population.[19] This is accomplished by examining the number of nuclei that have diminished fluorescent intensities after incubation with BrdU. Examination of the effect of PHA on young and old donor lymphocyte cultures revealed that 4.5% of the cell population is stimulated each hour to enter cell replication in young donor lymphocyte cultures, compared with only 2.8% in old donor cultures.[60] Thus, the BrdU techniques have revealed that with aging, fewer human lymphocytes respond to PHA, and those cells that do respond have diminished cell replication rates.

IN VIVO STUDIES

Although in vitro studies can provide insight into a variety of biological processes, it is important to complement these studies with investigations of cell populations in vivo. Ideally, these studies should be performed on human subjects. However, since this is impractical in most cases, laboratory animals are utilized. Although primates are the closest phylogenetic species to man, these animals are extremely difficult to work with and are exceedingly expensive. Most studies have utilized the laboratory

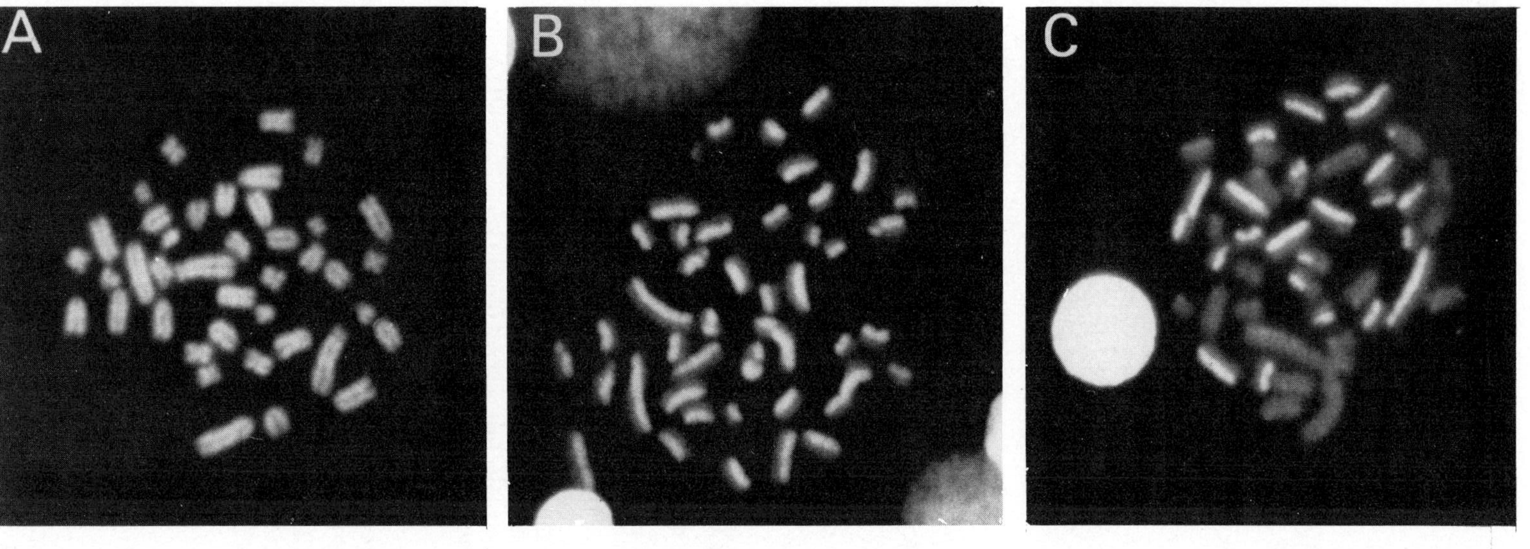

FIGURE 5. Metaphase cells stained with Hoechst 33258 and examined by fluorescent microscopy after one (A), two (B), and three (C) replications in the presence of BrdU. (From Schneider, E. L., Sternberg, H., and Tice, R., *Proc. Natl. Acad. Sci. U.S.A.*, 74, 2041, 1977. With permission.)

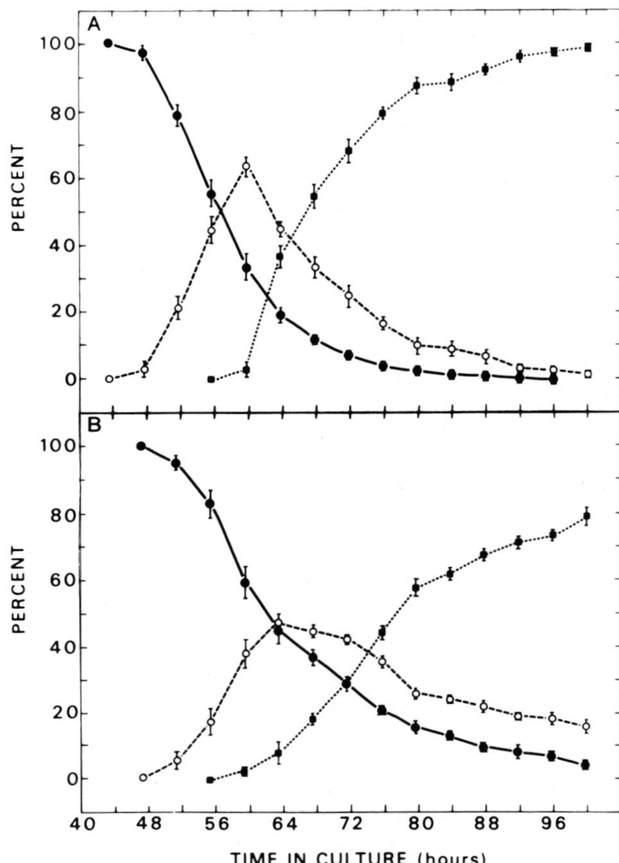

FIGURE 6. Examination of cellular replication kinetics in PHA-stimulated lymphocyte cultures from four young (A) and four old (B) human subjects. Closed circles are first, open circles are second, and closed squares are third and subsequent replication cycle cells. Each point represents the mean and each bar the standard error of the mean of the results from four cultures. (From Tice, R., Schneider, E. L., and Rary, J. M., *Exp. Cell Res.*, 102, 232, 1976. With permission.)

Table 3
COMPARISON OF PHA RESPONSIVENESS AND CELL-CYCLE DURATION FOR LYMPHOCYTES FROM YOUNG AND AGED HUMAN SUBJECTS[60]

	PHA stimulation rate	Cell cycle duration (hr)		
		Minimum	Mean	Maximum
Young	4.5%/hr	10.6	12.3	15.6
Old	2.8%/hr	10.0	15.0	25.0

Table 4
EFFECT OF AGING ON CHRONIC CELL REPLICATION IN VIVO

Tissue or cell type	Technique	Observations	Ref.
Skin	Graft of parental to Fl hybrid	Survival through several animals (10.25 years)	61
Mammary epithelium	Serial transplants into gland-free fat pads	Survival through at least 6 transplants (6 years)	62, 63
Bone marrow hemato-poetic cells	Injected into lethally irradiated host mice	Colony formation declined with number of transfers	64
	Injected into lethally irradiated mice	^{3}H-thymidine incorporation decreased with number of transfers	65
	Injected into genetically anemic histocompatible mice	Survival and function for at least 73 months	66

mouse and rat which have a well-defined life span, are relatively inexpensive to maintain, easy to work with, and share many chromosomal gene sequences with man (Table 4).

Chronic Cell Replication

Skin

The first attempt to examine the total proliferative capacity of a mammalian cell population in vivo was the serial transplantation of skin.[61] By grafting parental skin onto Fl hybrids, the transplanted skin could be identified (by means of hair color), and its survival followed through many serial transplants. With this technique, Krohn was able to maintain one skin transplant through several animals to a total in vivo life span of 10.25 years, far exceeding the life span of the mouse.[61] However, the interpretation of these studies was clouded by the possibility of host cells invading and populating the transplanted skin.

Mammary Epithelium

In a most elegant system, Daniel et al. were able to serially transplant mammary epithelium into gland free fat pads of recipient mice.[62] They were able to serially transplant this mammary tissue for at least 6 transplant generations and for periods of time ranging up to 6 years, again exceeding the life span of these mice by at least twofold. In these experiments, Daniel noted a decline in the proliferative rate of the transplanted tissue which seemed to be related to the number of previous transplantations, rather than to the in vivo life span of these cells.[63]

Hematopoetic Cells

Till and McCulloch[64] developed an elegant system for studying stem cell populations. In this system, bone marrow cells from syngeneic donors are injected into lethally irradiated host mice. Nine to 14 days after receiving bone marrow, the host animal spleens have macroscopic hematopoetic colonies in their spleen which can be rapidly identified and enumerated. Utilizing this technique, it was demonstrated that the ability to form colonies declined as a function of the number of transfers. Using radiolabeled nucleotide precursors, Cudkowitz et al.[65] demonstrated that the rate of DNA synthesis also declined as a function of serial transplantations.

Harrison[66] has developed a system where lethal radiation is unnecessary. Genetically anemic mice (W/W^v) are used as bone marrow recipients. Bone marrow transplantation from histocompatible C57BL/6J mice cure the anemia in these animals. Bone marrow can then be serially transplanted to W/W^v mice and the functional abilities of the transplanted cells examined by their ability to maintain normal red blood counts. Utilizing this technique, Harrison was able to demonstrate that donor C57BL/6J bone marrow cells were able to survive and function effectively for as long as 73 months. Thus, it is again demonstrated that in vivo cell populations can survive well past the life span of the intact animal. However, the functional ability of these cells declined as a function of transplantation.[66]

Acute Cell Replication

Studies of acute cellular replication in vivo are extremely difficult. They rely on the incorporation of tritiated thymidine into cells and the identification of the percent of labeled mitosis by autoradiography. Besides the technical difficulties of the technique, the tritiated thymidine used in these studies may inhibit cellular replication. However, results from these studies are important in that they provide the first insights into the behavior of cell populations in vivo (Table 5).

GI Tract Cells

The first approach to examining the effect of aging on cellular proliferation was undertaken by Lesher et al.[67,68] They indirectly measured cellular proliferation in GI tract cells by measuring the transit time for tritiated thymidine-labeled cells to pass from the crypt cell layer to extrusion at the tips of the intestinal villi.[67,68] In their studies of cells from the duodenum, ilium, and jejunum of young, middle-aged, and old mice, they found a decline in the generation time as a function of aging at all small intestinal sites examined. In addition, with aging there appears to be an increased heterogeneity of cell generation times. These studies were extended by Thrasher and Greulich[69] who found that the G1 phase of the cell cycle appeared to be lengthened while G2, S, and M phases did not appear to be altered as a function of aging. In addition, these authors demonstrated that fewer crypt cells are proliferating in the older animals.[70]

Examination of other GI tract cells, such as colonic[71] and esophageal[72] cell populations, also reveal a decreased rate of cellular proliferation in older cell populations.

Liver Cells

The vast majority of liver cells, the hepatocytes, are a nondividing cell population that can be stimulated to replicate by partial hepatectomy. Examination of the effect of aging on liver regeneration indicates that in older animals there is (1) a longer lag period before the initiation of DNA synthesis, (2) slower replacement of lost hepatic cells, (3) greater asynchrony of cells entering the mitotic cycle, and (4) less tolerance to hepatectomy in that a 10% loss of liver tissue in old rats results in the same kind of response elucidated by a 40% loss in younger animals.[73] These studies also indicate a progressive impairment in the regenerative capabilities of liver with aging.

Salivary Gland Cells

DNA synthesis can be stimulated in rat salivary glands by a single injection of isoproteranol. In a series of experiments, Adelman et al.[74] demonstrated that with aging fewer cells were stimulated by isoproteranol and the time required before initiation of DNA synthesis (lag phase) was lengthened.

Table 5
EFFECT OF AGING ON ACUTE CELL REPLICATION IN VIVO

Tissue or cell type	Observation	Ref.
GI	Decreased generation time in small intestinal crypt cells	67, 68
	Lengthened G_1 phase of cell cycle	69
	Diminished number of proliferating cells	70
Colon	Decreased cell proliferation	71
Esophagus	Decreased cell proliferation	72
Liver (after partial hepatectomy)	Longer lag before initiation of DNA synthesis; slower generation of new liver cells; increased asynchrony of cells entering mitotic cycle	73 73 73
Salivary gland (after isoproterenol stimulation)	Decreased number of cells with DNA synthesis; increased time required before initiation of DNA synthesis	74 74

CONCLUSIONS

Does Human Cellular Replication In Vivo Decline with Aging?

There is little direct evidence for a decline in human cellular replication in vivo with aging. Perhaps the best data are the results of Grove and co-workers[9] which indicate a substantial delay in wound healing as a function of human aging. Aside from this unpublished data, most studies of cell replication were conducted on human cell populations in tissue culture or on rodent cell populations in vivo. However, the preponderance of this data indicates that in both in vivo and in vitro cell populations, a significant decline in cellular proliferation occurs as a function of aging. In addition, an increased heterogeneity of individual cell replication times is also observed with aging. Increasing numbers of aging replicating cells appear to accumulate in the G1 phase of the cell cycle.

Does This Decline in Cellular Proliferation with Aging Have Functional Importance?

It is clear from transplantation studies in vivo that replicating cell populations outlive their host organisms.[9] Therefore, we do not age and die from a Hayflick phenomenon occurring in vivo, i.e., from running out of cell replications. However, this does not diminish the contribution of a decline in the replicative abilities of cell populations to aging of the organism. The clearest example of how a decline in cellular replicative abilities can be related to diminished function with age occurs in the immune system. Although the mechanisms for the decline in immune response with aging have not been fully elucidated, the work of Albright and Makinodan[4] indicates that decreased cellular proliferation may be an important component to this decline.

There is no doubt that further studies are needed to assess the importance of the decline in cellular replication that occurs with aging. Particular systems that should be explored, besides the obviously important immune system, are skin wound healing, response to blood loss, and GI cell replacement.

SUMMARY

While there is little data to indicate a decline in DNA replication in human cells in vivo, the preponderance of data derived from in vitro studies of human cells and in vivo studies of rodent cell populations indicates that cell replication is impaired as a function of aging. Studies of human diploid cells have indicated that cellular replication declines both as a function of serial in vitro passage (in vitro aging) and donor aging. In vivo, a decline in cellular replication has also been demonstrated in a variety of cell populations. Both in vivo and in vitro, this decline occurs in the number of replicating cells as well as in the replication rate of the dividing cell population. The functional importance of this decline in cellular replication with aging is best seen in the immune system where a loss of proliferative capability may contribute to the decline in immune response observed with aging. In the future, research should be directed at elucidating the mechanisms for this decline and at seeking approaches to reverse this lost function.

REFERENCES

1. **Makinodan, T. and Peterson, W. J.,** Growth and senescence of the primary antibody forming potential of the spleen, *J. Immunol.,* 94, 886, 1964.
2. **Walford, R. L.,** *The Immunologic Theory of Aging,* Munksgaard, Copenhagen, 1969.
3. **Adler, W. H., Jones, K. H., and Nariguchi, H.,** Aging and immune function, in *Recent Advances in Clinical Immunology,* Thompson, R. A., Ed., Churchill Livingstone, Edinburgh, 1977, 77.
4. **Albright, J. W. and Makinodan, T.,** Decline in the growth potential of spleen-colonizing bone marrow stem cells of long-lived aging mice, *J. Exp. Med.,* 144, 1204, 1976.
5. **Dougherty, J. and Rosenblatt, L.,** Changes in the hemogram of the beagle with age, *J. Gerontol.,* 20, 131, 1965.
6. **Finch, C. and Foster, J.,** Hematologic and serum electrolyte values of the C57BL/6J male mouse in maturity and senescence, *Lab. Anim. Sci.,* 23, 339, 1973.
7. **Dram, D., Senula, G., and Schneider, E. L.,** Unpublished data, 1979.
8. **Doberauer, W.,** Effect of age on wound healing process, *Gerontol. Clin.,* 41, 112, 1962.
9. **Grove, G.,** personal communication, 1979.
10. **Ebeling, A.,** Measurement of the growth of tissues in vitro, *J. Exp. Med.,* 34, 231, 1921.
11. **Parker, R. C.,** *Methods of Tissue Culture,* Harper & Row, New York.
12. **Swim, H. E. and Parker, R. F.,** Culture characteristics of human fibroblasts propagated serially, *Am. J. Hyg.,* 66, 235, 1957.
13. **Hayflick, L. and Moorhead, P.,** The serial cultivation of human diploid cell strains, *Exp. Cell Res.,* 25, 585, 1961.
14. **Hayflick, L.,** The limited in vitro lifetime of human diploid cell strains, *Exp. Cell Res.,* 37, 614, 1965.
15. **Dell'Orco, R. T., Mertens, J. G., and Kruse, P. F., Jr.,** Doubling potential, calendar time, and donor age of human diploid cells in culture, *Exp. Cell Res.,* 84, 363, 1974.
16. **Cristofalo, V. J. and Sharf, B. B.,** Cellular senescence and DNA synthesis, *Exp. Cell Res.,* 76, 419, 1973.
17. **Macieira-Coelho, A.,** Are nondividing cells present in aging cell cultures? *Nature,* 248, 421, 1974.
18. **Mitsui, Y.,** personal communication, 1979.
19. **Schneider, E. L., Tice, R. R., and Kram, D.,** Bromodeoxyuridine-differential chromatid staining technique: a new approach to examining sister chromatid exchange and cell replication kinetics, in *Methods in Cell Biology,* Prescott, D., Ed., Academic Press, New York, 1978, 379.
20. **Bowman, P. D., Meck, R. L., and Daniel, C. W.,** Aging of human fibroblasts in vitro, *Exp. Cell Res.,* 93, 184, 1975.
21. **Mitsui, Y. and Schneider, E. L.,** Relationship between cell replication and volume in senescent human diploid fibroblasts, *Mech. Ageing Dev.,* 5, 45, 1976.
22. **Schneider, E. L. and Fowlkes, B. J.,** Measurement of DNA content and cell volume in senescent human fibroblasts utilizing flow multiparameter single cell analysis, *Exp. Cell Res.,* 98, 298, 1976.
23. **Yanishevsky, R., Mendelsohn, M. L., Mayall, B. H., and Cristofalo, V. J.,** Proliferative capacity and DNA content of aging human diploid cells in culture: a cytophotometric and autoradiographic analysis, *J. Cell. Physiol.,* 84, 165, 1974.

24. **Grove, G. L., Kress, E. D., and Cristofalo, V. J.,** The cell cycle and thymidine incorporation during aging in vitro, *J. Cell Biol.*, 70, 133, 1976.
25. **Mitsui, Y. and Schneider, E. L.,** Characterization of fractionated human diploid fibroblast cell populations, *Exp. Cell Res.*, 103, 23, 1976.
26. **Mitsui, Y., Smith, J., and Schneider, E. L.,** Unpublished data, 1979.
27. **Absher, P. M., Absher, R. G., and Barnes, W. D.,** Genealogy of clones of diploid fibroblasts, *Exp. Cell Res.*, 88, 95, 1974.
28. **Bell, E., Marek, L. F., Levinstone, D. S., Merrill, C., Sher, S., Young, I. T., Eden, M.,** Loss of division potential in vitro: aging or differentiation?, *Science*, 202, 1158, 1978.
29. **Smith, J. R. and Hayflick, L.,** Variation in the life span of clones derived from human diploid cell strains, *J. Cell Biol.*, 62, 48, 1974.
30. **Smith, J. R., Pereira-Smith, O. M., and Good, P. I.,** Colony size distribution as a measure of age in cultured human cells, *Mech. Ageing Dev.*, 6, 283, 1977.
31. **Martin, G. M., Sprague, C. A., Norwood, T. H., Pendergrass, W. R., Bornstein, P., Hoehn, H., and Arend, W. P.,** Do hyperplastoid cell lines differentiate themselves to death?, *Adv. Exp. Med. Biol.*, 53, 67, 1975.
32. **Martin, G. M., Norwood, T. H., and Hoehn, H.,** Somatic cell genetic investigations of clonal senescence, in *The Molecular Biology of the Mammalian Genetic Apparatus*, unpublished data, 1977.
33. **Stein, G.,** Personal communication, 1979.
34. **Littlefield, J. W.,** Attempted hybridizations with senescent human fibroblasts, *J. Cell. Physiol.*, 82, 129, 1973.
35. **Wright, W. E. and Hayflick, L.,** Nuclear control of cellular aging demonstrated by hybridization of anucleate and whole cultured normal fibroblasts, *Exp. Cell Res.*, 96, 113, 1975.
36. **Muggleton-Harris, A., and Hayflick, L.,** Cellular aging studied by the reconstruction of replicating cells from nuclei and cytoplasms isolated from normal human diploid cells, *Exp. Cell Res.*, 103, 321, 1976.
37. **Todaro, G. J. and Green, H.,** Serum albumin supplemented medium for long-term cultivation of mammalian fibroblast strains, *Proc. Soc. Exp. Biol. Med.*, 116, 688, 1964.
38. **Macieira-Coelho, A.,** Action of cortisone on human fibroblasts in vitro, *Experientia*, 22, 390, 1966.
39. **Cristofalo, V. J.,** Metabolic aspects of aging in diploid human cells, in *Aging in Cell and Tissue Culture*, Holecková, E., and Cristofalo, V. J., Eds., Plenum Press, New York, 1970, 83.
40. **Schneider, E. L., Braunschweiger, K., and Mitsui, Y.,** The effect of serum batch on the in vitro life spans of cell cultures derived from old and young human donors, *Exp. Cell Res.*, 115, 47, 1978.
41. **Packer, L. and Smith, J. R.,** Extension of the life span of cultured normal human diploid cells by vitamin E, *Proc. Natl. Acad Sci. U.S.A.*, 71, 4763, 1974.
42. **Packer, L. and Smith, J. R.,** Extension of the life span of cultured normal human diploid cells by vitamin E: a reevaluation, *Proc. Natl. Acad. Sci. U.S.A.*, 74, 1640, 1977.
43. **Schneider, E. L., Mitsui, Y., Au, K. S., and Shorr, S. S.,** Tissue-specific differences in cultured human diploid fibroblasts, *Exp. Cell Res.*, 108, 1, 1977.
44. **Goldstein, S., Littlefield, J. W., and Soeldner, J. S.,** Diabetes mellitus and aging: diminished plating efficiency of cultured human fibroblasts, *Proc. Natl. Acad. Sci. U.S.A.*, 64, 155, 1969.
45. **Martin, G. M., Sprague, C. A., and Epstein, C. J.,** Replicative life span of cultivated human cells: effect of donor age, tissue, and genotype, *Lab. Invest.*, 23, 86, 1970.
46. **Schneider, E. L. and Mitsui, Y.,** The relationship between in vitro cellular aging and in vivo human age, *Proc. Natl. Acad. Sci. U.S.A.*, 73, 3584, 1976.
47. **LeGuilly, Y., Lenoir, P., and Bourel, M.,** Long-term cultures of human adult liver cells: morphological changes related to in vitro senescence and effect of donor's age on growth potential, *Gerontologia*, 19, 303, 1973.
48. **Rheinwald, J. G. and Green, H.,** Epidermal growth factor and the multiplication of cultured human epidermal keratinocytes, *Nature*, 265, 421, 1977.
49. **Schneider, E. L. and Epstein, C. J.,** Replication rate and life span of cultured human fibroblasts in Down's syndrome, *Proc. Soc. Exp. Biol. Med.*, 141, 1092, 1972.
50. **Smith, J. R., Pereira-Smith, O. M., and Schneider, E. L.,** Colony size distributions as a measure of in vivo and in vitro aging, *Proc. Natl. Acad. Sci. U.S.A.*, 75, 1353, 1978.
51. **Pisciotta, A. V., Westring, D. W., DePrey, C., and Walsh, B.,** Mitogenic effect of phytohemagglutinin at different ages, *Nature (London)*, 215, 193, 1967.
52. **Hallgren, H. M., Buckley, C . E., Gilbertson, V. A., and Yunis, E. J.,** Lymphocyte phytohemagglutinin responsiveness, immunoglobulins, and autoantibodies in aging humans, *J. Immunol.*, 111, 1101, 1973.
53. **Foad, B. S. I., Adams, Y., Yamaguchi, Y., and Litwin, A.,** Phytomitogen response of peripheral blood lymphocytes in young and older subjects, *Clin. Exp. Immunol.*, 17, 657, 1974.
54. **Weksler, M. E. and Hutteroth, T. H.,** Impaired lymphocyte function in aged humans, *J. Clin. Invest.*, 53, 99, 1974.

55. **Inkeles, B., Judith, B., Kuntz, M. M., Kadish, A. S., and Weksler, M. E.**, Immunologic studies of aging. III. Cytokinetic basis for the impaired response of lymphocytes from aged humans to plant lectins, *J. Exp. Med.*, 145, 1176, 1977.
56. **Latt, S. A.**, Microfluorometric detection of deoxyribonucleic acid replication in human metaphase chromosomes, *Proc. Natl. Acad. Sci. U.S.A.*, 70, 3395, 1973.
57. **Perry, P. and Wolff, S.**, A new Giemsa method for the differential staining of sister chromatids, *Nature*, 251, 156, 1974.
58. **Schneider, E. L., Sternberg, H., and Tice, R.**, In vivo analysis of cellular replication, *Proc. Natl. Acad. Sci. U.S.A.*, 74, 2041, 1977.
59. **Tice, R., Schneider, E. L., and Rary, J. M.**, The utilization of bromodeoxyuridine incorporation into DNA for the analysis of cellular kinetics, *Exp. Cell Res.*, 102, 232, 1976.
60. **Tice, R., Schneider, E. L., Kram, D., and Thorne, P.**, Cytogenetic analysis of the impaired proliferative response of peripheral lymphocytes from aged human to PHA, *J. Exp. Med.*, 149, 1029, 1979.
61. **Krohn, P. L.**, Review lectures on senescence. II. Heterochronic transplantation in the study of aging, *Proc. R. Soc. London*, 157, 128, 1962.
62. **Daniel, C. W., deOme, K. B., Young, J. T., Blair, P. B., and Faulkin, L. J., Jr.**, The in vivo life span of normal and preneoplastic mouse mammary glands: a serial transplantation study, *Proc. Natl. Acad. Sci. U.S.A.*, 61, 53, 1968.
63. **Daniel, C. W.**, Cell longevity in vivo, in *Handbook of the Biology of Aging*, Finch, C. and Hayflick, L., Eds., Van Nostrand Reinhold, New York, 1977, 122.
64. **Till, J. E. and McCulloch, E. A.**, A direct measurement of the radiation sensitivity of normal mouse bone marrow cells, *Radiat. Res.*, 14, 213, 1961.
65. **Cudkowicz, G., Upton, A. C., and Shearer, G. M.**, Lymphocyte content and proliferative capacity of serially transplanted mouse bone marrow, *Nature*, 201, 165, 1964.
66. **Harrison, D. E.**, Normal production of erythrocytes by mouse marrow continuous for 73 months, *Proc. Natl. Acad. Sci. U.S.A.*, 70, 3184, 1973.
67. **Lesher, S., Fry, R. J. M., and Kohn H. I.**, Age and the generation time of the mouse duodenal epithelial cell, *Exp. Cell Res.*, 24, 334, 1961.
68. **Lesher, S., Fry, R. J. M., and Kohn, H. I.**, Aging and the generation cycle of intestinal epithelial cells in the mouse, *Gerontologia*, 5, 176, 1961.
69. **Thrasher, J. D. and Greulich, R. C.**, The duodenal progenitor population. I. Age-related increase in the duration of the cryptal progenitor cycle, *J. Exp. Zool.*, 159, 39, 1965.
70. **Thrasher, J. D. and Greulich, R. C.**, The duodenal progenitor population. II. Age-related changes in size and distribution, *J. Exp. Zool.*, 159, 39, 1965.
71. **Thrasher, J. D.**, Age and the cell cycle of the mouse colonic epithelium, *Anat. Rec.*, 157, 621, 1967.
72. **Thrasher, J. D.**, Age and the cell cycle of the mouse esophageal epithelium, *Exp. Gerontol.*, 6, 19, 1971.
73. **Bucher, N. L. R. and Swaffield, M. N.**, The rate of incorporation of labelled thymidine into the deoxyribonucleic acid of regenerating rat liver in relation to the amount of liver excised, *Cancer Res.*, 24, 1611, 1964.
74. **Adelman, R. C., Stein, G., Roth, G. S., and Englander, D.**, Age-dependent regulation of mammalian DNA synthesis and cell proliferation in vivo, *Mech. Aging Dev.*, 1, 49, 1972.

DNA DAMAGE AND REPAIR IN AGING MAMMALS

Jerry R. Williams and Kerry L. Dearfield

INTRODUCTION

It seems accurate at this time to state that there is no body of data which disqualifies altered DNA structure or function as a possible underlying mechanism of the aging process, but neither is there such an extensive body of data as to insure this premise to be universally or even widely accepted. Recent advances in understanding mutation, the structure of DNA within chromatin, and the role which DNA repair processes play in mutation in mammalian cells establish a much wider range of possible mechanisms by which mutations or other DNA or chromatin damage might arise and be expressed in somatic cells. Knowledge of the types, quantity, and quality of DNA damage and repair which occur in various somatic cells *in situ* and the sequelae of such processes is limited. Nonetheless, the body of evidence implicating changes in the prevalence of DNA damage or changes in rates of DNA repair associated with aging is becoming more impressive, and it is to the compilation of that data that this section is directed.

Existing data in three major areas will be described: (1) changes in the DNA or chromatin of mammalian cells as their host organism ages, or in mammalian cells as they senesce in vitro; (2) DNA repair activities observed in these same cells initiated by agents which damage DNA and are mutagenic when assayed in appropriate systems; and (3) evidence of accelerated aging in human beings who have or are hypothesized to have defects in molecular processes which repair DNA.

This section will eschew the description of several lines of research, which although important in the eventual evaluation of the relationship between DNA damage and repair processes and in vivo aging, are at this point somewhat speculative. Major among such research areas are (1) the effects of DNA damage by exogenous mutagens and the manifestation of their in vivo sequelae in the tissues of mammals and other organisms, (2) radiation-induced life shortening or extension, and (3) the comparative effects of mutagens on the life span of organisms of different DNA content. These data and more general and speculative descriptions are discussed elsewhere.[1-5]

Before presenting the selected data, it is necessary to describe both the mechanisms by which damage is induced in DNA and cells repair DNA. Although there is still disagreement as to the biological relevance for mammalian cells of different DNA repair activities that are better documented in microorganisms, the types of repair seem similar. More detailed evaluations of DNA repair mechanisms in general are offered.[6-10]

Mechanisms for Induction of DNA/Chromatin Damage

The term spontaneous mutation is misleading because no mutation is truly spontaneous. Certain types of DNA damage, however, do occur spontaneously, but these damages do not transmutate one nucleotide to another. Rather, spontaneous damage or damage induced by endogenous or exogenous agents changes a nucleotide from its intelligible form to a biologically unintelligible form, i.e., to a form which is not exactly complementary to any other nucleotide. This altered form may be substrate for the various repair systems; mutations may then occur by misrepair or use of the damaged nucleotide as template for replication. The use of altered and unintelligible nucleotides as a template for replication may occur either during semiconservative synthesis in a replicating cell or repair synthesis. In the following discussion, types of damage will be examined as possible substrates for DNA repair activities. The types of damage which will be described should be considered as examples only, as it seems clear that knowledge of the spectrum of DNA/chromatin damage is rather incomplete.

Spontaneous Damage

Although DNA is — as its biological function implies — a basically stable structure, spontaneous damage occurs. A good example of such damage is the spontaneous rupture of the N-glycosidic bond in pyrimidine and especially purine nucleotides.[11] The resulting lesion is termed a site without base. Such a common spontaneous rupture, perhaps in the range of 10^2 to 10^3 ruptures per mammalian cell per day[11] would require efficient repair for evolutionary stability. This type of spontaneous DNA damage is the most common, and as will be discussed subsequently, the resulting site without base is a condition which appears to be an intermediate state during excision repair of a wide variety of DNA damages.

Another type of spontaneous damage would be typified by the spontaneous deamination of cytosine to uracil within the DNA polymer.[12] The resulting presence of uracil in the DNA sequence is specific substrate for an N-glycosylase which cleaves the N-glycosidic bond, again producing a site without base.[13] It is interesting to note that bacterial strains which are deficient for this activity are mutation-prone at other loci.[14]

The measurement of relative rates at which spontaneous damage occurs in the DNA of long- compared to short-lived species or aged compared to young individuals has not been made, although the prime dependence of the rupture of the N-glycosidic bond upon temperature would suggest these rates would be similar. It is possible to speculate, however, that higher order structure of DNA might perturb the rate of induction of damage since it clearly affects DNA repair, albeit by different mechanisms. Higher order DNA/chromatin structure restricts (probably by controlling access) the repair of exogenously induced DNA damage.[15,16] This control varies between short- and long-lived species (Williams, unpublished data). Thus, it is possible to speculate that the intimate association between DNA and protein in the nucleosome may also possibly alter the molecular energy states such that induction rates for spontaneous damage may vary from region to region within a genome or even vary between species. Until more precise measurement of the incidence and prevalence of spontaneous damage is possible, the role of such damage in aging must remain conjectural.

In summary, spontaneous damage occurs at substantial rates in the DNA of cells, particularly the production of sites without base. Although it is possible that these rates may vary slightly in species of different life spans, this is not likely. What is clear, however, is that spontaneous damage continually produces a DNA repair substrate such that metabolic control of the quantity or fidelity of repair could control the rate of mutation in cells of different species and at different rates during the life span. Thus, the control of DNA repair fidelity could in turn control an intrinsic rate of mutation and possibly cellular function, providing a candidate for an intrinsic mutator such as proposed by Burnet[17] under developmental or time-dependent control.

Endogenously Induced Damage

At least two types of damage can be cited which originate from within a somatic cell, and these serve as examples for endogenously induced DNA damage. Nonspecific DNA or chromatin damage can be induced by chemical alteration through interaction with reactive species such as free radicals. It is conceivable that such damage could be intrinsically controlled by the induction of enzymes such as superoxide dismutase or the control of internal concentrations of antioxidants. A second example of a mechanism of endogenously originating damage is that of endonuclease attack. This type of enzyme can be of lysosomal or nuclear origin, can have great specificity, and has been demonstrated to be implicated in sudden cell death in cultured systems.[18]

It is possible to hypothesize that either the rate of induction of these two types of damage or their repair could be under developmental or time-dependent control. Again, there is no body of evidence which presents or convincingly demonstrates any causal relationship between endogenous induction of damage or its repair and the aging process.

Exogenously Induced Damage

Organisms are exposed to two types of exogenously produced agents which can induce DNA damage. The first, best known, and most important is ionizing radiation. The exposure from cosmic and γ-rays, produced by internal and external emitters, is fairly uniform throughout the soma and in rate of exposure through time. Thus, short- and long-lived organisms exist in the same radiation environment. If the results of this type of damage are associated with aging, it must be the cellular response to the damage, rather than in its induction.

UV light is another form of radiation which has been demonstrated to cause DNA damage (most prevalently in the form of pyrimidine dimers) and induce DNA repair processes. Unlike ionizing radiation, however, UV radiation, principally from the sun, does not penetrate beyond the outer layers of the skin.

The second example of damage is included only for completeness; this is damage induced by certain chemicals in food and other phases of the environment. Clearly, some chemicals within the natural environment induce DNA damage and subsequent repair activities as does UV radiation. However, again these chemicals do not provide an equal distribution throughout the organism since most chemicals appear to be tissue-specific. Once within the body, these substances can be mutagenic in cells which are penetrated. Since aging appears to occur in all components of the soma, agents which are tissue-specific can be summarily discounted as being the proximal agent in the aging process.

Mechanisms of DNA Repair in Cells

Figure 1 illustrates general patterns of DNA repair. Several statements can be made from this illustration. Excision repair — the general process by which damaged portions of DNA are removed — appears to be the dominant mechanism of repair. Excision repair is a generic term now considered to encompass: (1) base insertion with no scission of the polynucleotide strand, (2) nucleotide(s) insertion via incision by the sequential action of a specific N-glycosylase and AP endonuclease, and (3) nucleotide(s) insertion via incision by a specific or general endonuclease which incises the phosphodiester backbone directly prior to excision and resynthesis of one or more nucleotides. The alternate pathways of excision repair by which a particular damage is repaired is at least partially dependent upon the chemical nature of the damage.

Evidence suggests that different types of initial DNA lesions are repaired at different rates[19] and result in repaired "patches" of different length.[20,21] Further, studies in cells from several human syndromes presumed to represent deficiency in some aspect of excision repair indicate that each syndrome is sensitive to a separate type of DNA damage, indicating that the defective repair systems are disjointed. (These syndromes will be discussed later.) These several lines of evidence suggest multiple pathways for excision repair, with selection determined by the initial lesion. Thus, the block in Figure 1 which represents "endonuclease, exonuclease, polymerase, ligase" includes the several pathways which accomplish excision repair. Although each of these actions are necessary for complete repair, the interrelationship between the control of these activities and the initial lesion is unknown.

The types of DNA damage at the left in Figure 1 illustrate the general categories of damage. Two of these — the site without base and the pyrimidine dimer — have special

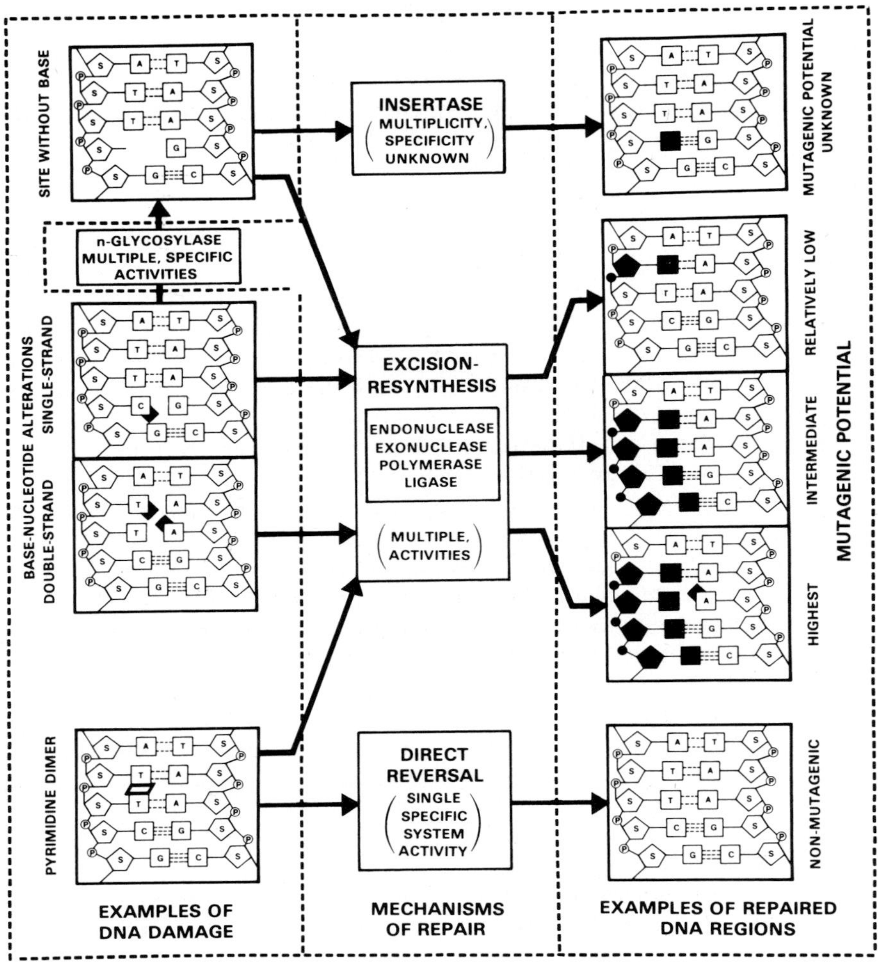

FIGURE 1. Schema for DNA repair mechanisms in mammalian cells.

biological implications and two or more pathways by which they can be repaired. As described earlier, the site without base is the most prevalent form of spontaneous damage incurred by DNA and has probably been continually produced during evolution. The pyrimidine dimer is also a damage which has been present from the early evolution of our biosystem (it was especially prevalent before the establishment of the ozone layer), and by necessity must have been overcome by repair in order for DNA to maintain the fidelity required for biological evolution to occur. From Figure 1 it is clear that both of these important damages can be repaired by excision.

The other two types of damage illustrated in the left column represent those which involve alteration of a base(s) on a single strand and damage on both strands of the DNA. In the latter case, repair replication of an excised base(s) or nucleotide(s) may require use of a damaged base as template. Such replication on damaged template may be an exceptionally error-prone process. The right column represents examples of repaired regions of the DNA and speculates on the possible fidelity of repair. This speculation is based on the simple proposition that the probility for mutation is dependent upon the number of nucleotides inserted and the damaged or undamaged condition of the template; it is intended to be suggestive rather than rigorous. If, for instance, different repair pathways require different polymerase activities, then longer repair patches would not necessarily be more mutagenic.

Repair systems which are speculated to require four DNA strands for possible interchange between homologous DNA sequences have not been included, primarily because nondividing tissue ages, but does not replicate its DNA. Upon the demonstration that homologous chromosomes in postmitotic tissue synapse, these repair systems would need to be considered.

Before proceeding to a description of manifestation of DNA damage and a compilation of existing aging data, six statements are provided to act as caveats against overinterpretation of data:

1 The relationship between the quantity of DNA repair and the quality of DNA repair is not known.
2. Chromatin structure alters and perhaps controls at least certain activities in DNA repair.
3. DNA repair appears to be lesion-specific to a high degree, both as to quantity and quality.
4. Inducible processes probably can alter the mutational and cytotoxic potential of DNA repair.
5. DNA can be replicated with major damage present, and DNA damage can persist in both dividing and nondividing cells for significant periods of time.
6. DNA repair occurring at low levels of damage (noncytotoxic) is probably qualitatively different from those at higher levels of damage.

In summary, modification of the effectiveness of DNA repair could produce deterioration in the fidelity of DNA which could in turn cause aging in somatic cells. Such modification could occur by the differential occurrence of DNA repair in either selected regions or all of the genome. It is also hypothetically possible that alteration of the fidelity of repair could produce the differential effect necessary for different rates of aging. An example of such a mechanism is the inducible, error-prone alteration of polymerase fidelity described by Radman.[22] In either case, our knowledge of the in vivo functioning of the various repair systems described in Figure 1 is so limited at this point that any detailed speculation is premature.

Tissue Manifestation of DNA/Chromatin Damage

These previous sections have described the multiple processes involved in the possible induction of DNA damage and its repair. The processes which, subsequent to these events, manifest altered or damaged DNA as observable changes at the cellular, tissue, or organismal level are not well-characterized. It is clear that agents which damage DNA can induce both cytotoxicity and changes in phenotypic expression in individual cells, and also induce necrotic failure and decreased function in tissues, but the several processes involved in this manifestation of damage have been rather refractory to study. To a large extent, this difficulty stems from the inability to selectively alter a single parameter in a treated tissue or cell population. An evaluation of the literature on the tissue response in animals treated with DNA damaging agents is beyond the scope of the present discussion, although it is important to emphasize that this information is an essential part of evaluating the theory which attempts to relate DNA damage to the deterioration in tissue function which is observed during aging. Those experiments which have been based on the measurement of age-associated tissue function in animals treated with mutagens are confounded by lack of knowledge in this area.

ALTERATION OF DNA OR CHROMATIN STRUCTURE IN MAMMALIAN CELLS AGING IN VIVO OR SENESCING IN VITRO

Table 1 is a compilation of reported experiments which have compared the prevalence of altered DNA or chromatin structure between cells from mammals of different ages, life spans, and stages of in vitro senescence.

Evidence is included that indicates any alteration in the chromatin structure, varying from DNA strand breaks to acetylation of histone proteins. The methods of interrogation vary from physical-chemical assays to the quantity of enzymatic substrate available, to exogenously supplied nucleases.

This table (as well as Table 2 discussed subsequently) includes data from studies performed on cells both in vivo and in vitro. This permits comparison of these two types of data; however, is not intended to be a critical evaluation through DNA damage and repair of in vitro senescence as a model for in vivo aging as proposed by Hayflick.[23] As far as possible, an attempt has been made to preserve the exact wording used by the various authors to describe experimental design and results.

DNA REPAIR ACTIVITIES OF MAMMALIAN CELLS AGING IN VIVO AND CELLS SENESCING IN VITRO

Table 2 is a compilation of experiments wherein cells from aging mammals, cells from mammals of different life spans, or cells at different stages of in vitro senescence are challenged by physical or chemical agents which produce DNA damage. Thus, these data reflect the ability or capacity of challenged cells to perform repair of the induced lesions. Considering DNA repair as a series of enzymatic activities, all of the experiments describe the sudden presentation of a large amount of substrate to the repair system.

All reported measurements reflect repair endpoints which are, as was discussed previously, difficult to interpret as to biological relevance. That is, a quantity of accomplished repair or the observation of a possible sequelae of repair such as sister chromatid exchanges or chromosome aberrations are exceptionally difficult to interpret in terms of mutation, cytotoxicity, or other endpoints of altered cellular or tissue function.

AGING IN HUMAN BEINGS THOUGHT TO BE DNA REPAIR-DEFICIENT

If defects in DNA repair mechanisms induce or accelerate the aging process, human beings with inherent errors in such mechanisms should exhibit characteristics of accelerated aging. This simple rationale can be evaluated directly by examining indices of aging in such individuals. Martin has evaluated several indices of aging in individuals with a wide range of genetic disease, including those diseases believed to be associated with DNA repair deficiency.[102]

Several inherited disease states have been identified which, to varying degrees, have been demonstrated or hypothesized to have DNA repair defects. These diseases are xeroderma pigmentosum (XP), ataxia telangiectasia (AT), Fanconi's anemia (FA), Bloom's syndrome (BS), Cockayne's syndrome (CS), Werner's syndrome (WS), Hutchinson-Gilford progeria syndrome (PG), and retinoblastoma (RB). The degree of certainty in placing each of these syndromes into the class of DNA repair-deficient diseases varies from excellent for XP, to good for AT and FA, to fair for BS, CS, and RB, to poor for WS and PG.

Table 1
ALTERATION OF DNA/CHROMATIN STRUCTURE

Technique of measurement	Cell type	Degree of change in parameter	Ref.
DNA Strand Breaks of Unknown Etiology[a]			
DNA template activity measured with DNA polymerase and autoradiography	Fixed brain, liver, and heart tissues from young and senescent mice	Greater incorporation of dNMP into nuclei of 30 to 35-month-old mice than 3 to 4-month-old mice	24
Sedimentation velocities in alkali; viscometry	Isolated liver nuclei from rats of increasing ages	A tenfold decrease in molecular weight with increasing age; most significant decrease in rats younger than 400 days	25
Alkaline sucrose gradient sedimentation	Thigh muscles from Wistar rats of increasing ages	DNA structure decreases in molecular weight from 1—28 days of age	26
	Internal granular layer neurons from cerebella of beagle dogs of increasing ages	DNA structure decreases in molecular weight from 7 weeks to 10 years of age	27
	Livers from mice of increasing ages	Decreased molecular weight with age, particularly between 1 and 14 months; total net increase of 3.2×10^4 DNA scissions per cell	28
DNA Strand Breaks of Unknown Etiology; Also, Single-Stranded Regions of DNA[a]			
CsCl density gradient and alkaline sucrose gradient sedimentations; single-strand-specific nuclease S_1 sensitivity	Myocardial cells from CBF_1 mice of increasing ages	Age-associated increase in single-stranded gaps shown by (1) broad bands of DNA in CsCl gradients of old mice (20, 25, 30 months old), a narrow peak for young mice (6, 15 months old); (2) multimodal dispersion in 30-month-old mice vs. monodisperse for 6-month-old mice on alkaline sucrose gradients; and (3) S_1 sensitivity increased from 6 to 20 to 30 months of age (digests 2.6%, 12.8%, and 15.1% DNA, respectively)	29
Alkaline sucrose gradient sedimentation and single-strand-specific nuclease S_1 sensitivity	Cell lysate of brain from CBF_1 mice of increasing ages	Gradients of 6-month samples show monodisperse sedimentation patterns; 30 months show polydisperse patterns; S_1 sensitivity begins at 20 months of age, maximizes at 30 months (14.2% total genome digested) from a minimum at 6—15 months (2.2—2.0% digested)	30
Alkaline sucrose gradient sedimentation	Retinal photoreceptors from rabbits of increasing ages	Age-associated decrease in molecular weight from 6 weeks to 7 years of age	31

Table 1 (continued)
ALTERATION OF DNA/CHROMATIN STRUCTURE

Technique of measurement	Cell type	Degree of change in parameter	Ref.
		Single-Stranded Regions of DNA[a]	
Single-strand-specific nuclease S_1 sensitivity	Livers from CBF_1 mice of increasing ages	Increasing S_1 sensitivity to 14—25% of total genome after 20 months of age (from 20 to 30 months) from no sensitivity during 1—15 months of age	33
	Pre- and post-menopausal human ovaries	No difference in S_1 sensitivity between pre- and postmenopausal ovaries	34
Single-strand-specific nuclease S_1 sensitivity; isopyknic density gradient-centrifugation; thermal stability	Livers from male C57B1/6 mice of increasing ages	No age-associated increase in single-stranded DNA	35
Immunofluorescence using anti-cytidine antibody	Brain cells, hepatocytes, and gastric mucosal cells of dd-strain mice	Age-associated increase of single-stranded regions in DNA of brain and liver cells from young 4-week-old to senescent 1-year-old mice; no such increase in gastric mucosal cells	36
		Chromosome Aberrations[a]	
Cytogenetic examination	Livers from female CF_1 mice of increasing ages	Age-associated increase of aberrations reaching 22% abnormalities at 10 months of age	37
	Livers from female C57BL/6J and A/HEJ mice of increasing ages	The development of aberrations is inversely proportional to the life expectancy seen with these two strains	38
	Livers from registered beagles of increasing ages	Age-associated increase of aberrations reaching 16% abnormalities at 8 years of age	39
	Bone marrow from male albino rats (Wistar) of increasing ages	Progressive increase of aberration frequency reaching 15% abnormalities at 30 months of age from 2—4% abnormalities at 10 months of age	40
	Human leukocytes from males and females of increasing ages	Higher frequency of hypodiploidy in females aged 75—95 years than 15—35 years; marked loss of G-chromosomes in males aged 78—90 years compared to 20—32 years	41
	Swine leukocytes from animals of increasing ages	Slight increase of spontaneous chromosome deletions at 24 weeks of age and persisting among older animals	42

	Liver from Moen-Chase strain guinea pigs of increasing ages	Age-associated increase of aberrations intermediate to mice and beagles; 22 and 16% abnormalities, respectively (cf. mice and beagle references, this table)	43
	Human lymphocytes from males and females of increasing ages	Increased aberration (acentric fragments) frequency in aged groups 60—79 years of age	44
	Bone marrow from mouse and rat strains of increasing ages	No age-associated increases of chromosome aberrations	45
	Human leukocytes of males and females of increasing ages	No increased aberration frequency in groups of newborn, 20—30 years, and over 60 years of age; a tenfold increase of chromosome aberrations observed in premature babies	46
	Liver from Chinese hamsters of increasing ages	Age-associated increase of aberrations from 74—1100 days of age regardless of the stage of the cell cycle	47
	Human leukocytes from individuals of increasing ages	Age-associated increase in level of aneuploidy and structural abnormalities in aged (ages 62—96 years) rather than young persons (ages 10—13)	48
	Human lymphocytes from males and females of increasing ages	Increase of breaks per mitosis by two-fold for ages over 40 years vs. ages under 40 years	49
	Human peripheral lymphocytes from males and females of increasing ages	Age-associated increase in aneuploidy in females and males (ages 0—89 years); increase in hypodiploidy and hyperdiploidy seen more markedly in females	50
	Human peripheral lymphocytes from males and females of increasing ages	Age-associated increase in aberrant cells, cells with chromatid fragments, and with chromosome fragments in females aged from 20—29 years to 60—70 years; males aged 20—50 years showed no differences	51
		DNA Cross-Linking[a]	
Tritium feeding, tissue degradation, and UV absorption measurements	Brain and liver from rat offspring of different ages	Age-associated increase in frequency of DNA-protein-RNA complexes	52

Table 1 (continued)
ALTERATION OF DNA/CHROMATIN STRUCTURE

Technique of measurement	Cell type	Degree of change in parameter	Ref.
Structural Changes in Chromatin[a]			
Solubilizing chromatin preparations and assaying for chromatin components	Liver from Wistar rats of increasing ages	Age-associated decrease of acid proteins in 3- and 30-month-old rats and of RNA in 12- and 30-month-old rats from 1-month-old rats; amounts of histones remain unchanged	53
	Cardiac muscle from dogs of increasing ages	No age-associated changes of protein/DNA and RNA/DNA ratios in chromatin; no major change in the binding of protein to DNA with age	54
	Liver from female C57BL/6J mice of increasing ages	Age-associated increase in proportion of histones relative to nonhistones, decrease in RNA content of chromatin, and small increase in total chromatin proteins	55
	Submandibular glands from male Sprague-Dawley rats of increasing ages	Age-associated (from 2 to 12 months of age) increase of histone extractability suggests less tenacious histone binding to DNA in older chromatin; histone content of young and old chromatin in submandibular glands is similar, but reduced amount of nonhistone chromosomal protein found in 12-month-old chromatin	56
Urea high-resolution of polyacrylamide gel electrophoresis	Livers from Osborn-Mendel and Sprague-Dawley strain rats and C57/BL mice	No apparent age-associated change in proportion of any histone fraction of mouse and rat liver	57
Tritiated acetate and ^{32}P-ATP incorporation and liquid scintillation counting	Liver from C57/6J mice of increasing ages	Age-associated increase in rate of acetylation from young (2 months) to old (29 months) mice, but no difference in rate of phosphorylation of liver nuclear proteins	58
Tritiated acetate incorporation and liquid scintillation counting	Liver and thymus histones from male Sprague-Dawley rats of increasing ages	Linear decrease of liver histone acetylation from 1 (690 cpm) to 16 months of age (350 cpm) and remains at this level until maximum age of 24 months; thymus histone acetylation shows a cyclic acetylation process with a minimum at 8 months of age	59

Micrococcal nuclease digestion and gel electrophoresis	Human neuronal nuclei from autopic cerebral cortices of brains of increasing ages	Age-associated increase in nucleosomal repeat length (in linker region) from 170 (±18) base pairs in young group (23—36 years) to 199 (±8) base pairs in old group (78—85 years); decrease in amount DNA digested (80% nuclear DNA in young vs. 60% in old)	60
Micrococcal nuclease and DNAse I digestion	Nuclei from liver, brain, and heart of C57BL mice	Nucleosomal organization similar in all 3 tissues regardless of age; rate and extent of digestion, size of DNA repeat unit and nucleosome core do not significantly differ with age	61
Tritiated acetate incorporation and polyacrylamide gel electrophoresis	Histones from liver of CD male rats	Incorporation declined with age up to 24 months, then leveled; H4 histone predominantly labeled in 2-month rats and H3 histone more highly labeled in 12-, 16-, and 24-month rats	62
Extraction, fractionation, and subsequent separation by SDS-disc polyacrylamide gel electrophoresis of nonhistone chromatin (NHC) protein	Livers from Mill Hill CBA strain mice and Sprague-Dawley strain rats of increasing ages	Age-associated increase in number and quantities of high molecular weight, water soluble NHC proteins; differences in salt-soluble NHC proteins (0.35 *M* NaCl) also evident, though not very different in a lower concentration of salt (0.14 *M* NaCl).	63
	Chromosome Aberrations[b]		
Cytogenetic examination	Human fetal lung diploid cells (WI-38)	Increase in polyploidy, aneuploidy, and frequency of dicentrics seen from passage 40 as cells senesced	64
	Male fetal lung fibroblast strain MRC-5	Increase in polyploidy at passage 50 (to 5.7% at passage 60), and in aneuploidy and chromosome abnormalities at passage 60 (to 43 and 14%, respectively)	65
	Human fetal lung diploid cells (WI-38)	Increased frequency of dicentrics (to 24.1%) in late senescent cells (passage 55); aneuploidy and polyploidy also increased during senescence	66
	Human embryo lung fibroblast-like and human embryo kidney epitheloid lines	Significant increase in polyploid cells in early passages following explantation, low levels of all aberrations in mid-passages, and increases in polyploidy and breakage-type aberrations associated with senescence	67
	DNA Cross-Linking[b]		
Elution of DNA by alkaline solutions	Human fetal lung diploid cells (WI-38)	No increase of DNA cross-links as cells senesce	68

Table 1 (continued)
ALTERATION OF DNA/CHROMATIN STRUCTURE

Technique of measurement	Cell type	Degree of change in parameter	Ref.
Sister Chromatid Exchange[b]			
Bromodeoxyuridine differential staining	Human fetal lung diploid cells (IMR-90)	No difference in baseline levels of SCE as a function of passage number	69
Structural Changes in Chromatin[b]			
Incorporation of radioactivity and liquid scintillation counting	Human fetal lung diploid cells (WI-38)	Decrease in rate of histone acetylation with increasing passage number (17th to 52nd population doubling), but no change in the histone/DNA ratio	70

[a] Aging in vivo.
[b] Senescing in vitro.

Table 2
DNA REPAIR ACTIVITIES

Inducing agent	Type of damage	Cell type	Differences in repair activities	Ref.
		Aging In Vivo		
UV light[a]	Thymine dimers and/or other UV-induced alterations	Sprague-Dawley rat myocardial cells	Primary cultures from newborn animals perform unscheduled DNA synthesis (UDS); cultures from adult animals do not undergo UDS	71
	Thymine dimers and/or other UV-induced alterations	Mouse embryonic fibroblasts (BALB/c)	Embryos of 13—15 days gestation perform UDS more so than embryos of 17—19 days gestation (later stages of development); subsequent in vitro studies of these cells exhibited a decrease in excision repair as a function of increasing passages	72
	Thymine dimers and/or other UV-induced alterations	Human peripheral leukocytes from individuals of increasing ages	Decrease of 30% of average DNA repair capacity in cells from 90-year-old individuals than in 20-year-olds as measured by UV-induced [^{3}H]thymidine uptake	73
X-radiation[b]	Chromosome aberrations	Swine leukocytes from animals of increasing ages	No age-associated increase in chromosome-type aberrations; an increase in chromatid-type aberrations with advancing age seen in scored metaphases	42
	Chromosome aberrations	Bone marrow of mouse and rat strains of increasing ages	Similar initial amounts of radiation damage and recoveries from induced chromosome aberrations in young and old animals seen in scored metaphases	45
	Chromosome aberrations	Human lymphocytes from males and females of increasing ages	Age-associated decrease in dicentric yield (0.4% per year); frequency of acentric fragments, rings, and intercalary deletions independent of age	44
	DNA single-strand breaks	Internal granular layer neurons from cerebella of beagle dogs of increasing ages	No age-associated decrease in ability of cells to rejoin single-strand breaks	27
	DNA single-strand breaks	Retinal photoreceptors from New Zealand white rabbits of increasing ages	No age-associated alteration in ability of cells to rejoin single-strand breaks	31

Table 2 (continued)
DNA REPAIR ACTIVITIES

Inducing agent	Type of damage	Cell type	Differences in repair activities	Ref.
	DNA single-strand breaks	Liver and cerebellum from male C57BL/6 mice of increasing ages	Similar amounts of radiation-induced DNA scission repair in hepatic and cerebellum cells of young (2 months) and old (22 months) mice	74
	DNA single-strand breaks	Liver, heart, kidney, and spleen from male white Sprague-Dawley rats of increasing ages	Distinct reduction in relative repair with increasing age (from 6 months, 18—20 months, to 32—34 months) in liver, heart, and kidney; spleen cells showed no difference in older groups	75
Vinblastine	Chromosome aberrations	Bone marrow of mouse and rat strains of increasing ages	No age-associated increase of aberration frequency compared to untreated controls seen with scoring metaphases	45
Thio-tepa and degranol	Chromosome aberrations	Human peripheral lymphocytes from males and females of increasing ages	Age-associated increase in aberration frequency with higher mutagen doses; greater frequency difference between ages (newborn, young of 23 mean years of age, and elderly of 70 mean years)	76
1,2-Dimethylhydrizine hydrochloride (DMH)	DNA alkylation	Intestinal mucosal cells from male CFN rats of increasing ages	Considerable repair occurred by 24 hr after carcinogen treatment in young animals; relatively little repair seen by alkaline sucrose gradient centrifugation after 40 hr in old animals	77
Bleomycin	DNA strand breaks	Liver nuclei from pathogen-free Fisher rats of increasing ages	Old (19 months) rats do not respond with increased tritiated thymidine uptake to same extent as mature rats (4 months); up to 50% reduction at high bleomycin concentrations; sucrose density profiles show bleomycin induces breaks in mature and old cells to same extent	78
	DNA strand breaks	Human peripheral lymphocytes of males and females of increasing ages	Age-associated increase of sensitivity to bleomycin suggests age-related alteration in DNA	79
4-Nitroquinoline 1-oxide, ethylnitrosourea, and methylmethane sulphonic acid	Chemical carcinogen induced	Retinal ganglion cells from male Wistar rats of increasing ages	The 3 carcinogens showed similar dose-dependent effects, but no age-associated changes in UDS	80
	Chemical carcinogen induced	Ganglion cells of Mekada fish of increasing ages	No age-associated changes in UDS	81

Mitomycin C, N-acetoxy-2-acetyl-aminofluorene	Sister chromatid exchange (SCE)	Bone marrow from male C57Bl/6J mice and female Wistar rats; human skin fibroblasts, all of increasing ages	Age-associated decrease of induced SCEs as a function of donor age (in vivo aging) with BrdUrd differential staining; an increase in chromosome aberrations with age also noted	82, 83
Cyclophosphamide, mitomycin C, doxorubicin	Sister chromatid exchange (SCE)	Bone marrow from male C57Bl/6J mice	At low concentrations of DNA-damaging agent, young and old cell populations demonstrate similar levels of induced SCEs; at higher mutagen concentrations, induced SCEs were significantly reduced (approximately 30%) in old cell populations	84
			Senescing In Vitro	
UV light	Thymine dimers and/or other UV-induced alterations	Human skin fibroblasts	Early and intermediate passage cells show similar levels of UDS and a slight decrease in late-passage cells; no differences in UV sensitivity of early passages of cells from fetal, newborn, young, and elderly donors	85
	Thymine dimers and/or other UV-induced alterations	Human fetal lung diploid cells (WI-38)	Early, intermediate, and almost senescent cells have similar repair capacities measured with isopyknic centrifugation; a 35% loss of capacity in senescent cells	86
	Thymine dimers and/or other UV-induced alterations	Cells obtained by biopsy from animals of varying life spans; human fetal lung diploid cells (WI-38)	Parallel relationship between repair capacity and maximum life span of various animals; many late-passage WI-38 cells show much less UDS than do early-passage cells	87
	Thymine dimers and/or other UV-induced alterations	Mouse embryonic fibroblasts (BALB/c)	Loss of dimer excision in late passages (7—9) from early passages	88
	Thymine dimers and/or other UV-induced alterations	Hamster embryo cells	Repair measured by UDS decreases until no longer detected as cells reached senescence	89
	Thymine dimers and/or other UV-induced alterations	Human fetal lung diploid cells (WI-38)	Repair capacity showed a fourfold decline in specific activity and a twofold decline in repair activity from young to old cultures measured by UDS and fluorescence	90

Table 2 (continued)
DNA REPAIR ACTIVITIES

Inducing agent	Type of damage	Cell type	Differences in repair activities	Ref.
	Thymine dimers and/or other UV-induced alterations	Human fetal lung diploid cells (WI-38)	UDS of cells from passage 18 through 36 and 48 decreases to a low or almost undetectable amount of UDS in passage 60	91
	Thymine dimers and/or other UV-induced alterations	Embryonic fibroblasts from 3 inbred mouse strains (N2B, C_3Hf, and CBA/H)	Capacity of repair synthesis correlates to maximal expected life span; ability to perform UDS exhibits age-associated decline (a measurable reduction after only 3 generations in early passages in 1 line)	92
	Pyrimidine dimers	Hamster embryo cells	Rate of removal of endonuclease-sensitive sites declined during senescence	93
X-radiation	DNA single-strand breaks	Diploid skin fibroblasts from biopsy of normal humans	Similar rate of DNA repair throughout in vitro life span outside very early passage (slightly more rapid) until a decline in rejoining rate appeared with senescence	94—96
	DNA single-strand breaks	Human progeroid cells	Significantly less rate of DNA repair in progeroid cells than normal diploid cells possibly due to accelerated in vitro senescence	95
	DNA single-strand breaks	Human progeroid cells	No inherent defect in DNA repair	97
	DNA single-strand breaks	Human fetal lung diploid cells (WI-38)	No age-associated repair decline from young (passage 27) to old (passage 55) cells	98
	DNA single-strand breaks	Hamster embryo cells	Rate of rejoining of strand breaks and repair measured by UDS declined until no longer detected as cells reached senescence	89
	DNA single-strand breaks	Human fetal lung diploid cells (WI-38)	Rates of strand rejoining for young (Phase II) and old (Phase III) cells are normal	99
	DNA single-strand breaks	Human fetal lung diploid cells (WI-38)	Decrease of UDS in cells from passage 18 through 48, to small amount of UDS in passage 60	91
X-radiation; osmium tetroxide oxidation	5,6-dihydroxydihydrothymine (t′) residues	Isolated nuclei and nuclear sonicates from human fetal lung diploid cells (WI-38)	Total loss of excision of t′ residues in old cells (over 42 passages) compared to young and intermediate aged cells (15—25 and 26—42 passages, respectively)	100

Mitomycin C, N-acetoxy-2-acetyl-aminofluorene, ethyl-methane-sulfonate	Sister chromatid exchange (SCE)	Human fetal lung diploid cells (IMR-90, WI-38)	Age-associated decrease of induced SCEs as a function of serial passage (in vitro aging)	101

[a] Predominantly 254 nm.
[b] X- or γ-rays: any minimally ionizing radiation.

XP has been the most widely studied of these diseases.[103] Defects in DNA repair in XP cells have been measured by loss of UV endonuclease sites,[104] unscheduled DNA synthesis (UDS),[105] and repair replication measured by photolysis of BrdUrd and isopyknic gradients.[106] Cells from people with AT have been shown to both remove γ-damaged bases more slowly than normal cells[107] and exhibit reduced levels of UDS.[108] Evidence implicating FA consists of poor support of γ-irradiated and UV-irradiated adenovirus,[109] reduced excision of pyrimidine dimers at high UV doses,[110] and increased sensitivity to DNA cross-linking agents.[111] Few patients with CS have been studied, but fibroblasts show increased UV-sensitivity, reduced UDS, and reduced ^{3}H-dTdR incorporation.[112] PG has been implicated as a repair-deficient disease from measurements of rates of rejoining of γ-induced DNA strand breaks[94,95] and reduced levels of γ-irradiated adenovirus growth on progeroid cells.[113] BS and WS are both possible repair-deficient diseases, as cells from patients exhibit a high frequency of chromosomal aberrations,[114,115] and in the case of BS, the chromosomes have been shown to be more sensitive to radiation[114] and the cells have shown slightly greater sensitivity to UVL.[116] Although hereditary RB has not demonstrated characteristics of accelerated aging, individuals with this genetic predisposition for malignant eye tumors are postulated to be deficient in DNA repair. Skin fibroblasts from hereditary RB patients appear to have increased X-ray sensitivity over normal controls or sporadic RB.[117,118]

Martin has examined the characteristics of aging in a variety of diseases in great detail. We have extracted primarily from his tables aspects of aging associated with each of the known or suspected DNA repair-deficient diseases. These data are presented in Table 3.

SUMMARY AND CONCLUSIONS

Table 1 lists 47 studies comparing prevalence of altered DNA or chromatin structure in aging or senescing cells. Of these, 33 indicated that there was a demonstrable change in at least some cells of aging mammals; 7 reported no observed change; 5 observed a change in DNA or chromatin structure in cells senescing in vitro; and 2 were negative in similar experiments.

In toto, these data are convincing that DNA/chromatin structure, at least in nondividing cells, changes during aging. The changes range from DNA strand scissions to subtle alterations in chromatin proteins. It does not seem possible at this time to associate these changes with a mechanism by which such damage might have been induced. Thus, it is not possible to suggest whether these changes underlie the physiological detriments associated with age, or whether they are a concomitant of a more basic process.

Table 2 describes data which should indicate whether altered DNA structure may result from altered DNA repair capacity. In this table of 19 experiments, 10 indicated cellular DNA repair or sequalae of DNA repair in vivo, decreased with age, or increased with maximum life span. Seven studies were negative, and in two there were positive results in some cell populations and negative results in others. The major problem in interpreting these data is the lack of experimental confidence in interpreting the biological relevance of the endpoints measured. This is especially true for measurements in cells senescing in vitro. Even though the observations of altered repair are more numerous than negative observations (15 of 18 positive, 3 of 18 negative), the meaning in terms of aging in vivo is not at all clear.

Table 3 is primarily an augmented tabular presentation of the thoughts of Martin,[102] and indicates that there are aspects of accelerated aging in individuals with DNA repair deficiencies. It is not surprising that these various individuals show evidence of aging in only a limited way. Indeed, since cells from these individuals are sensitive to specific

Table 3
DNA REPAIR-DEFICIENT DISEASES

Characteristics associated with aging	Repair-deficient diseases[a]						
	XP	AT	FA	BS	CS	WS	PG
Loci of potential relevance to the "intrinsic mutagenesis" theory of aging (DNA polymerases, repair enzymes, "scavenger" proteases, metabolic activators and inactivators, macromolecular effects on frequencies of mutations, and rearrangements)	x	x	x	x	x	x	x
Increased frequency of "nonconstitutive chromosomal aberrations"	x	x	x	x		x	
Increased susceptibility to neoplasms that are highly characteristic of aging populations	x	x	x	x		x	
Possibility of a defect in a stem-cell population or the kinetics of stem-cell proliferation						x	x
Premature graying and/or loss of hair		x				x	x
Dementia and/or relevant degenerative neuropatholgy	x	x			x		
Increased depositions of lipofuscin pigments					x		
Diabetes mellitus		x	x		x	x	
Lipid metabolism disorder					x		x
Hypogonadism		x		x	x	x	x
Hypertension					x		x
Degenerative vascular disease					x	x	x
Osteoporosis					x	x	x
Cataracts (may overlap with senile cataracts)					x	x	
Regional fibrosis	x	x		x	x	x	x
Variations in amounts and/or distributions of adipose tissues					x	x	x
Glucose intolerance and/or insulin resistance		o	o		o	o	o
Atherosclerosis						o	o
Poikiloderma	+	+					
Hyporeflexia	+	+					

Note: XP = xeroderma pigmentosum; AT = ataxia telangiectasia; FA = Fanconi's anemia; BS = Bloom's syndrome; CS = Cockayne's syndrome; WS = Werner's syndrome; and PG = Hutchinson-Gilford progeria syndrome.

[a] Information from x: Martin;[102] o: Goldstein;[119] +: Kraemer.[120]

or narrow ranges of DNA damage, tissues should show accelerated aging only if they experience such damage. Thus, patients with XP whose cells are sensitive to UV light-induced damage evidence accelerated aging in their skin which is exposed to the sun; such increased aging is not detected in internal organs.

In conclusion it seems that on the basis of both the compiled evidence and the biological role of the DNA molecule in directing cellular activity, DNA damage must remain a preferred candidate for the basic mechanism of aging. The acceptance of DNA damage as the prime cause of aging will depend first upon the ability to establish an exact hypothesis which traces DNA damage from its induction through attempted repair, to eventual manifestation in the aging tissue. This exact hypothesis must then be demonstrated to occur in vivo, and finally will be accepted only when a defined and specific manipulation of DNA damage in vivo alters the life span of the host organism.

Within the limits of present knowledge of both DNA/chromatin damage and repair in vivo and the cellular basis of aging, there is no mutual incompatibility. Deterioration in DNA and/or chromatin structure could underly the aging process.

ACKNOWLEDGMENT

The authors are supported by grants AG-01735 and AG-01736 from the National Institute on Aging.

REFERENCES

1. **Bergsma, D. and Harrison, D., Eds.,** *Genetic Effects on Aging,* Alan R. Liss, New York, 1978.
2. **Schneider, E., Ed.,** *The Genetics of Aging,* Plenum Press, New York, 1978.
3. **Strehler, B.,** *Time, Cells and Aging,* 2nd ed., Academic Press, New York, 1977.
4. **Comfort, A.,** *The Biology of Senescence,* Elsevier, New York, 1979.
5. **Rockstein, M., Ed.,** *Theoretical Aspects of Aging,* Academic Press, New York, 1974.
6. **Hanawalt, P., Cooper, P., Ganesan, A., and Smith, C. A.,** DNA repair in bacteria and mammalian cells, *Annu. Rev. Biochem.,* 48, 783, 1979.
7. **Beers, R. F., Jr., Herriott, R. M., and Tilghman, R. C., Eds.,** *Molecular and Cellular Repair Processes,* Johns Hopkins University Press, Baltimore, 1972.
8. **Hanawalt, P., Friedberg, E., and Fox, C. F., Eds.,** *DNA Repair Mechanisms,* Academic Press, New York, 1978.
9. **Nichols, W. and Murphy, D., Eds.,** *DNA Repair Processes,* Symposia Specialists, Miami, 1977.
10. **Hanawalt, P. and Setlow, R., Eds.,** *Molecular Mechanisms for Repair of DNA,* (Parts A and B), Plenum Press, New York, 1975.
11. **Lindahl, T.,** DNA repair enzymes acting on spontaneous lesions in DNA, in *DNA Repair Processes,* Nichols, W. and Murphy, D., Eds., Symposia Specialists, Miami, 1977, 225.
12. **Lindahl, T. and Hyberg, B.,** Heat-induced deamination of cytosine residues in deoxyribonucleic acid, *Biochemistry,* 13, 3405, 1974.
13. **Wovcha, M. and Warner, H.,** Synthesis and nucleolytic degradation of uracil-containing deoxyribonucleic acid by *Escherichia coli* deoxyribonucleic acid polymerase I, *J. Biol. Chem.,* 248, 1746, 1973.
14. **Duncan, B. and Weiss, B.,** Uracil-DNA glycosylase mutants are mutators, in *DNA Repair Mechanisms,* Hanawalt, P., Friedberg, E., and Fox, C. F., Eds., Academic Press, New York, 1978, 183.
15. **Cleaver, J. E.,** Nucleosome structure controls rates of excision repair in DNA of human cells, *Nature,* 270, 451, 1977.
16. **Smerdon, M. and Lieberman, M.,** Distribution of UV-induced DNA repair synthesis in human chromatin, in *DNA Repair Mechanisms,* Hanawalt, P., Friedberg, E., and Fox, C. F., Eds., Academic Press, New York, 1978, 327.
17. **Burnet, F. M.,** *Intrinsic Mutagenesis: A Genetic Approach to Aging,* John Wiley & Sons, New York, 1974.

18. **Williams, J., Little, J., and Shipley, W.,** Association of mammalian cell death with a specific endonucleolytic degradation of DNA, *Nature,* 252, 754, 1974.
19. **Williams, J. R.,** Role of DNA repair in cell inactivation, aging, and transformation: a selective review, a speculative model, *Adv. Radiat. Biol.,* 6, 161, 1976.
20. **Regan, J. D., Setlow, R. B., and Ley, R. D.,** Normal and defective repair of damaged DNA in human cells: a sensitive assay utilizing the photolysis of bromodeoxyuridine, *Proc. Natl. Acad. Sci. U.S.A.,* 68, 708, 1971.
21. **Regan, J. D. and Setlow, R. B.,** Two forms of repair in the DNA of human cells damaged by chemical carcinogens and mutagens, *Cancer Res.,* 34, 3318, 1974.
22. **Radman, M.,** SOS repair hypothesis: phenomenology of an inducible DNA repair which is accompanied by mutagenesis, in *Molecular Mechanisms for Repair of DNA,* Hanawalt, P. C. and Setlow, R. B., Eds., Plenum Press, New York, 1975, 355.
23. **Hayflick, L.,** The limited *in vitro* life span of human diploid cell strains, *Exp. Cell Res.,* 37, 614, 1965.
24. **Price, G., Modak S., and Makinodan, T.,** Age-associated changes in the DNA of mouse tissue, *Science,* 171, 917, 1971.
25. **Massie, H., Baird, M., Nicolosi, R., and Samis, H.,** Changes in the structure of rat liver DNA in relation to age, *Arch. Biochem. Biophys.,* 153, 736, 1972.
26. **Karran, P. and Ormerod, M.,** Is the ability to repair damage to DNA related to the proliferative capacity of a cell? The rejoining of X-ray produced strand breaks, *Biochim. Biophys. Acta,* 299, 54, 1973.
27. **Wheeler, K. and Lett, J.,** On the possibility that DNA repair is related to age in nondividing cells, *Proc. Natl. Acad. Sci. U.S.A.,* 71, 1862, 1974.
28. **Ono, T., Okada, S., and Sugahara, T.,** Comparative studies of DNA size in various tissues of mice during the aging process, *Exp. Gerontol.,* 11, 127, 1976.
29. **Chetsanga, C., Tuttle, M., and Jacoboni, A.,** Changes in structural integrity of heart DNA from aging mice, *Life Sci.,* 18, 1405, 1976.
30. **Chetsanga, C., Tuttle, M., Jacoboni, A., and Johnson, C.,** Age-associated structural alterations in senescent mouse brain DNA, *Biochim. Biophys. Acta,* 474, 180, 1977.
31. **Lett, J.,** Cellular senescence and the capacity for rejoining DNA strand breaks, in *DNA Repair Processes,* Nichols, W. and Murphy, D., Eds., Symposia Specialists, Miami, 1977, 89.
32. **Cheah, K. and Osborne, D.,** DNA lesions occur with loss of viability in embryos of aging rye seed, *Nature,* 272, 593, 1978.
33. **Chetsanga, C., Boyd, V., Peterson, L., and Rushlow, K.,** Single-stranded regions in DNA of old mice, *Nature,* 253, 130, 1975.
34. **Sheid, B., Pedrinan, L., Lu, T., and Nelson, J.,** Single-stranded regions in DNA from pre- and postmenopausal human ovaries, *Biochem. Biophys. Res. Commun.,* 66, 1131, 1975.
35. **Dean, R. and Cutler, R.,** Absence of significant age-dependent increase of single-stranded DNA extracted from mouse liver nuclei, *Exp. Gerontol.,* 13, 287, 1978.
36. **Nakanishi, K., Shima, A., Fukuda, M., and Fujita, S.,** Age-associated increase of single-stranded regions in the DNA of mouse brain and liver cells, *Mech. Ageing Dev.,* 10, 273, 1979.
37. **Stevenson, K. and Curtis, H.,** Chromosome aberrations in irradiated and nitrogen mustard-treated mice, *Radiat. Res.,* 15, 774, 1961.
38. **Crowley, C. and Curtis, H.,** The development of somatic mutations in mice with age, *Proc. Natl. Acad. Sci. U.S.A.,* 49, 626, 1963.
39. **Curtis, H., Leith, J., and Tilley, J.,** Chromosome aberrations in liver cells of dogs of different ages, *J. Gerontol.,* 21, 268, 1966.
40. **Chlebovsky, D., Praslicka, M., and Horak, J.,** Chromosome aberrations: increased incidence in bone marrow of continuously irradiated rats, *Science,* 153, 195, 1966.
41. **Jarvik, L. and Kato, T.,** Chromosome examinations in aged twins, *Am. J. Hum. Genet.,* 22, 562, 1970.
42. **McFee, A., Banner, M., and Sherrill, M.,** Influence of animal age on radiation-induced chromosome aberrations in swine leukocytes, *Radiat. Res.,* 41, 425, 1970.
43. **Curtis, H. and Miller, K.,** Chromosome aberrations in liver cells of guinea pigs, *J. Gerontol.,* 26, 292, 1971.
44. **Liniecki, J., Bajerska, A., and Andryszek, C.,** Chromosomal aberrations in human lymphocytes irradiated *in vitro* from donors (males-females) of varying age, *Int. J. Radiat. Biol.,* 19, 349, 1971.
45. **Curtis, H. and Tilley, J.,** The life span of dividing mammalian cells *in vivo, J. Gerontol.,* 26, 1, 1971.
46. **Bochkov, N.,** Spontaneous chromosome aberrations in human somatic cells, *Humangenetik,* 16, 159, 1972.
47. **Brooks, A., Mead, D., and Peters, R.,** Effect of aging on the frequency of metaphase chromosome aberrations in the liver of Chinese hamster, *J. Gerontol.,* 28, 452, 1973.

48. **Mattevi, M. and Salzano, F.,** Senescence and human chromosome changes, *Humangenetik*, 27, 1, 1975.
49. **Ayme, S., Mattei, J., Mattei, M., Aurran, Y., and Giraud, F.,** Nonrandom distribution of chromosome breaks in cultured lymphocytes of normal subjects, *Hum. Genet.*, 31, 161, 1976.
50. **Galloway, S. and Buckston, K.,** Aneuploidy and aging: chromosome studies on a random sample of the population using G-banding, *Cytogenet. Cell Genet.*, 20, 78, 1978.
51. **Ivanov, B., Praskova, L., Mileva, M., Bulanova, M., and Georgieva, I.,** Spontaneous chromosomal aberration levels in human peripheral lymphocytes, *Mutat. Res.*, 52, 421, 1978.
52. **Acharya, P.,** The isolation and partial characterizatin of age-correlated oligodeoxyribonucleotide with covalently linked aspartyl-glutamyl-polypeptides, *Johns Hopkins Med. J. Suppl.*, 1, 254, 1972.
53. **Zhelabosovskaya, S. and Berydyshev, G.,** Composition, template activity, and thermostability of the liver chromatin in rats of various age, *Exp. Gerontol.*, 7, 313, 1972.
54. **Shirey, T. and Sobel, H.,** Compositional and transcriptional properties of chromatins isolated from cardiac muscle of young-mature and old dogs, *Exp. Gerontol.*, 7, 15, 1972.
55. **O'Meara, A. and Herrmann, R.,** A modified mouse liver chromatin preparation displaying age-related differences in salt dissociation and template activity, *Biochim. Biophys. Acta*, 269, 419, 1972.
56. **Stein, G., Wang, P., and Adelman, R.,** Age-dependent changes in the structure and function of mammalian chromatin. I. Variations in chromatin template activity, *Exp. Gerontol.*, 8, 123, 1973.
57. **Carter, D. and Chae, C.,** Composition of liver histones in aging rat and mouse, *J. Gerontol.*, 30, 28, 1975.
58. **Liew, C. and Gornall, A.,** Covalent modification of nuclear proteins during aging, *Fed. Proc.* 34, 186, 1975.
59. **Petricevic, M.,** Temporal changes in histone acetylation, *Mech. Ageing Dev.*, 8, 241, 1978.
60. **Ermini, M., Moret, M., Reichmeier, K., and Dunne, T.,** Age-dependent structural changes in human neuronal chromatin, *Aktuel Gerontol.*, 8, 675, 1978.
61. **Gaubatz, J., Eliis, M., and Chalkley, R.,** Nuclease digestion studies of mouse chromatin as a function of age, *J. Gerontol.*, 34, 672, 1979.
62. **O'Meara, A. and Pochron, S.,** Age-related effects on the incorporation of acetate into rat liver histones, *Biochim. Biophys. Acta*, 586, 391, 1979.
63. **Medvedev, Z., Medvedeva, M., and Robson, L.,** Age-related changes of the pattern of nonhistone chromatin proteins from rat and mouse liver chromatin, *Gerontology*, 25, 219, 1979.
64. **Saksela, E. and Moorhead, P.,** Aneuploidy in the degenerative phase of serial cultivation of human cell strains, *Proc. Natl. Acad. Sci. U.S.A.*, 50, 390, 1963.
65. **Thompson, K. and Holliday, R.,** Chromosome changes during the *in vitro* aging of MRC-5 human fibroblasts, *Exp. Cell Res.*, 96, 1, 1975.
66. **Benn, P.,** Specific chromosome aberrations in senescent fibroblast cell lines derived from human embryos, *Am. J. Hum. Genet.*, 28, 465, 1976.
67. **Miller, R., Nichols, W., Pottash, J., and Aronson, M.,** *In vitro* aging. Cytogenetic comparison of diploid human fibroblast and epitheloid cell lines, *Exp. Cell Res.*, 110, 63, 1977.
68. **Bradley, M., Erickson, L., and Kohn, K.,** Normal DNA strand rejoining and absence of DNA cross-linking in progeroid and aging human cells, *Mutat. Res.*, 37, 279, 1976.
69. **Schneider, E. and Kram, D.,** Examination of the effect of aging on cell replication, in *DNA Repair Processes*, Nichols, W. and Murphy, D., Eds., Symposia Specialists, Miami, 1977, 177.
70. **Ryan, J. and Cristofalo, V.,** Histone acetylation during aging of human cells in culture, *Biochem. Biophys. Res. Commun.*, 48, 735, 1972.
71. **Lampidis, T. and Schaiberger, G.,** Age-related loss of DNA repair synthesis in isolated rat myocardial cells, *Exp. Cell Res.*, 96, 412, 1975.
72. **Peleg, L., Ray, E., and Ben Ishai, R.,** Changing capacity for DNA excision repair in mouse embryonic cells *in vitro, Exp. Cell Res.*, 104, 301, 1976.
73. **Lambert, B., Ringborg, Y., and Skoog, L.,** Age-related decrease of ultraviolet light-induced DNA repair synthesis in human peripheral leukocytes, *Cancer Res.*, 39, 2792, 1979.
74. **Ono, T. and Okada, S.,** Does the capacity to rejoin radiation-induced DNA breaks decline in senescent mice? *Int. J. Radiat. Biol.*, 33, 403, 1978.
75. **Niedermuller, H., Hofecker, G., and Knent, A.,** Gerontological investigations of the nucleic acid metabolism in the rat. II. DNA repair capacity in different ages, *Aktuel Gerontol.*, 8, 253, 1978.
76. **Bochkov, N. and Kuleskov, N.,** Age sensitivity of human chromosomes to alkylating agents, *Mutat. Res.*, 14, 345, 1972.
77. **Kanagalingam, K. and Balis, M.,** *In vivo* repair of rat intestinal DNA damage by alkylating agents, *Cancer*, 36, 2364, 1975.
78. **Ove, P. and Coltzee, M.,** A difference in bleomycin-induced DNA synthesis between liver nuclei from mature and old rats, *Mech. Ageing Dev.*, 8, 363, 1978.
79. **Seshadri, R., Morley A., Trainor, K., and Sorrell, J.,** Sensitivity of human lymphocytes to bleomycin increases with age, *Experientia*, 35, 233, 1979.

80. **Ishikawa, T., Takayama, S., and Kitagawa, T.,** DNA repair synthesis in rat retinal ganglion cells treated with chemical carcinogens or ultraviolet light *in vitro,* with special reference to aging and repair level, *J. Natl. Cancer Inst.,* 61, 1101, 1978.
81. **Ishikawa, T., Takayama, S., and Kitagawa, T.,** Autoradiographic demonstration of DNA repair synthesis in ganglion cells of aquarium fish at various age *in vivo, Virchows Arch. B: Cell Pathol.,* 28, 235, 1978.
82. **Kram, D., Schneider, E., Tice R., and Gianas, P.,** Aging and sister chromatid exchange. I. The effect of aging on mitomycin C-induced sister chromatid exchange of frequencies in mouse and rat bone marrow cells *in vivo, Exp. Cell Res.,* 114, 471, 1978.
83. **Schneider, E. and Gilman, B.,** Sister chromatid exchanges and aging. III. The effect of donor age on mutagen-induced sister chromatid exchange in human diploid fibroblasts, *Hum. Genet.,* 46, 57, 1979.
84. **Nakanishi, R., Kram, D., and Schneider, E.,** Aging and sister chromatid exchange. IV. Reduced frequencies of mutagen-induced sister chromatid exchanges *in vivo* in mouse bone marrow cells with aging, *Cytogenet. Cell Genet.,* 24, 61, 1979.
85. **Goldstein, S.,** The role of DNA repair in aging of cultured fibroblasts from xeroderma pigmentosum and normals, *Proc. Soc. Exp. Biol. Med.,* 137, 730, 1971.
86. **Painter, R., Clarkson, J., and Young, B.,** Ultraviolet-induced repair replication in aging diploid human cells (WI-38), *Radiat. Res.,* 56, 560, 1973.
87. **Hart, R. and Setlow, R.,** Correlation between deoxyribonucleic acid excision repair and life span in a number of mammalian species, *Proc. Natl. Acad. Sci. U.S.A.,* 71, 2169, 1974.
88. **Ben-Ishai, R. and Peleg, L.,** Excision repair in primary cultures of mouse embryo cells and its decline in progressive passages and established cell lines, in *Molecular Mechanisms for Repair of DNA,* Hanawalt, P. and Setlow, R., Eds., Plenum Press, New York, 1975, 607.
89. **Williams, J. and Little, J.,** Correlation of DNA repair and *in vitro* growth potential in hamster embryo cells (abstract) 1975; cited in Little, J., Relationship between DNA repair capacity and cellular aging, *Gerontology,* 22, 28, 1976.
90. **Bowman, P., Meek, R., and Daniel, C.,** Decreased unscheduled DNA synthesis in nondividing aged WI-38 cells, *Mech. Ageing Dev.,* 5, 251, 1976.
91. **Hart, R. and Setlow, R.,** DNA repair in late-passage human cells, *Mech. Ageing Dev.,* 5, 67, 1976.
92. **Paffenholz, V.,** Correlation between DNA repair of embryonic fibroblasts and different life span of 3 inbred mouse strains, *Mech. Ageing Dev.,* 7, 131, 1978.
93. **Olson, F., Ritter, M., Little, J., and Williams, J.,** Excision repair of ultraviolet light-induced DNA damage through the life span of cultured embryonic Syrian hamster cells, *Mech. Ageing Dev.,* in press.
94. **Epstein, J., Williams, J., and Little, J.,** Deficient DNA repair in progeria and senescent human cells, *Radiat. Res.,* 55, 527, 1973.
95. **Epstein, J., Williams, J., and Little, J.,** Rate of DNA repair in progeric and normal human fibroblasts, *Biochem. Biophys. Res. Commun.,* 59, 850, 1974.
96. **Little, J., Epstein, J., and Williams, J.,** Repair of DNA strand breaks in progeric fibroblasts and aging diploid cells, in *Molecular Mechanisms for Repair of DNA,* Hanawalt, P. and Setlow, R., Eds., Plenum Press, New York, 1975, 793.
97. **Regan, J. and Setlow, R.,** DNA repair in human progeroid cells, *Biochem. Biophys. Res. Commun.,* 59, 858, 1974.
98. **Clarkson, J. and Painter, R.,** Repair of X-ray damage in aging WI-38 cells, *Mutat. Res.,* 23, 107, 1974.
99. **Bradley, M., Erickson, L., and Kohn, K.,** Normal DNA strand rejoining and absence of DNA cross-linking in progeroid and aging human cells, *Mutat. Res.,* 37, 279, 1976.
100. **Mattern, M. and Cerutti, P.,** Age-dependent excision repair of damaged thymidine from irradiated DNA by isolated nuclei from human fibroblasts, *Nature,* 254, 450, 1975.
101. **Schneider, E. and Monticone, R.,** Aging and sister chromatid exchange. II. The effect of the *in vitro* passage level of human fetal lung fibroblasts on baseline and mutagen-induced sister chromatid exchange frequencies, *Exp. Cell Res.,* 115, 269, 1978.
102. **Martin, G.,** Genetic syndromes in man with potential relevance to the pathobiology of aging, in *Genetic Effects on Aging,* Bergsma, D. and Harrison, D., Eds., Alan R. Liss, Inc., New York, 1978, 5.
103. **Setlow, R.,** Repair-deficient human disorders and cancer, *Nature,* 271, 713, 1978.
104. **Paterson, M., Lohman, P., and Sluyter, M.,** Use of a UV endonuclease from *Micrococcus luteus* to monitor the progress of DNA repair in UV-irradiated human cells, *Mutat. Res.,* 19, 245, 1973.
105. **Cleaver, J. and Bootsma, D.,** Xeroderma pigmentosum: biochemical and genetic characteristics, *Annu. Rev. Genet.,* 9, 19, 1975.
106. **Cleaver, J.,** Repair processes for photochemical damage in mammalian cells, *Adv. Radiat. Biol.,* 4, 1, 1974.

107. **Paterson, M., Smith, B., Lohman, P., Anderson, A., and Fishman, L.,** Defective excision repair of γ-ray-damaged DNA in human (Ataxia telangiectasia) fibroblasts, *Nature,* 260, 444, 1976.
108. **Paterson, M., Smith, B., Knight, P., and Anderson, A.,** Ataxia telangiectasia: an inherited human disease involving radiosensitivity, malignancy, and defective DNA repair, in *Research in Photobiology,* Castellani, A., Ed., Plenum Press, New York, 1977, 207.
109. **Rainbow, A. and Howes, M.,**Defective repair of ultraviolet and gamma-ray-damaged DNA in Fanconi's anemia, *Int. J. Radiat. Biol.,* 31, 191, 1977.
110. **Poon, P., O'Brien, R., and Parker, J.,** Defective DNA repair in Fanconi's anemia, *Nature,* 250, 223, 1974.
111. **Sasaki, M. and Tonomura, A.,** A high susceptibility of Fanconi's anemia to chromosome breakage by DNA cross-linking agents, *Cancer Res.,* 33, 1829, 1973.
112. **Wade, M., Chu, E., and Schmickel, R.,** Ultraviolet light sensitivity and deficiency in DNA polymerase activity in cultured skin fibroblasts from patients with Cockayne syndrome, *Mutat. Res.,* 46, 162, 1977.
113. **Rainbow, A. and Howes, M.,** Decreased repair of gamma-ray-damaged DNA in progeria, *Biochem. Biophys. Res. Commun.,* 74, 714, 1977.
114. **Higurashi, M. and Conen, P.,** *In vitro* chromosomal radiosensitivity, in Chromosomal breakage syndromes, *Cancer,* 32, 380, 1973.
115. **Hoehn, H., Bryant, E., Au, K., Norwood, T., Boman, H., and Martin, G.,** Variegated translocation mosaicism in human skin fibroblast cultures, *Cytogenet. Cell Genet.,* 15, 282, 1975.
116. **Giannelli, F., Benson, P., Pawsey, S., and Polani, P.,** Ultraviolet light sensitivity and delayed DNA-chain maturation in Bloom's syndrome fibroblasts, *Nature,* 265, 466, 1977.
117. **Weichselbaum, R., Nove, J., and Little, J.,** Skin fibroblasts from a D-deletion type retinoblastoma patient are abnormally X-ray sensitive, *Nature,* 266, 726, 1977.
118. **Weichselbaum, R., Nove, J., and Little, J.,** X-ray sensitivity of diploid fibroblasts from patients with hereditary or sporadic retinoblastoma, *Proc. Natl. Acad. Sci. U.S.A.,* 75, 3962, 1978.
119. **Goldstein, S.,** Human genetic disorders that feature premature onset and accelerated progression of biological aging, in *The Genetics of Aging,* Schneider, E., Ed., Plenum Press, New York, 1978, 171.
120. **Kraemer, K.,** Progressive degenerative diseases associated with defective DNA repair: xeroderma pigmentosum and ataxia telangiectasia, in *DNA Repair Processes,* Nichols, W. and Murphy, D., Eds., Symposia Specialists, Miami, 1977, 37.

Transcription

RNA SYNTHESIS

Morton Rothstein
and Sarah C. Seifert

INTRODUCTION

The purpose of this section is to summarize published data of the effects of age on the transcription of genetic information. Any change, programmed or random, would have major effects on the function of a given organism. Accordingly, changes in template activity of DNA as well as activities of enzymes involved in RNA synthesis are considered.

DOSAGE

There have been a number of investigations into the possibility of age-related loss of transcriptional ability. One approach involves the idea that there may be age-related changes in the amount of reiterated DNA or gene dosage. However, as shown in Table 1, studies on gene dosage and change of types of DNA do not show any consistent relationships to aging. These studies have not ruled out the possibility that even a partial loss of function of one or two critical genes could create an irreversible cascading effect which would develop into what we know as aging. Such changes may be far too small to be determined by the methods currently available.

CHANGES IN CHROMATIN

Changes in gene expression could result not only from changes in DNA itself, but also possibly from alterations in chromatin structure. Research in this area has involved a number of straightforward approaches: a search for changes in the amount of protein (histone or nonhistone) in the chromatin of young vs. old animals; the effect of such changes, if any, on the thermal stability or template activity of the chromatin; the possible differential dissociation of proteins from chromatin at various salt concentrations; the possibility of qualitative changes in the proteins associated with chromatin. The information listed in Table 2 is contradictory and confusing. It has been pointed out[53] that the study of chromatin can be complicated by contamination with proteases, nucleases, and other basic proteins which co-migrate with histones. As these problems became more apparent, procedures were developed to deal with them. Therefore, the isolation and analysis of chromatin became more reliable about the beginning of the 1970s. If attention is restricted to papers published after 1970, the apparent effects of increased age on chromatin properties are much more consistent; most reports agree that the amounts of histone, nonhistone, and RNA in chromatin do not change with age.

One approach used by a number of investigators is the extraction of chromatin with various concentrations of salts or detergents in an attempt to determine if proteins are removed differentially according to the age of the donors. Results from such studies are summarized in Table 3. Unfortunately, the salt extraction procedures seem to offer no clearer answers than the studies on intact chromatin. The binding of proteins to DNA has been reported to be stronger, the same as, and weaker in older animals. Perhaps that result should be expected: chromatin preparations which have different properties to start with might show different results upon treatment with salt or deter-

Table 1
CHANGES IN GENE DOSAGE AND DNA FRACTIONS WITH AGE

Animal	Age	Tissue	Component	Effect of age	Ref.
Dog	1—10 years	Heart, brain, muscle	r-RNA genes	D	1
	1—10 years	Spleen, liver, kidney	r-RNA genes	NC	1
Human	18—20, 64—75 years	Cardiac tissue	r-RNA	D	2
Mouse	42, 810 days	Brain	Reiterated DNA	NC	3
Human	8 months, 72 years	Brain	Reiterated DNA	NC	3
Mouse		Liver	Reiterated DNA	D	4
			Unique DNA	D	
	35—788 days	Brain	r-RNA genes	NC	5
	35—788 days	Liver	r-RNA genes	I	
Human	0.2—67 years	Brain	r-RNA genes	NC	5
	0.7—75 years	Liver	r-RNA genes	NC[a]	
Mouse		Liver	DNA fraction[b]	NC → I	6
		Brain	DNA fraction[b]	NC → I	
		Brain, kidney, spleen	Satellite DNA	NC	7
		Liver	Satellite DNA	I → NC[c]	

Note: I = increase with age; D = decrease; NC = no change; NC → I = no change from young to mature, then an increase.

[a] Trend seems down, then back to "young" value.
[b] Spontaneously reassociating fraction.
[c] Increased until 455 days, then no further change.

gent. Certainly at this time no conclusions can be reached relating the binding of proteins to DNA and the aging process.

Another approach to the idea that chromatin in old organisms becomes altered has been to examine the nature of the proteins removed by various reagents, typically salt or detergents. Again, the results are varied (Table 4). However, if attention is again restricted to papers published after 1970, the results are in general agreement; chromatin-associated proteins do not change significantly with age. Whether or not small changes in acetylation, phosphorylation, or other modification of invididual histone occur with age has not been clearly established. However, it seems clear that the histones do not alter dramatically with age, either in quantity or quality.

RNA SYNTHESIS

A number of reports deal with the RNA content of various animal tissues at different ages; they are summarized elsewhere in this handbook. There are obvious limitations in the extent to which such information can be used to reach inferences concerning rates of RNA synthesis. Attempts to measure RNA synthesis in vivo or in intact cells are hampered by the problems of isotope dilution considered in detail in Richardson's section on protein synthesis. In the case of RNA, the problem is further complicated by the fact that none of the nucleosides usually employed as labeled precursors are on the *de novo* pathway to nucleoside triphosphates. Furthermore, significant amounts of cytosine and adenosine can be incorporated into acid-insoluble material by exchange of the −CCA terminus of tRNA. Avoidance of these difficulties by use of isolated

Table 2
EFFECTS OF INCREASED AGE ON CHROMATIN PROPERTIES

Animal	Tissue	Ages	Preparation	Protein	Histone	NHP	RNA	T_m	Template activity[a]	Remarks	Ref.
Mouse	Brain	3 days—30 months	Chromatin: washed nuclei and low speed dispersion; used soluble portion which compared well with whole nucleoprotein	D → I				D → I			8
Bovine	Thymus	2 months vs. 10 years	Nucleoprotein: older procedure[9]	NC			I	I	D	No change in DNA base composition	
			Nucleoprotein: later procedure;[11] DNA (obtained without isolation of nuclei)	NC[b]			NC	NC	NC	This procedure gives a preparation containing less extraneous NHP and RNA	10
Mouse	Prostate	6 vs. 30 months	Chromatin: washed nuclei	D		D[c]			D		12
	Lung			D		D			D		
	Liver			NC		D			NC		
Rat	Kidney	6—35 months	Soluble chromatin: sheared	D			D			Base composition of RNA in liver chromatin altered at 6 vs. 14 months; RNA and protein content varies with different tissues	13
	Liver	206, 512, 965 days	Chromatin: crude						NC[d]		
	Liver		Chromatin: sheared	NC					NC	The sheared chromatin showed much higher template activity	14

Table 2 (continued)
EFFECTS OF INCREASED AGE ON CHROMATIN PROPERTIES

Animal	Tissue	Ages	Preparation	Protein	Histone	NHP	RNA	T_m	Template activity[a]	Remarks	Ref.
Dog	Cardiac muscle	1—16 years	Chromatin: nuclei (Triton X-100), mild shearing	NC			NC[e]		NC	Gel electrophoresis showed no change in pattern of chromosomal proteins; considerable fluctuation in protein/DNA and RNA/DNA from sample to sample	15
Rat	Liver	1—30 months	Chromatin: solubilized		NC	D	D	I	D		16
Mouse	Liver	3.6, 13.7, 21.4 months	Chromatin: nuclei agitated gently	NC	I	D	D		NC[f]	Total protein content unchanged but shifted to more histone and less NHP; no RNAse activity	17
Rat	Submandibular gland	2 vs. 12 months	Chromatin: washed nuclei (Triton X-100)		NC	D			I	Preparations demonstrably contained no RNAse or protease activity	18
	Liver		Chromatin: as above		NC	NC			NC		18
	Submandibular		DNA (submandibular)						NC		

Mouse	Brain	Av. 3.4, 11.6, 18.7 months	Chromatin: washed nuclei, slight agitation	NC → D	D → +				19
	Liver	6, 20, 31 months	Chromatin: purified nuclei (Triton X-100)	NC[g]	NC[h] → + NC		D	When homologous RNA polymerase was used for template activity, ''young'' polymerase was more active with ''young'' chromatin and ''old'' polymerase with ''old'' chromatin; the ''young- young'' and ''old-old'' activities were comparable	20
	Kidney			NC[g]	NC → I	NC	D		
	Brain			NC[g]	NC → I	NC	D		
Rat	Liver regenerating	2, 25, 29 months	Chromatin: *in situ*				D		21
	Liver						NC		
Mouse	Liver	3—30 months	Nuclei	NC	NC	NC	NC	Nuclei prepared to minimize nucleolysis; no change with age in repeat length or core size	22
	Heart		Nucleosomes						
	Brain								

Note: I = increase with age: D = decrease; NC = no change; D → I = decrease from young to mature, then an increase; NC → I = no change from young to mature, then an increase, etc.

[a] RNA polymerase from *E. coli.*
[b] Stated by authors does not appear in their table of results.
[c] ''Acid proteins''.
[d] The data in the authors' table shows a significant increase for mature and old vs. young animals.
[e] Authors report no gross change. However, the data show an increase in old vs. mature groups of animals.
[f] The template activities are measured after dissociation in various salt concentrations. Template activity at the initial points (no salt) is unchanged.
[g] The author claims a slight increase in the 31-month-old mice.
[h] The author indicates that the figures for the 31-month-old animals show an increase. However, statistical data are not given.

Table 3
STUDIES ON SALT-EXTRACTED CHROMATIN

Species	Tissue	Age	Conditions	Effect of age: Removal of histone control	Effect of age: Change in template activity	Ref.
Dog	Cardiac muscle	1—16 years	1.25 *M* NaCl	NC		15
Mouse	Liver	3.6, 13.7, 21.4 months	0.01 *M*—3.0 *M* NaCl	D:0.01—1.0 *M* NC:1.0—3.0 *M*	NC:3.04	17
Rat	Submandibular glands	2, 12 months	0-0.01 *M* sodium deoxycholate	I	NC	18
	Liver	1—30 months	0-2.5 *M* NaCl	NC:0—1.0 *M* D:1.0—2.5 *M*	NC:1—12 months D:30 months	16

Note: I = increase with age; D = decrease; NC = no change.

Table 4
CHROMATIN-ASSOCIATED PROTEINS

Species	Tissue	Age	Procedure	Difference with age	Ref.
Rat	Liver	6, 12, 26—28 months	Acid extraction Sephadex® G-75	NC: total content D: arginine-rich/arginine-poor	23
Cow	Thymus	<2 months, >10 months	See Ref. 23	D: arginine-rich/arginine-poor[a]	25
Chicken	Brain, liver, erythrocytes	4—8-day embryo, 1 year	Acid extraction	NC: total histones D: NHP	26
Dog	Cardiac muscle	1—2, 8—9, 11—16 years	Acid and SDS extraction Acrylamide gel electrophoresis	NC: histones NC: NHP	15
Mouse	Brain	3 days—30 months		D → I T_m D→I: protein:DNA ratio	8
	Liver, kidney, brain	6, 20, 31 months	See Ref. 26	NC	20
Rat and mouse	Liver	3—25 months	Gel electrophoresis	NC: total histones NC: various histones (F_1, F_{2b}, F_{2a1}, F_{2a2}, F_3)	28
Rat	Spleen, kidney	3, 13—14 weeks, 14—15 months, 20—22 months	Amino acid analyzer	I: total residues	29
	Intestines	3, 13—14 weeks, 14—15 months, 20—22 months	Amino acid analyzer	D: total residues	29
Human	WI-38 fibroblasts	17—18 41—48 passages	Incorporation of L-(^{3}H) tryptophan	NC: NHP	30

Note: I = increase with age; D = decrease; NC = no change; D → I = decrease from young to mature, then an increase.

[a] Methods yield considerable cross contamination of different histone fractions.

nuclei or purified enzymes can introduce errors resulting from loss of controlling factors, differences in stability or extractability of individual enzymes, etc. Virtually all of the published work on effects of aging on RNA synthesis (Table 5) suffers from one or another of these deficiencies; therefore, it is difficult to arrive at firm generalizations from these varied and conflicting data.

Obviously, the rate of synthesis of RNA may depend not only on the basic structure of DNA, but also on the enzymes specifically involved in its synthesis. Therefore, age-related deficiencies in RNA polymerases would be of primary importance to studies of aging. At this time, there are few reports which deal with changes in enzyme activity. Again, the results listed in Table 6 are contradictory, and no general conclusions are apparent.

CONCLUSION

It takes little study of the above material to conclude that research in the area of nucleic acids has not brought to light any readily interpretable age-related changes. In fact, the available information does not even tell us where not to look, since conflicting data do not permit dismissal of negative results. Nonetheless, one cannot dismiss the previous work as unimportant. To a large degree, many of the ideas behind the research are still valid. It seems clear that in many cases we simply need more precise techniques: if age-related changes occur, they are subtle ones and are not easily detectable. It therefore remains for future investigators to solve the problem of the role of gene expression in aging. Surely the key lies here. The molecular changes described in other sections of this handbook can best be interpreted as *results* of aging rather than *causes*. This statement, of course, represents only the authors' opinion. Devotees of specialized areas of investigation often prefer to consider their field of primary importance until conclusive evidence to the contrary is available; partisan polemics probably cannot be avoided. Nonetheless, it is doubtful that anyone would deny an important role for nucleic acids in the aging process.

Table 5
RNA SYNTHESIS

Animal	Tissue	Ages	Determination	Effect of age	Ref.
Mouse and rat	Muscle, liver, kidney	110—127, 838—894 days	^{3}H-cytidine incorporation	I	31
	Neurons	110—127, 838—894 days	^{3}H-cytidine incorporation	D → NC	31
Rat	Liver	1, 30 months	^{32}P-UMP incorporation into acid-insoluble material	D	32
	Marrow	12, 24 months	^{14}C-orotic acid incorporation	NC	33
	Several tissues	3, 10, 22 months	^{14}C-U incorporation	I in general, but varied with age and tissue	34
	Liver, brain	5, 22 months	^{14}C-ATP incorporation into acid-insoluble material	NC	35
	Brain	12, 24 months	^{14}C-orotic acid and H-L-leucine injected intraperitoneally and turnover assessed by loss of label	NC: mitochondrial RNA NC: soluble RNA	36
	Liver, kidney, lung, spleen, intestinal mucosa	12, 24 months	^{14}C-orotic acid incorporation	NC: ribosome turnover	37
	Lung, intestinal mucosa	12, 24 months	^{14}C-orotic acid incorporation	NC: soluble RNA	37
	Spleen, liver, kidney	12, 24 months	^{14}C-orotic acid incorporation	D: soluble RNA	37
	Striatum, other brain regions	2, 10, 20 months	See Ref. 38	D: (striatum) D → I: other brain regions	39
	Liver	2, 4, 6, 13, 22, 31 months	^{3}H-UMP incorporation into acid-insoluble material	I: 3—6 months D:10—31 months	40
	Liver	0.75—24 months	^{3}H-uridine incorporation	D	41
	Hepatocytes	6, 12, 18, 30 months	^{3}H-orotic acid incorporation	D	42

Table 5 (continued)
RNA SYNTHESIS

Animal	Tissue	Ages	Determination	Effect of age	Ref.
Mouse	Liver, prostate	6, 30 months	^{3}H-UTP incorporation	D (particularly rRNA)	13
	Liver, muscle	8—9, 25—28 months	^{3}H-uridine incorporation by isolated nuclei	D	43
	Brain	10—13, 29—30 months	See Ref. 44	NC: hypothalmus, cerebellum, hippocampus, septum D: striatum	45
	Liver, kidney, brain	6, 20, 30 months	^{3}H-UTP incorporation	D when use *E. coli* RNA polymerase NC when use mouse RNA polymerase	20
	Liver, kidney, brain	2—4, 5—16, 19—28 months	Phenol-chloroform extraction of RNA followed by polyacrilamide gel electrophoresis	D: ratio of 28s to 18s rRNA in cytoplasm	46
Human	Embryo, lung fibroblasts	5th, 17th passage	^{3}H-UTP incorporation into acid-insoluble material	NC	47
	WI-38 fibroblasts	17—18, 41—48 passages	^{3}H-Uridine incorporation into acid-insoluble material	NC	30
	WI-38 fibroblasts	21—25, 41—45 passages	^{3}H-Uridine incorporation into acid-insoluble material	Slight I both tRNA and rRNA	48

Note: I = increase with age; D = decrease; NC = no change; D → I = decrease from young to mature, then an increase, etc.

TABLE 6
RNA POLYMERASE LEVELS

Animal	Tissue	Ages	Procedure	Effect of age	Ref.
Rat	Liver	1 day—1 year	^{14}C-ATP incorporation	I:polymerase I I:polymerase II	49
	Liver	3, 4, 6, 13, 22, 31 months	^{3}H-UMP incorporation into acid-insoluble material	NC	40
	Heart	21—30 months	^{3}H-UMP incorporation	D:polymerase I D:polymerase II NC:polymerase III	50
Mouse (BALB/c)	Spleen	3—8, 24—30 months		NC:high molecular weight polymerase D:low molecular weight polymerase	51
Mouse (BC3F1)	Liver, kidney, spleen	3—8, 24— 30 months		NC	51
Mouse	Liver, brain	18, 25, 29 months 23—31 months	^{3}H-UMP incorporation	NC	52
	Liver, prostate, lung	6, 30 months	^{3}H-UTP incorporation into acid-insoluble material	D:liver, prostate NC:lung	13
	Liver	8—9, 25—28 months	^{3}H-uridine incorporation by isolated nuclei	D:polymerase I D:polymerase II	43

Note: I = increase with age; D = decrease; and NC = no change.

REFERENCES

1. **Johnson, R. W., Chrisp, C., and Strehler, B. L.,** Selective loss of ribosomal RNA genes during the aging of postmitotic tissues, *Mech. Ageing Dev.*, 1, 183, 1972.
2. **Johnson, L. K., Johnson, R. W., and Strehler, B. L.,** Cardiac hypertrophy, aging, and changes in cardiac ribosomal RNA gene dosage in man, *J. Mol. Cell Cardiol.*, 7, 125, 1975.
3. **Cutler, R. G.,** Redundancy of information content in the genome of mammalian species as a protective mechanism determining aging rate, *Mech. Ageing Dev.*, 2, 381, 1974.
4. **Cutler, R. G.,** Transcription of unique and reiterated DNA sequences in mouse liver and brain tissues as a function of age, *Exp. Gerontol.*, 10, 37, 1975.
5. **Gaubatz, J., Prashad, N., and Cutler, R. G.,** Ribosomal RNA gene dosage as a function of tissue and age for mouse and human, *Biochim. Biophys. Acta*, 418, 358, 1976.
6. **Herrmann, R. L., Dowling, L., Russell, A. P., and Bick, M. D.,** Age-related changes in a spontaneously reassociating fraction of mouse DNA, *Mech. Ageing Dev.*, 4, 181, 1975.
7. **Prashad, N. and Culter, R. G.,** Percent satellite DNA as a function of tissue and age of mice, *Biochim. Biophys. Acta*, 418, 1, 1976.
8. **Kurtz, D. I. and Sinex, F. M.,** Age-related differences in the association of brain DNA and nuclear protein, *Biochim. Biophys. Acta*, 145, 840, 1967.
9. **Zubay, G. and Doty, P.,** The isolation and properties of deoxyribonucleoprotein particles containing single nucleic acid molecules, *J. Mol. Biol.*, 1, 1, 1959.
10. **Von Hahn, H. P.,** Age-dependent thermal denaturation and viscosity of crude and purified DNA prepared from bovine thymus, *Gerontologia*, 8, 123, 1963.
11. **Bonner, J. and Huang, R. C.,** Properties of chromasomal nucleohistone, *J. Mol. Biol.*, 6, 169, 1963.
12. **Pyhtila, M. J. and Sherman, F. G.,** Age-associated studies on thermal stability and template effectiveness of DNA and nucleoproteins from beef thymus, *Biochem. Biophys. Res. Commun.*, 31, 340, 1968.
13. **Mainwaring, W. I. P.,** Changes in the ribonucleic acid metabolism of aging mouse tissues with particular reference to the prostate gland, *Biochem. J.*, 110, 79, 1968.

14. **Samis, H. V., Jr., Poccia, D. L., and Wulff, V. J.**, The effect of salt extraction and heat-denaturation on the behavior of rat liver chromatin, *Biochem. Biophys. Acta*, 166, 410, 1968.
15. **Shirey, T. L. and Sobel, H.**, Composition and transcriptional properties of chromatins isolated from cardiac muscle of young-mature and old dogs, *Exp. Gerontol.*, 7, 15, 1972.
16. **Berdyshev, G. D. and Zhelabovskaya, S. M.**, Composition, template properties, and thermostability of liver chromatin from rats of various age at deproteinization by NaCl solutions, *Exp. Gerontol.*, 7, 321, 1972.
17. **O'Meara, A. R. and Herrmann, R. L.**, A modified mouse liver chromatin preparation displaying age-related differences in salt dissociation and template activity, *Biochim. Biophys. Acta*, 269, 419, 1972.
18. **Stein, G. S., Wang, P. L., and Adelman, R. G.**, Age-dependent changes in the structure and function of mammalian chromatin, *Exp. Gerontol.*, 8, 123, 1973.
19. **Kurtz, D. I., Russell, A. P., and Sinex, F. M.**, Multiple peaks in the derivative melting curve of chromatin from animals of varying age, *Mech. Ageing Dev.*, 3, 37, 1974.
20. **Hill, B. T.**, Influence of age on chromatin transcription in murine tissues using an heterologous and an homologous RNA polymerase, *Gerontology*, 22, 111, 1976.
21. **Pieri, C., Zs-Nagy, I., Guili, C., Zs-Nagy, V., and Bertoni-Freddari, C.**, Age-dependent increase of thermal stability of *in situ* chromatin of rat liver and its reversal after hepatectomy, *Experientia*, 32, 891, 1976.
22. **Gaubatz, J., Ellis, M., and Chalkley, R.**, Nuclease digestion studies of mouse chromatin as a function of age, *J. Gerontol.*, 34, 672, 1979.
23. **Von Hahn, H. P., Miller, J., and Eichhorn, G. L.**, Age-related alterations in the structure of nucleoprotein, *Gerontolgia*, 15, 293, 1969.
24. **Johns, E. W.**, Studies on histones. VII. Preparative methods for histone fractionation from calf thymus, *Biochem. J.*, 92, 55, 1964.
25. **Pyhtila, M. J. and Sherman, F. G.**, Studies on the histones and DNA of calf and old cow thymus, *J. Gerontol.*, 23, 450, 1968.
26. **Dingman, C. W. and Sporn, M. B.**, Isolation and characterization of nuclear complexes of deoxyribonucleic acid, ribonucleic acid, and protein from embryonic and adult tissues of the chicken, *J. Biol. Chem.*, 239, 3483, 1964.
27. **Paul, J. and Gilmour, R. S.**, Template activity of DNA is restricted in chromatin, *J. Mol. Biol.*, 16, 242, 1966.
28. **Carter, D. B. and Chae, C. B.**, Composition of liver histones in aging rat and mouse, *J. Gerontol.*, 30, 28, 1975.
29. **Salser, J. S. and Balis, M. E.**, Alterations in deoxyribonucleic acid-bound amino acids with age and sex, *J. Gerontol.*, 27, 1, 1972.
30. **Stein, G. S. and Burtner, D. L.**, Gene activation of human diploid cells age-dependent modifications in the stability of messenger RNAs for nonhistone chromosomal proteins, *Biochim. Biophys. Acta*, 390, 56, 1975.
31. **Wulff, V. J., Samis, H. V. Jr., and Falzone, J. A. Jr.**, The metobolism of ribonucleic acid in young and old rodents, *Adv. Gerontol. Res.*, 2, 37, 1967.
32. **Devi, A., Lindsay, P., Raina, P, L., and Sardar, N. K.**, Effect of age on some aspects of the synthesis of ribonucleic acid, *Nature, (London)*, 212, 474, 1966.
33. **Menzies, R. A., Press, G. D., and Strehler, B. L.**, Nucleic acid synthesis by old and young adult rat marrow *in vitro, Biochim. Biophys. Acta*, 145, 178, 1967.
34. **Kanungo, M. S., Koul, O., and Reddy, K. R.**, Concomitant studies on RNA and protein synthesis in tissues of rats of various ages, *Exp. Gerontol.*, 5, 261, 1970.
35. **Gibas, M. A. and Harman, D.**, Ribonucleic acid synthesis by nuclei isolated from rats of different ages, *J. Gerontol.*, 25, 105, 1970.
36. **Menzies, R. A. and Gold, P. H.**, The apparent turnover of mitochondria, ribosomes, and sRNA of the brain in young adult and aged rats, *J. Neurochem.*, 19, 1671, 1972.
37. **Menzies, R. A., Mishra, R. K., and Gold, P. H.**, The turnover of ribosomes and soluble RNA in a variety of tissues of young adult and aged rats, *Mech. Ageing Dev.*, 1, 117, 1972.
38. **Schmidt, G. and Thannhauser, S. J.**, A method for the determination of deoxyribonucleic acid, ribonucleic acid, and phosphoproteins in animal tissues, *J. Biol. Chem.*, 161, 83, 1945.
39. **Shaskan, E. G.**, Brain regional spermidine and spermine levels in relation to RNA and DNA in aging rat brain, *J. Neurochem.*, 28, 509, 1977.
40. **Castle, T., Katz, A., and Richardson, A.**, Comparison of RNA synthesis by liver nuclei from rats of various ages, *Mech. Ageing Dev.*, 8, 383, 1978.
41. **Collins, J. M.**, RNA synthesis in rat liver cells with different RNA contents, *J. Biol. Chem.*, 253, 5773, 1978.
42. **Kreamer, W., Zorich, N., Liu, D. S. H., and Richardson, A.**, Effect of age on RNA synthesis by rat hepatocytes, *Exp. Gerontol.*, 14, 27, 1979.

43. **Britton, V. S., Sherman, F. G., and Florini, J. R.,** Effect of age on RNA synthesis by nuclei and soluble RNA polymerases from liver and muscle of C57Bl/6J mice, *J. Gerontol.*, 27, 188, 1972.
44. **Ogur, M. and Rosen, G.,** The nucleic acids of plant tissues. I. The extraction and estimation of desoxypentose nucleic acid and pentose nucleic acid, *Arch. Biochem.*, 25, 262, 1950.
45. **Chaconas, G. and Finch, C. E.,** The effect of aging on RNA/DNA ratios in brain regions of the C57BL/6J male mouse, *J. Neurochem.*, 21, 1469, 1973.
46. **Mori, U., Mizuno, D., and Goto, S.,** Increase in the ratio of 18s RNA to 28s RNA in the cytoplasm of mouse tissues during aging, *Mech. Ageing Dev.*, 8, 285, 1978.
47. **Hill, B. T.,** A lack of correlation between decline in growth capacity and nuclear RNA synthesizing activity in aging human embryonic cells in culture, *Mech. Ageing Dev.* 5, 267, 1976.
48. **Schneider, E. L., Mitsui, Y., Tice, R., Shorr, S. S., and Braunschweiger, K.,** Alteration in cellular RNAs during the in vitro life span of cultured human diploid fibroblasts. II. Synthesis and processing of RNA, *Mech. Ageing Dev.*, 4, 449, 1975.
49. **Novello, F. and Stripe, F.,** Simultaneous assay of RNA polymerase I and II in nuclei isolated from resting and growing rat liver with the use of α-amanitin, *FEBS Lett.*, 8, 57, 1970.
50. **Benson, R. W.,** RNA polymerase activities in heart tissue of aging mice, *Exp. Gerontol.*, 13, 305, 1978.
51. **Barton, R. W. and Yang, W. K.,** Low molecular weight DNA polymerase decreased activity in spleens of old Balb/c mice, *Mech. Ageing Dev.*, 4, 123, 1975.
52. **Benson, R. W. and Harker, C. W.,** RNA polymerase activities in liver and brain tissue of aging mice, *J. Gerontol.*, 33, 323, 1978.
53. **Chalkley, R.,** personal communication.

POSTTRANSCRIPTIONAL MODIFICATION OF RNA IN AGING ORGANISMS

Laura L. Mays

The main cytoplasmic RNAs characteristic of eukaryotic cells are the ribosomal RNAs, typically, 28s, 18s, 5.8s, and 5s, the transfer RNAs, and messenger RNAs of various sizes. There is convincing evidence for posttranscriptional modification of each of these types of RNA, but both the extent and types of modification vary widely from RNA to RNA.[1-3] Only a little evidence has been accumulated relating to RNA modification in aging organisms. With the exception of turnover data, that evidence is restricted to modification of transfer RNA. The evidence at hand is incomplete and often indirect, but there is reason to believe that the posttranscriptional modification of RNA may change during aging.

Of the four classes of evidence presented, base analysis is the most direct method used. To date, the Randerath analytical method has been applied only to unfractionated tRNA populations,[4] and hardly any analysis of the important hypermodified bases next to the anticodons has yet been performed.[5] Indirect evidence includes isoacceptor analysis on reverse-phase chromatography columns,[6-9,14] amino acylation capacity measurements,[6-8,10,11,15] analysis of turnover rates,[13] and assays of the modification enzymes.[11,15,16] Reverse-phase chromatography of a tRNA can be shown to differ with modification differences,[17,18] but modification does not always change the pattern.[5] When modification levels of tRNAs change, small changes in the ratios of isoacceptors are more characteristic than the appearance or disappearance of isoacceptor peaks.[17,18]

Table 1
BASE ANALYSIS OF TRANSFER RNA

Aging organism(s) studied	Ages compared	Modifications studied	Findings	Ref.
Wheat	Apical leaf and basal leaf	Y base of $tRNA^{phe}$	Apical (nongrowing) tissue had 1/100 the level of Y base, and was inactive in poly(U)-directed polyphenylalanine synthesis	5
Aedes aegypti (mosquito)	10 and 30 days (50% survivorship)	ψ, hU, m^1A + m^6A, rT, m^5C, m^1G, m^2G, m^2_2G, m^7G	No significant differences	4
Female C57BL/6J mice	12 and 30 months (50% survivorship)	ψ, hU, m^1A + m^6A, m^1G, m^2G, m^2_2G, m^7G, m^3C, m^5C, rT, m^3U	Conclusions state no significant differences; data show possible small decrease in m^1G	4

Note: Y is a hypermodified tricyclic imidazo derivative of guanine occurring only in phenylalanine tRNA adjacent to the anticodon; $tRNA^{phe}$ is the transfer RNA specific for the amino acid phenylalanine; ψ is pseudouridine; hU is hydrouridine; m^1A and similar formats indicate methylased derivatives (the superscript number refers to the location of the methyl group, in this case, 1-methyl adenine); and rT is ribothymidine.

Table 2
REVERSE-PHASE CHROMATOGRAPHY OF TRANSFER RNA

Aging organism and tissue(s) studied	Ages compared	Isoacceptors studied	RPC system(s) used	Experimental conditions and findings	Ref.
Turbatrix aceti (vinegar eel)	2 days after hydroxyurea (75% < 11 days old) and 21 days after hydroxyurea (virtually all >20 days old)	With single peaks: phe, ile, his, val, asn, pro, lys; with multiple peaks: ala, met, leu, ser, glu, asp, arg, tyr	RPC-2 and RPC-4	Arg isoacceptors: ratio of major to minor isoacceptors decreased 35%; tyr isoacceptors: second major isoacceptor decreased 50%; findings with same synthetase,[a] using N-2-hydroxyethylpiperazine-N′-2-ephanesulphonic acid (HEPES) buffer and checking for mitochondrial origin of tRNAs	6
Aedes aegypti	7 and 30 days (50% survivorship)	Lys, ala, phe, val, met, leu, thr, tyr	RPC-5	Changes in ratios of peaks for val, met, leu, thr, and tyr isoacceptors	7
BC3F1 mice, pathogen-free; liver, some brain	5—9 and 28—36 months (10% survivorship)	Arg, asp, glu, his, leu, lys, phe, ser	RPC-2, some RPC-5	Stated to have no significant isoacceptor differences; peak ratios clearly differ by small amounts in figures, especially for glu, his, and lys (not normalized, so difficult to evaluate); for liver, synthetases[a] were from same age preparation	8

Table 2 (continued) REVERSE-PHASE CHROMATOGRAPHY OF TRANSFER RNA

Aging organism and tissue(s) studied	Ages compared	Isoacceptors studied	RPC system(s) used	Experimental conditions and findings	Ref.
				as tRNAs; for brain, young synthetases[a] only were used	
Soybean cotyledons	5 and 21 days (about maximum life span)	Leu	Not stated	With 5 day synthetases,[a] decreased major isoacceptor 2, sharp increases in minor isoacceptors 5 and 6; synthetases decrease in parallel, and at 21 days are high in acylation ability with isoacceptors 5 and 6, but low in acylation ability with isoacceptors 1—4	9
Male Sprague-Dawley rats	3 and 24 months	Lys, ser, phe	RPC-5	With young synthetase,[a] minor isoacceptor 4 for lys increased; changes in proportion of a minor phe isoacceptor and 2 of 7 ser isoacceptors	10
Male Charles River rats; livers and spleens	2 and 11 months	Not acylated	RPC-2	Measured the absorbance to radioactivity ratios after in vivo labeling with 14C methyl groups; adult liver tRNA showed lower methylation across all	11

				absorbance peaks; adult splenic tRNA had lower methylation unequally distributed among the absorbance peaks	
Pea leaves	Green, intermediate, and yellow leaves	Leu	RPC-2	Isoacceptors 5 and 6 for leucine are preferentially lost during senescence (isoacceptor 5 is particularly high in chloroplasts)	14
Drosophila melanogaster	5 and 35 days	Ser, leu, asp, asn, his, tyr	RPC-5	Serine and leucine isoacceptor ratios unchanged; the rest have larger proportions of those isoacceptors containing modified base Q (generally early eluting forms) in old animals	21
Drosophila melanogaster (Samarkand and Oregon R wild types; two mutant stocks)	0—1 day with either 13—14 or 20—21 days; in some cases, 6- to 7-day-old flies were used for old data points; ratios for tyrosine isoacceptors given at 8 data points between 0 and 21 days for each of the 4 stocks	Tyr, his, asp, asn	RPC-5	In general, the Q containing isoacceptors increased in proportion during aging, but the increase was not linear with age; the Samarkand stocks increased more rapidly than the Oregon R stocks; Q^+ and Q^- tRNAs accepted amino acids and functioned in EMC virus RNA translation equally well	22

[a] Amino acyl tRNA synthetases — catalyze attachment of amino acid to the cognate tRNA with concomitant breakdown of ATP to AMP and inorganic pyrophosphate.

Table 3
AMINO ACYLATION CAPACITY (CHARGING) OF TRANSFER RNA

Aging organism and tissue(s)	Ages compared	Amino acids studied	Amino acyl tRNA synthetase source	Experimental conditions and findings	Ref.
Turbatrix aceti (vinegar eel)	2 days after hydroxyurea (75%< 11 days) and 21 days after hydroxyurea (virtually all >20 days old)	Phe, ile, his, val, asn, pro, lys, ala, met, leu, ser, glu, asp, arg, tyr	Young	Old tRNA charged only 50% the extent of young tRNA	6
BC3F_1 mice; liver	5—9 and 28—36 months (10% survivorship)	Asp, glu, his, leu, lys, phe, ser, arg, tyr	Synthetases from same age as tRNAs; age stated to make no difference in synthetase activity	Young was 1.4 times old except for arg (1.34 times old) and tyr (1.22 times old); study included only 1 preparation of each age; Mg^{+2}/ATP optimized	8
BC3F_1 mice; brain	5—9 and 28—36 months (10% survivorship)	Arg, asp, his, leu, lys, phe, ser	Young synthetases	Young was 0.6 times old except for asp (0.72 times old); only 1 preparation of each age; Mg^{+2}/ATP optimized	8
Soybean cotyledons	5 and 21 days (maximum life span)	Leu	Young synthetase;[a] old synthetase[a]	36.6±3 pmol/A260[b] young tRNA 18.2±2 pmol/A260[b] old tRNA 11.0±1 pmol/A260[b] young tRNA 6.0±1 pmol/A260[b] old tRNA	9
Male Charles River rats; spleens	2 months (young) and 9 months old (adult)	Ile, arg, ala, leu, tyr, thr, ser, met, lys, val	Both homologous and heterologous mixtures tested; young synthetases were more active than adult synthetases with either tRNA	All amino acylation capacities low in older animals; with young synthetases, the adult tRNA had between 0.48 (val) and 0.92 (ser) of the young capacity; with adult synthetases, the adult tRNA had between 0.38 (val) and 0.85 (arg) of the young capacity	11

Male Sprague-Dawley rats; livers	3 and 24 months	Lys, ser, leu, phe, val	Young	All amino acid acylation capacities low in old animals; lys at 58% of young, ser at 50% of young, leu at 34% of young, phe at 25% of young, and val at 15% of young	12
Male Sprague-Dawley rats; livers	3 and 24 months	All except cys, asn, glu	Young	Low acceptance by average of 64% in old tRNA purified from whole tissue; low acceptance by only 7% in old tRNA purified from high-speed supernatants	10
Drosophila melanogaster	5, 27, and 35 days	Gly, ile, thr, val, pro, ala, arg, ser, leu	Both homologous and heterologous mixtures tested; young synthetases were more active than old synthetases with some tRNAs; with others the different synthetases had equal potency	All the amino acylation capacities were lower in old flies; with young synthetases, old tRNA had from 49 (leu) to 91% (arg) of the young capacity; with old synthetase, old tRNA had from 20 (arg) to 88% (val) of the young acylation capacity; heat treatment to separate nicked molecules did not affect old ser, gly, and val tRNAs differently than young	21

[a] Amino acyl tRNA synthetases.
[b] Absorbance unit at 260 nm, roughly equivalent to 0.05 mg of tRNA.

Table 4
TURNOVER OF RIBOSOMAL RNA AND SOLUBLE RNA

Aging organism and tissue(s) studied	Ages compared	Type of RNA fraction	Findings	Ref.
Male Wistar rats; liver, kidney, lung, spleen, and intestinal mucosa	12 and 24 months	Ribosomal RNA[a]	No age-associated turnover differences; $t_{1/2}$ liver = 5.89 days, $t_{1/2}$ kidney = 6.53 days, $t_{1/2}$ lung = 8.98 days, $t_{1/2}$ spleen = 8.61 days, and $t_{1/2}$ intestinal mucosa = 8.13 days	13
Male Wistar rats; lung, intestinal mucosa, spleen, liver, and kidney	12 and 24 months	Soluble RNA[b]	No differences for lung ($t_{1/2}$ = 8.75 days) or intestinal mucosa ($t_{1/2}$ = 1 and 11.4 days); spleen: young adult $t_{1/2}$ = 6.46 days, aged $t_{1/2}$ = 8.29 days; liver: young adult $t_{1/2}$ = 4.59 days, aged $t_{1/2}$ = 5.34 and 1.1—1.2 days; kidney: young adult $t_{1/2}$ = 4.99 days, aged $t_{1/2}$ = 1.1—1.2 and 9.51 days	13
WI-38 cultured human diploid fibroblasts; PAL-II fetal lung fibroblasts	Passages 5—9, 20—24, 25—29, 30—34, 35—39, 40—44, 45—49, 50—54, and 55—59 (PAL-II used for 5—9; WI-38 used for remainder)	Total RNA; formation of ribosomal RNAs (28s, 18s) and tRNAs (4s) identified on polyacrylamide gels; poly A RNA (putative mRNAs)	Up to passage 39, RNA/DNA ratio is near 2; RNA content increase then begins and continues to passage 55—59, RNA/DNA = 8.41; uridine (3H/14C) double labeling, followed by electrophoresis of RNAs, showed parallel patterns in 28s, 18s, and 4s RNA regions for senescent and presenescent cells; similarly, double labeling in poly A fraction indicated parallel patterns for senescent and presenescent RNA region oligo(dT) chromatography	23

WI-38 cultured human diploid fibroblasts	27 and 42 passages	Formation of total RNA; ribosomal (28s, 18s) and transfer (4s) RNAs identified on polyacrylamide gels	Uridine incorporation was lower (cpm $\times 10^{-7}$ per mg RNA/6 hr incorporation was 8 for early passage cells, but 4 for late passage cells); uridine pools were the same for the two ages; ratios of 3H uridine incorporation into 28s/18s RNA and 28s + 18s/4s RNA were almost identical for the two ages; pulse chase experiment showed 45s + 32s rRNA precursors are converted to rRNAs at similar rates in the two types of cultures	24

[a] Ribosomal subunits were isolated by 30,000 rpm, 2 hr centrifugation of sodium deoxycholate-treated postmitochondrial supernatant in a type 30 rotor in a Spinco L centrifuge (followed by washing to remove debris), and repeated precipitation.

[b] Soluble RNA is small, cytoplasmic RNA usually consisting largely of tRNAs. It was isolated from the supernatant from the 30,000 rpm centrifugation described above.

Table 5
ASSAYS OF MODIFICATION ENZYMES AND SUBSTRATES

Aging organism and tissue(s) used	Ages compared	Type of modification substrate	Type of assay	Findings	Ref.
Charles River rats; spleens and livers	3 and 11 months	Natural (rat spleen or rat liver) tRNA	In vivo methylation labeling	Methyl label incorporation:young spleens, 275 cpm/A_{260}; adult spleens, 184 cpm/A_{260}; Young livers, 133 cpm/A_{260}; adult livers, 88 cpm/A_{260}; identified labeled derivatives from in vivo labeling of liver tRNAs: me^5C,[a] rT,[b] m^7G, m^2_2G, and m^1A	11
Charles River rats; livers and spleens	3 and 11 months	*E. coli* tRNA (heterologous tRNA, undermethylated with respect to eukaryotic tRNA methyl transferases)	In vitro, kinetic rather than saturation, 3 A_{260}[c] of tRNA with 1.2 mg of cytosol protein as enzyme source	No differences in kinetics detected with either mature or undermethylated *E. coli* tRNA substrate using liver enzymes; spleen methylases were slightly slower in older animals	11
Male Sprague-Dawley rats; liver and kidney	3 and 12 months	*E. coli* B tRNA	In vitro, saturation of 1 μg of tRNA via increasing levels of cytosol protein as enzyme source	30% decrease in saturating tRNA methyltransferase activity of liver and 40% decrease in kidney as a result of the competitive activity of glycine N-methyl transferase, which increases in activity by 50%	15
Male C57Bl/6J mice; liver	12, 18, and 30 months	*E. coli* B tRNA	In vitro, saturation of 1 μg of tRNA	Linear decrease in saturating tRNA methyltransferase activity resulting from linear increase in competitive activity of glycine N-methyl transferase	15

Corn, WF9 X 38-11 single cross population; cob, stalk parenchyma, and first developed leaf	Cob; 0—11 days after silking; stalk parenchyma: fourth internode when plant was 4-ft tall, with sections 8-mm long representing older tissue as distance from intercalary meristem was increased; first developed leaf: 8—20 days after planting	100 μg of *E. coli* tRNA	In vitro	Overall, as a function of age, activity declined in all 3 tissues studied	16
Male Sprague-Dawley rats; liver, adrenal glands, lung, muscle, brain, cerebellum, and blood	3 and 30 months	Substrate, rather than enzyme, was measured	Content of S-adenosyl methionine by isotope dilution	S-adenosyl methionine content: μg / g wet wt; liver:[d] young 29.6 ± 2.2, old 19.4 ± 1.4; adrenals:[d] young 19.3 ± 0.7, old 15.1 ± 0.8; lung:[d] young 8.9 ± 0.4, old 7.2 ± 0.4; muscle: young 11.5 ± 1.0, old 10.7 ± 0.4; brain:[d] young 10.0 ± 0.3 old 8.7 ± 0.3; cerebellum: young 10.2 ± 0.2, old 9.5 ± 0.2; and blood: young 1.2 ± 0.1 old 1.0 ± 0.1; concomitant increases in catecholamine O-methyl transferase were noted in some tissues	19

[a] 5-Methyl cytosine; other methylated derivatives abbreviated using the same format.
[b] Ribothymidine (5-methyl uridine).
[c] One absorbance unit at 260 nm, approximately equivalent to 0.05 μg of tRNA.
[d] Statistically significant.

REFERENCES

1. **Kerr, S. J. and Borek, E.,** Regulation of tRNA methyl transferases in normal and neoplastic tissue, *Adv. Enzyme Regul.,* 11, 63, 1974.
2. **Perry, R.,** Processing of RNA, *Ann. Rev., Biochem.,* 45, 605, 1976.
3. **Heckle, W., Fenton, R., Wood, T., Merkel, C., and Lingrel, J.,** Methylated nucleosides in globin mRNA from mouse nucleated erythroid cells, *J. Biol. Chem.,* 252, 1964, 1977.
4. **Hoffman, J. L. and McCoy, M. T.,** Stability of the nucleoside composition of tRNA during biological ageing of mice and mosquitoes, *Nature (London),* 249, 558, 1974.
5. **Shugart, L.,** A possible age-related modification of phenylalanine transfer RNA from wheat tissue, *Exp. Gerontol.,* 7, 251, 1972.
6. **Reitz, M. S. and Sanadi, R.,** An aspect of translational control of protein synthesis in aging: changes in the isoaccepting forms of tRNA in *Turbatrix aceti, Exp. Gerontol.,* 7, 119, 1972.
7. **Hoffman, J. L.,** Quantitative and qualitative changes in mosquito tRNA as a function of age, *Fed. Proc.,* 31, 866, 1972.
8. **Frazer, J. and Yang, W.-K.,** Isoaccepting transfer ribonucleic acids in liver and brain of young and old BC3F mice, *Arch. Biochem. Biophys.,* 153, 610, 1972.
9. **Bick, M. and Strehler, B. L.,** Leucyl transfer RNA synthetase changes during soybean cotyledon senescence, *Proc. Natl. Acad. Sci. U.S.A.,* 68, 224, 1971.
10. **Mays, L. L., Lawrence, A. E., Ho, R. W., and Ackley, S.,** Age-related changes in function of transfer RNA from rat liver, *Fed. Proc.,* 38, 1984, 1979.
11. **Wust, C. and Rosen, L.,** Aminoacylation and methylation of tRNA as a function of age in the rat, *Exp. Gerontol.,* 7, 331, 1974.
12. **Zedalis-Readinger, J., Scott, J., Feigon, J., and Mays, L. L.,** Transfer RNA from livers of aging rats, *Age,* 1, 31, 1978.
13. **Menzies, R. A., Mishra, R. K., and Gold, P. H.,** The turnover of ribosomes and soluble RNA in a variety of tissues of young adult and aged rats, *Mech. Ageing Dev.,* 1, 117, 1972.
14. **Wright, R. D., Pillay, D. T. N., and Cherry, J.,** Changes in leucyl tRNA species of pea leaves during senescence and after zeatin treatment, *Mech. Ageing Dev.,* 1, 403, 1972/73.
15. **Mays, L. L., Borek, E., and Finch, C. E.,** Glycine N-methyltransferase is a regulatory enzyme which increases in ageing animals, *Nature (London),* 243, 411, 1973.
16. **BeMiller, J. N., Hoffmann, W. E., and Pappelis, A. J.,** Changes in tRNA methylase activity in senescing cob and stalk parenchyma tissue and the first developed leaf of corn (*Zea mays* L.), *Mech. Ageing Dev.,* 2, 363, 1973.
17. **Katze, J.,** Relation of cell type and cell density to the degree of posttranscriptional modification of $tRNA^{lys}$ and $tRNA^{phe}$, *Biochim. Biophys. Acta,* 407, 392, 1975.
18. **Kitchingman, G. R., Webb, E., and Fournier, M. J.,** Unique phenylalanine transfer ribonucleic acids in relaxed control *Escherichia coli:* genetic origin and some functional properties, *Biochemistry,* 15, 1848, 1976.
19. **Stramentinoli, G., Gualano, M., Catto, E., and Algeri, S.,** Tissue levels of S-Adenosyl methionine in aging rats, *J. Gerontol.,* 32, 392, 1977.
20. **Hosbach, H. A. and Kubli, E.,** Transfer RNA in ageing *Drosophila.* I. Extent of amino acylation, *Mech. Ageing Dev.,* 10, 131, 1979.
21. **Hosbach, H. A. and Kubli, E.,** Transfer RNA in ageing *Drosophila.* II. Isoacceptor patterns, *Mech. Ageing Dev.,* 10, 141, 1979.
22. **Owenby, R. K., Stulberg, M. P., and Jacobson, K. B.,** Alteration of the Q family of transfer RNAs in adult *Drosophila melanogaster* as a function of age, nutrition, and genotype, *Mech. Ageing Dev.,* 11, 91, 1979.
23. **Schneider, E. L. and Shorr, S. S.,** Alteration in cellular RNAs during the *in vitro* life span of cultured human diploid fibroblasts, *Cell,* 6, 179, 1975.
24. **Schneider, E. L., Mitsui, Y., Tice, R., Shorr, S. S., and Braunschweiger, K.,** Alteration in cellular RNAs during the *in vitro* life span of cultured human diploid fibroblasts. II. Synthesis and processing of RNA, *Mech. Ageing Dev.,* 4, 449, 1975.

Translation

THE RELATIONSHIP BETWEEN AGING AND PROTEIN SYNTHESIS

Arlan Richardson

INTRODUCTION

The natural life span of a living organism is believed to be at least partially under genetic control. Therefore, changes in the genetic apparatus and protein biosynthesis would be one of the primary mechanisms involved in aging. Over the past 10 to 15 years, a large number of investigators have studied the effect of aging on protein synthesis in a variety of organisms. The basic objective of this section is to provide readers with enough information about these studies so that they will be able to critically evaluate what effect aging has on protein synthesis. To accomplish this objective, the methods employed by each investigator to measure protein synthesis are described. In many studies, investigators have attempted to determine what effect aging has on protein synthesis by measuring the activity of an enzyme or enzymes in organisms of various ages (see also "Enzyme Levels in Animals of Various Ages"). However, the information gained about changes in protein synthesis from changes in enzyme activity is limited because the levels of most enzymes are determined by opposing processes, e.g., synthesis and degradation or secretion, and these processes can vary independently of each other during aging.[1,2] Therefore, studies of this type will not be considered in this review.

In almost all of the studies cited here, protein synthesis was measured by the incorporation of a labeled precursor (in most cases, a radioactively labeled amino acid) into protein or acid-insoluble material. The main difference in the methods employed in the studies described in this section was the types of systems used to measure protein synthesis, e.g., cell-free, slices, in vivo, etc. Using a cell-free system, an investigator can carefully control experimental conditions and minimize most of the problems encountered when protein synthesis is measured in whole cells or in vivo. In addition, a cell-free system allows an investigator to study the effects of aging on the various steps of protein synthesis or the molecular components involved in protein synthesis. However, the internal ultrastructure and organization found in a cell is absent in a cell-free system. Furthermore, the rate of protein synthesis observed in cell-free systems has been reported to be only 1% of the rate observed in vivo.[3,4] Therefore, a major consideration with a cell-free system is whether age-related changes observed in cell-free protein synthesis accurately reflect the changes that occur in vivo.

Although the use of the whole organism would be preferable when studying the influence of aging on protein synthesis, measuring protein synthesis accurately in vivo is very difficult because of problems encountered with the absorption of the labeled precursor, compartmentalization of the precursor, and competing reactions.[5,6] The rate of amino acid incorporation into protein by whole cells or in vivo can be measured with relative ease; however, this measurement is not an accurate measure of protein synthesis. To determine actual rates of protein synthesis in vivo with radioactively labeled amino acids, it is necessary to correct for changes in both amino acid transport and pool sizes that could occur with increasing age. The actual rate of protein synthesis (expressed as moles of amino acid incorporated into protein per unit time per unit of the organism) can be estimated by dividing the rate of amino acid incorporation by the specific activity of the amino acid in the precursor pool.[8] The major problem encountered in making such measurements is identification of the pool of amino acids that serve as the immediate precursor for protein synthesis. Traditionally, investigators assumed that the intracellular amino acid pool served as the immediate pool for protein

Table 1
EFFECT OF AGING ON PROTEIN SYNTHESIS IN PLANTS AND FUNGI

	Change	Ref.
Plants		
Corn *(Zea mays)*		
Cob parenchyma tissue	30% decrease	29
First developed leaf	30% decrease	29
Stalk parenchyma tissue	200% increase	29
Soybean (*Glycine max* var. Harosoy 63) cotyledons	90% decrease	30
Fungi		
Sclerotium bataticola		
Mycelia	40—53% decrease	35, 36
Rhizoctonia solani		
Mycelia	72—99% decrease	35—37
Cell-free system	50% decrease	35, 38

synthesis.[9] However, this view was challenged when Kipnis et al.[10] showed with diaphragm and lymph node cells that the incorporation of [^{14}C]-proline and [^{14}C]-glycine into protein was linear before the radioactivity in the intracellular proline and glycine pools had equilibrated. Similar results were obtained with heart[11] and kidney.[12] Kipnis et al.[10] proposed a functional heterogeneity of the intracellular amino acid pool, and suggested that amino acids used for protein synthesis were compartmentalized in a specific amino acid pool. Studies from Mortimore's laboratory [13,14] indicated that the intracellular valine pool in perfused rat liver was composed of two compartments: one that rapidly exchanged valine with the extracellular pool, and another that exchanged valine very slowly or not at all with the extracellular pool. Ward and Mortimore[14] suggested that the latter compartment was of lysosomal origin and derived its amino acids from intracellular proteolysis.

Several investigators[15-17] have proposed that the amino acids used for protein synthesis are derived from the extracellular amino acid pool. However, recent studies with perfused liver,[18] liver in vivo,[19,20] perfused heart,[21] and heart in vivo[22] demonstrate that the specific activity of the amino acid bound to tRNA is different from the specific activity of the amino acid in either the intracellular or extracellular pool. Currently, most investigators[18-24] believe that the amino acids used for protein synthesis either come from both the intracellular and extracellular amino acid pools, or from an intracellular compartment which rapidly exchanges amino acids with the extracellular amino acid pool. Due to the problems encountered in measuring the specific activity of the amino acid pool(s) that serve as the source of amino acids for protein synthesis, it is generally recommended that investigators measure the specific activity of the amino acid bound to tRNA (the immediate source of amino acids for protein synthesis) to accurately calculate the rate of protein synthesis in whole cells or in vivo.

PLANTS

Since several investigators[25-28] have reported that senescence in plants is accompanied by a decrease in ribosome and polyribosome content, it has been assumed that senescence is associated with a decline in the ability of plant tissues to synthesize protein. However, the effect of senescence on protein synthesis has been determined in only a few studies. BeMiller et al.[29] measured the effect of aging on the incorporation of [^{14}C]-leucine into acid-insoluble material by sections of various corn tissues (Table 1). In cob parenchyma tissue, [^{14}C]-leucine incorporation increased over threefold from the first to the ninth day after silking. The onset of cell death occurs 9 days after silking, and incorporation of [^{14}C]-leucine decreased 30% during this time. A 30% decrease in [^{14}C]-leucine incorporation was observed from 15 to 20 days after germination in the first developed leaf. The effect of aging on [^{14}C]-leucine incorporation by stalk parenchyma tissue was assessed using various sections of the stalk tissue. An increase in [^{14}C]-leucine incorporation was observed with increasing age in stalk tissue. BeMiller et al.[29] did not measure the specific activity of the leucine pool; therefore, it is not possible to establish if the age-related changes in [^{14}C]-leucine incorporation are due to changes in protein synthesis.

More recently, Pillay[30] measured the cell-free protein synthetic activity of soybean cotyledons harvested 1 to 10 days following germination (Table 1). Over a 90% decrease in polyuridylic acid-directed polyphenylalanine synthesis was observed; both ribosomal and supernatant factors isolated from cotyledon extracts were responsible for the decrease.[30]

In addition to the decrease in ribosome content,[25-28] other age-related changes in the protein synthetic apparatus have been observed; in plants, e.g., the amount of tRNA extracted from plant tissues decreases with age,[31] an age-related loss in the isoaccepting species of tRNA^{leu} occurs,[32] tRNA^{leu} charging decreases as a function of age,[31,33] and the structure of tRNA is modified during senescence.[31,34]

The effect of aging on the metabolism of fungi has been studied extensively by Gottlieb's laboratory.[35] Using whole cells prepared from mycelium ranging in age from 0 to 144 hr, Gottlieb et al.[36] measured the incorporation of [^{14}C]-leucine and [^{14}C]-phenylalanine into acid-insoluble material by either *Rhizoctonia solani* or *Sclerotium bataticola* (Table 1). A decrease in the incorporation of these two amino acids was observed in both fungi. Although the specific activity of the precusor pools of the leucine or phenylalanine were not measured, Gottlieb et al.[36] did measure the acid-soluble [^{14}C]-leucine and [^{14}C]-phenylalanine associated with the cells. The ratio of acid-soluble radioactivity to acid-insoluble radioactivity in the mycelium did not change with age in *S. bataticola;* therefore, the decrease in [^{14}C]-leucine and [^{14}C]-phenylalanine incorporation during aging in this fungus appears to be due to a decreased cell permeability to these amino acids. However, the ratio of acid-soluble radioactivity to acid-insoluble radioactivity increased during aging in *R. solani;* in this fungus, therefore, protein synthesis appears to decrease with increasing age. In a later study, Ricciardi et al.[37] reported that in vivo incorporation of [^{14}C]-phenylalanine into acid-insoluble material by mycelia from *R. solani* decreased over 99% from 1 to 8 days of age. This age-related decrease in [^{14}C]-phenylalanine incorporation was not due to a decreease in the ribosome content of the mycelium.[37] Using a cell-free system derived from the mycelia of different aged cultures of *R. solani,* Obrig and Gottlieb[38] have found that polyuridylic acid-directed polyphenylalanine synthesis decreased 50% from 0 to 6 days. The decreased polyphenylalanine synthesis was associated with the supernatant and ribosomal fractions of the mycelium extracts.[38] Ricciardi et al.[37] have shown that a shift of ribosomes from polyribosomes to 80S ribosomes occurred in *R. solani* as a function of age. It has been suggested that the age-related decline in protein synthesis and ribosomes aggregation to mRNA in *R. solani* is due to a defect in the initiation step of protein synthesis[37] or an increase in RNase activity in the mycelia.[39]

INVERTEBRATES

Almost all of the studies on the effect of aging on protein synthesis in invertebrates have been performed with insects. Although the initial study in 1966 by Clarke and Smith[40] indicated that protein synthesis increased during aging, most of the studies with insects have shown that protein synthesis declines with increasing age[41] (Table 2).

Table 2
EFFECT OF AGING ON PROTEIN SYNTHESIS IN INVERTEBRATES

	Change	Ref.
Insects		
Drosophila subobscura		
Whole insect	95% increase	40
Schistocera gergaria		
Wings	67% decrease	42
Drosophila melanogaster		
Ovaries	48% decrease	43
Thorax	20% increase	43
Musca domestica		
Isolated flight muscle	60—70% decrease	44
Drosophila melanogaster		
Whole insect	58—63% decrease	46
Phormia regina		
Whole insect	46—72% decrease	47
Nematodes		
Turbatrix aceti	80—90% decrease	51

In the initial study, Clark and Smith[40] reported that the in vivo incorporation of [^{3}H]-leucine into acid-insoluble material from whole insect homogenates increased 95% in 60-day-old *Drosophila sabobscura* compared to 20-day-old insects. However, Heslop[42] observed a continuous decrease in the in vivo incorporation of [^{14}C]-valine into protein by the wing of the locust *Schistocera gregaria* from 1 to 97 days after adult emergence. Using *Drosophilia melanogaster,* Wattiaux et al.[43] observed that the in vivo incorporation of [^{3}H]-leucine into protein extracted from the ovaries decreased 48% from 10 to 35 days; however, [^{3}H]-leucine incorporation into the thorax increased slightly. Rockstein and Baker[44] found that the in vitro incorporation of a mixture of radioactively labeled amino acids into protein by isolated flight muscle from *Musca domestica* L. decreased approximately 50% from 7 to 14 days of age. Although Clarke and Smith[40] showed that the total leucine pool did not change with age, none of the studies described above measured the specific activity of the amino acid precursor pool. Therefore, these studies do not establish that the age-related changes in amino acid incorporation into protein were due to changes in the rate of protein synthesis.

Using a method developed by Dinamarca and Levenbook[45] to measure the rates of protein synthesis in flies from the turnover rate of the amino acid precursor pool, two research groups have carefully determined what effect aging has on protein synthesis in insects. In both *D. melanogaster*[46] and *Phormia regina,*[47] a decrease in the rate of amino acid turnover and amino acid incorporation into protein was observed. Baumann and Chen[46] observed a 58 to 63% decrease in the incorporation of either [^{14}C]-lysine, [^{14}C]-glycine, or [^{14}C]-alanine by 50-day-old *D. melanogaster* compared to 3-day-old flies. The rate of [^{14}C]-alanine or [^{14}C]-leucine incorporation into acid-insoluble material by 37- to 40-day-old *P. regina* was 72 and 46% less than that observed for 5- to 6-day-old blowflies.[47] It appears that the increased [^{3}H]-leucine incorporation with age observed initially by Clarke and Smith[40] resulted from an age-related decrease in the turnover of amino acids, rather than an increased rate of protein synthesis.[47]

Age-related changes in the protein synthetic apparatus also have been observed in *D. melanogaster.* Baker and Schmidt[48] reported that the amount of 80S ribosomal material decreased during aging, and a change in the integrity of the protein-rRNA complex occurred during aging. Using tRNA and aminoacyl-tRNA synthetases isolated from 5-, 22-, and 35-day-old fruit flies, Hosbach and Kubli[49] observed an age-related decrease in the amino acid acceptor activity of tRNA regardless of the source of the aminoacyl-tRNA synthetases. For several amino acids, the aminoacyl-tRNA synthetase activity decreased with increasing age.

Although the nematode has become a valuable model for studies on aging,[50] only limited information is available on the effect of aging on protein synthesis in this organism (Table 2). Prasanna and Lane[51] reported that during aging the in vivo incorporation of [^{35}S]-methionine into acid-insoluble material decreased 80 to 90%; the ages of the nematodes were not reported. No age-related decrease in the transport of methionine, the methionine pool, or the specific activity of the methionine pool was observed. Therefore, the age-related decline in [^{35}S]-methionine appears to reflect a decline in protein synthesis. Wallach and Gershon[52] observed that the fraction of ribosomes in polyribosomes from homogenates of nematodes decreased 44% from 5 to 53 days of age, and the decrease was not due to RNase activity. Sundararaman and Cummings[53] reported a decrease in both the total amount of ribosomes per cell and the size of polyribosomes in aging *Paramecium aurelia*. An age-related decrease in the specific activity of elongation factor EF-1[54] and the aminoacylation of tRNA[55] also has been reported in nematodes.

RODENTS

Most of the research on the effect of aging on protein synthesis has been performed with rodents, the laboratory mouse or rat. These animals have a maximum life span of 3 to 4 years, depending on the strain and sex of the animals.[56] Although a variety of tissues from rodents have been employed in these studies, most investigators have used liver tissue. A comprehensive list of the reports describing the influence of age on liver protein synthesis is given in Table 3; it is grouped according to the system used to measure protein synthesis. It is evident that in the majority of studies, cell-free systems were employed. In a recent review, Buetow et al.[57] concluded that the present evidence indicates that the cell-free protein synthetic activity of liver microsomes decreases during senescence. Although Chen et al.[58] and Beauchene et al.[59] reported that cell-free protein synthesis did not decrease with increasing age, all other investigators have observed an age-related decrease in the cell-free protein synthetic activity of liver.[60-71] The decrease in cell-free protein synthesis was observed with systems employing the postmitochondrial supernatant[69] and microsomes[60-68] or ribosomes[61,71,78] supplemented with cell sap or pH 5 enzyme. Cell-free protein synthesis decreased with either endogenous mRNA[60-66,69] or exogenous mRNA[67,68,70,71] as the template. Using a purified cell-free system, Moldave et al.[71] recently demonstrated that the translation of globin mRNA by a liver system consisting of ribosomal subunits decreased with increasing age.[71]

Effects of aging on liver protein synthesis have also been studied using liver slices.[59,69] Beauchene et al.[59] observed that no age-related change in [^{14}C]-leucine incorporation occurred in liver slices prepared from mice or rats, but the specific activity of the leucine pool was not measured. More recently, Layman et al.[69] determined the rate of phenylalanine incorporation by rat liver slices from the specific activity of the acid-soluble phenylalanine associated with the liver slices. The rate of phenylalanine incorporation decreased 45% from 2 to 12 months of age.

Many of the reports describing the effect of aging on the in vivo incorporation of radioactively labeled amino acids into acid-insoluble material are conflicting.[72-77] Beauchene et al.[75] and Ove et al.[76] observed that no age-related change occurred in amino acid incorporation by the liver in vivo . On the other hand, Comolli et al.[74] reported a slight decrease in [^{3}H]-lysine incorporation, and Kanungo et al.[77] found that [^{14}C]-leucine incorporation increased with increasing age. However, the specific activ-

Table 3
EFFECT OF AGING ON PROTEIN SYNTHESIS BY THE LIVER FROM MICE OR RATS

	Change	Ages studied (months)	Ref.
	Total Protein Synthesis		
Cell-free			
Mice			
Microsomes	53% decrease	5—30	60
Rats			
Microsomes			
Endogenous mRNA	74% decrease	2—22	61
	64% decrease	2—25	62
	40% decrease	3—24	63
	20—40% decrease	12—31	64
	30% decrease	3—26	65
	10—20% decrease	3—24	66
	No change	1.5—24	58, 59
Polyuridylic acid	47% decrease	2—31	67
	21% decrease	11—28	68
Postmitochondrial Supernatant	56% decrease	1—18	69
Ribosomes			
Polyuridylic acid	30% decrease	3—12	70
Globin mRNA	30% decrease	3—30	71
Liver slices			
Mice	No change	3—28	59
Rats	45% decrease	2—12	69
	No change	10—28	59
Isolated hepatocytes			
Rats	64% decrease	1—18	73
	52% decrease	3—24	79, 80
	44% decrease	2.5—18	81
	18% increase	18—30	81
	77% increase	24—36	79, 80
In vivo			
Mice	0—37% increase	12—33	72
Rats	48% decrease	3—15	73
	18% decrease	1—26	74
	No change	11—28	75
	No change	1—20	76
	40—50% increase	10—22	77
	Albumin Synthesis		
Cell-free			
Rats	200% increase	1.5—24	58
Isolated hepatocytes			
Rats	61% decrease	3—24	80, 82
	300% increase	24—36	80, 82
In vivo			
Rats	30—40% increase	11—28	75
	64% increase	1.5—24	83
	67% increase	1—20	76

ity of the amino acid precusor pool was not determined in any of these studies. Using 12- to 15- and 31- to 33-month-old mice, Du et al.[72] compared the in vivo incorporation of [^{3}H]-leucine into various fractions of the liver. No age-related change in the leucine pool or uptake of [^{3}H]-leucine by the liver was observed. Their data indicated that the

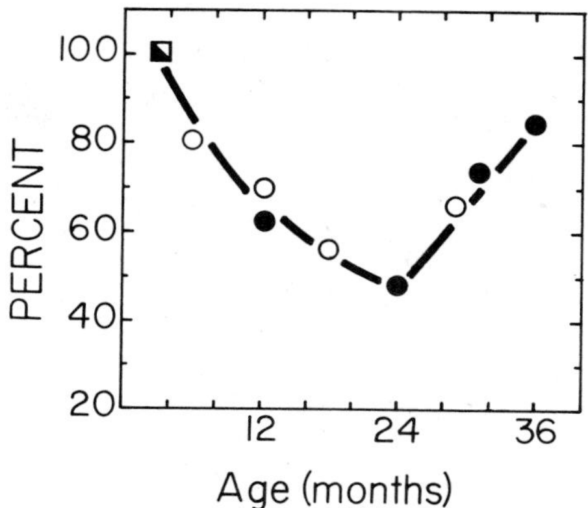

FIGURE 1. A comparison of the relative rates of protein synthesis by hepatocytes isolated from rats of various ages by van Bezooijen et al.[79] (●) and Coniglio et al.[81] (○). The rates of protein synthesis (pmol leucine per hr/mg protein or nmol valine per min/mg protein) by hepatocytes from rats of various ages in the two studies were normalized by expressing each value as a percent of the rate of protein synthesis observed for the 3-month-old rats (◪).

rate of [^{3}H]-leucine incorporation into most fractions of the liver did not change, or increased only slightly with increasing age. However, [^{3}H]-leucine incorporation into liver microsomes increased 37%. Using the specific activity of the valyl-tRNA, Ricca et al.[73] recently measured the in vivo rate of valine incorporation by the liver of 3- and 15-month-old rats. A 48% decrease in the rate of valine incorporation into protein was observed when this method of measuring amino acid incorporation was employed.

During the past few years, an increasing number of investigators have begun using suspensions of isolated hepatocytes to study various biochemical processes. The intracellular organization of the cell is maintained in isolated hepatocytes, and it appears that suspensions of hepatocytes are similar metabolically to the liver in vivo. The ability of an investigator to easily manipulate and control conditions with suspensions of hepatocytes makes this system ideal for studying a complex biochemical process like protein synthesis. Knook[78] and Ricca et al.[73] have shown that several changes that occur in the aging liver in vivo also occur in suspensions of hepatocytes. During the past 3 years, the laboratories of Knook[79,80] and Richardson[73,81] have independently studies the influence of aging on liver protein synthesis using suspensions of hepatocytes. van Bezooijen et al.[79] measured the rate of [^{14}C]-leucine incorporation into acid-insoluble material by hepatocytes isolated from 3-, 12-, 24-, 31-, and 36-month-old female WAG/Rij rats, and Coniglio et al.[81] actually determined the rate of valine incorporation from the specific activity of the valine pool by hepatocytes isolated from 2.5- to 4-, 6- to 7-, 12- to 13-, 18-, and 28- to 30-month-old male Fischer F344 rats. Although van Bezooijen et al.[79] did not measure the specific activity of the leucine pool, the rate of [^{14}C]-leucine incorporation measured by these investigators is probably a relatively accurate measure of protein synthesis because the intracellular and extracellular amino acid pools equilibrate rapidly in suspensions of isolated hepatocytes.[73] Thus, the results of these studies are comparable, and the relative rates of protein synthesis reported by van Bezooijen et al.[79] and Coniglio et al.[81] are presented in Figure 1. Liver protein synthesis exhibits a biphasic response as an animal ages.

Table 4
EFFECT OF AGING ON PROTEIN SYNTHESIS IN SKELETAL MUSCLE AND HEART OF MICE AND RATS

	Change	Ages studied (months)	Ref.
	Skeletal Muscle		
Cell-free			
Mice	16—32% decrease	1—10.5	89, 90
	80% increase	9—18	91
	60% decrease	18—29	91
Rats	33% decrease	—	88
In vivo			
Mice	52—65% decrease	1—10.5	89
Rats	15% decrease	10—22	77
	83% decrease	1—11	92
	Cardiac Muscle		
Cell-free			
Rats	32% decrease	3—24	93
Perfused heart			
Mice	300—400% increase	1—9	94
	50—60% decrease	8—27	94
	26% decrease	8—26	95
In vivo			
Mice	No change	12—33	72
Rats	150% increase	10—22	77
	46% decrease	3—24	93

[a] Weanling and adult rats were compared; no ages were given.

During the first 18 to 24 months of life, protein synthesis decreases approximately 50%. After 24 months of age, a continuous increase in the rate of protein synthesis occurs. Coniglio et al.[81] have suggested that the age-related increase in liver protein synthesis observed during senescence might be due to an increased synthesis of serum proteins by the liver to compensate for the increased urinary excretion of protein, which has been observed during senescence in rats.[75,84-87] This suggestion is supported by several investigators who have reported that albumin synthesis increases during aging (Table 3). Cell-free synthesis of albumin by liver microsomes increases twofold from 1.5 to 24 months of age.[58] The in vivo synthesis of albumin also has been shown to increase as a function of age.[75,76,83] Recently, albumin synthesis by hepatocytes has been shown to decrease from 3 to 24 months of age, and then increase threefold from 24 to 36 months of age.[80,82] The proportion of albumin synthesized to total protein synthesized was constant from 3 to 24 months of age; however, after 24 months of age, the proportion of albumin synthesized increased constantly.[79] Therefore, it appears that the increased protein synthesis by liver during senescence is at least partially due to an increased synthesis of the serum protein albumin.

The influence of age on the synthesis of other specific proteins by liver has been studied to a limited extent. Ove et al.[76] reported that the in vivo synthesis of ferritin increased from 1 to 20 months of age in rats. The synthesis of globulins by the liver in vivo does not appear to change from 1.5 to 24 months of age in rats.[83] Recently, Du et al.[72] reported that the in vivo synthesis of heme-containing proteins decreased 38% from 12 to 33 months of age in mice.

A list of the studies conducted to determine the effect of aging on skeletal and cardiac muscle protein synthesis is given in Table 4. Although several investigators[77,88,92] have studied protein synthesis in skeletal muscle as a function of age, the animals used in many of these studies were less than 1 year old.[88-90,92] The cell-free synthesis of protein by skeletal muscle has been measured with ribosomes prepared from detergent-treated microsomes using endogenous mRNA as the template. The cell-free protein synthetic activity of skeletal muscle appears to decrease rapidly after weaning.[88-90] Srivastava and Chaudhary[89] observed that the decrease occurred primarily during the first 3 months of life. Britton and Sherman[91] are the only investigators to determine the cell-free protein synthetic activity of skeletal muscle from old animals. Using muscle from the hind leg of mice, they observed an increase in cell-free protein synthesis from 9 to 18 months of age. From 18 to 29 months of age, cell-free protein synthesis decreased 60%.

Although all published reports currently available indicate that the in vivo incorporation of radioactively labeled amino acids into acid-insoluble material decreases as a function of age in skeletal muscle,[77,89,92] one must be cautious in assuming that these results mean that protein synthesis in skeletal muscle decreases during senescence. Srivastava and Chaudhary[89] and Kanungo et al.[77] observed a decrease in [^{14}C]-leucine incorporation with increasing age; however, the specific activity of the leucine pool in the skeletal muscle was not determined in these two studies. Using constant intravenous infusion of [^{14}C]-tyrosine, Millward et al.[92] accurately measured the rate of tyrosine incorporation from the specific activity of the free tyrosine pool, by the grastocnemius and quadricep muscles from rats of various ages. However, the oldest rats used in this study were 11 months of age, and the decrease in muscle protein synthesis occurred during the first 4 months of life.

More information is available on the effect of aging on cardiac muscle protein synthesis than on skeletal muscle protein synthesis because the investigators studying cardian protein synthesis have used a wide range of ages in their studies. Using ribosomes and cell sap prepared from cardiac tissue of rats, Meerson et al.[93] observed that cell-free protein synthesis decreased 32% from 3 to 24 months of age. The results of studies on the effect of aging on the in vivo incorporation of radioactively labeled amino acids into cardiac tissue are contradictory. Using rats, Kanungo et al.[77] reported that the in vivo incorporation of [^{14}C]-leucine increased with age, while Meerson et al.[93] observed an age-related decrease in the incorporation of a mixture of radioactively labeled amino acids. The specific activities of the amino acid precursor pools were not determined in either of these studies. Du et al.[72] measured the in vivo incorporation of [^{3}H]-leucine by various fractions of cardiac tissue from 12- and 33-month-old mice, as well as the leucine pool and [^{3}H]-leucine uptake by cardiac tissue. They found that no age-related change occurred in any of these parameters.

The most informative study on the effect of aging on cardiac protein synthesis was performed by Geary and Florini[94] and Florini and co-workers.[95] Using perfused hearts from mice of various ages, [^{3}H]-leucine incorporation into acid-insoluble material was observed to decrease continuously from 1 to 27 months of age. However, the specific activity of the intracellular leucine pool in the perfused hearts varied as a function of age. When the rate of leucine incorporation was determined from the specific activity of the leucine pool, a nonlinear change in the rate of leucine incorporation was observed from 1 to 27 months of age.[94] The rate of leucine incorporation by perfused hearts from mice of various ages is shown in Figure 2. During maturation, leucine incorporation increased; however, leucine incorporation by perfused hearts decreased during senescence.

Using mice,[96-103] rats,[104-116] and chickens,[117,118] it has been well-established that brain protein synthesis decreases during development and maturation. However, there are

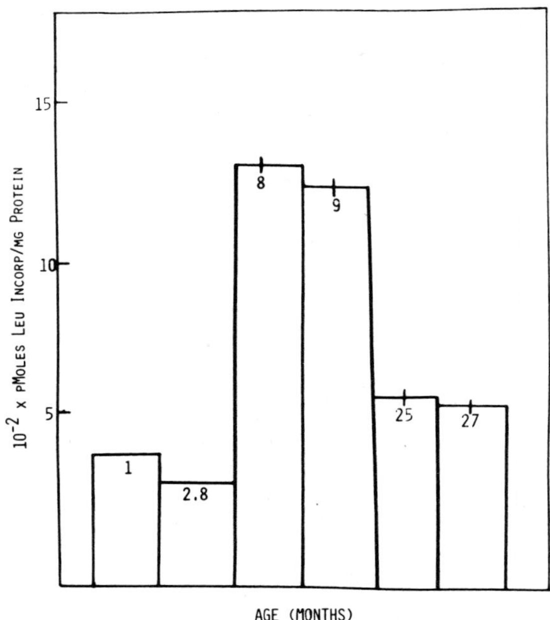

FIGURE 2. The effect of age on the rate of leucine incorporation by perfused heart. (From Geary, S. and Florini, J. R., *J. Gerontol.*, 27, 325, 1972. With permission.)

only a few investigators who have studied brain protein synthesis in old animals (Table 5). Using the postmitochondrial supernatant from whole rat brain, Ekstrom et al.[119] observed a 56% decrease in cell-free protein synthesis from 6 to 32 months of age. This decrease occurred primarily from 6 to 14 months of age. After 14 months of age, cell-free protein synthesis decreased only 15%. The incorporation of radioactively labeled amino acids into acid-insoluble material by brain slices from animals of various ages has also been compared.[120,121] McMartin and Schedlbauer[120] reported that [^{14}C]-leucine incorporation by brain slices from 5-, 12-, 18-, and 25-month-old mice was the same. Orrego and Lipmann[121] observed a 30% decrease in [^{14}C]-valine incorporation from 3 to 24 months of age in rats; however, from their data, this decrease does not appear to be statistically significant. Since the specific activity of the amino acid precursor pool was not determined in either study and Dunlop et al.[115] have found that age-related changes in brain protein synthesis observed with brain slices do not represent the changes that occur in brain protein synthesis in vivo, the information gained from the studies using brain slices is limited.

Several investigators[77,122-124] have compared the in vivo incorporation of radioactively labeled amino acids into acid-insoluble material by young and old animals. Using mice, Finch[122] and Gordon and Finch[123] found that the in vivo incorporation of either [^{3}H]-tyrosine or [^{3}H]-leucine by the brain of adult and senescent mice was the same. Kanungo et al.[77] also observed that the in vivo incorporation of [^{14}C]-leucine by brain did not change with age in rats. Although Finch[122] and Gordon and Finch[123] measured the radioactivity in the acid-soluble fraction of brain and blood plasma, none of the investigators cited above determined the specific activity of the amino acid precursor pools in the brain. By injecting animals with "flooding" amounts of a radioactively labeled amino acid, Dunlop et al.[115,116] have shown that the in vivo rate of protein synthesis by the brain can be measured accurately because the specific activity of the

Table 5
EFFECT OF AGING ON PROTEIN SYNTHESIS BY TISSUES OTHER THAN LIVER AND MUSCLE FROM MICE AND RATS

	Change	Ages studied (months)	Ref.
	Brain		
Cell-free			
Rats	56% decrease	6—32	119
Brain slices			
Mice	No change	5—25	120
Rats	30% decrease	3—24	121
In vivo			
Mice	No change	10—30	122
	No change	9—28	123
Rats	20% decrease	3—23	124
	No change	10—22	77
	Kidney (Rats)		
Cell-free	74—91% decrease	3—31	125
In vivo	0—15% decrease	11—28	75
	100% increase	10—22	77
	Testes (Rats)		
Cell-free	47% decrease	3—30	126
In vivo	800% increase	10—22	77
	Spleen (Rats)		
In vivo	100% increase	10—22	77

amino acid pool in the brain approaches that of the radioactively labeled amino acid administered. In addition, the specific activity of the amino acid precursor pool in the brain remains constant for several hours. Using this system, Dunlop et al.[115] found that valine incorporation by the cerebral hemispheres and cerebellum decreased from 2 to 10 months of age in rats.[115] However, Dunlop et al. did not study rats older than 10 months of age. Recently, Dwyer and Wasterlain[124] used the system developed by Dunlop et al.[115,116] to measure lysine incorporation by various brain regions from 3-, 11-, and 23-month-old rats. A statistically significant decrease in the in vivo incorporation of lysine was observed from 3 to 23 months of age in the forebrain, cerebellum, and brain stem.

The present information indicates that during brain development, a rapid and large decrease in brain protein synthesis occurs. However, it appears that brain protein synthesis continues to decline, albeit at a slower rate, after maturation.[119,124]

The effect of aging on protein synthesis in tissues other than liver, muscle, or brain has only been studied to a limited extent. A list of the tissues studied and the influence of aging on protein synthesis by these tissues is given in Table 5. Cell-free protein synthesis by the postmitochondrial supernatant from either kidney[125] or testes[126] decreased with increasing age. However, Kanungo et al.[77] observed an age-related increase in the incorporation of [^{3}H]-leucine by these tissues and also the spleen. On the other hand, Beauchene et al.[75] reported that the in vivo incorporation of [^{3}H]-leucine by kidney from rats decreased slightly from 11 to 28 months of age. Again, it should

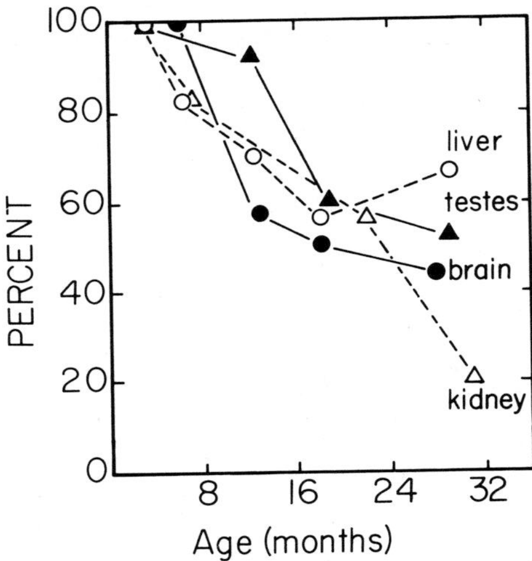

FIGURE 3. The effect of age on protein synthesis by various tissues from Fischer F344 rats. The protein synthetic activity at the various ages is expressed as a percent of that observed for 3- to 4-month-old rats for the liver[81] (○——○), kidney[125] (△——△), and testes[126] (▲——▲), and as a percent of that observed for 6-month-old rats for brain[119] (●——●).

be noted that the specific activity of the leucine pools in these tissues was not determined by either Kanungo et al.[77] or Beauchene et al.[75]

There are a few investigators who have studied the effect of aging on the synthesis of specific proteins in tissues other than liver. Using kinetic analysis of 3-amino 1,2,4 triazole perturbation of normal catalyase levels, Haining and Legan[127] reported that the synthesis of catalyase decreased almost 75% from 1.5 to 30 months of age in rat kidney. The synthesis of collagen by skin and tail tissue from 3- and 20- to 24-month-old rats was determined by Niedermuller et al.[128] who reported an age-related decrease in the synthesis of tropocollagen and the labile and stabile polymer forms of collagen.

It is evident from Tables 3, 4, and 5 that most studies with rodents have shown that protein synthesis decreases with increasing age. The effect of aging on the protein synthetic activity of various tissues of one strain of rats in compared in Figure 3. Cell-free protein synthesis by brain,[119] kidney,[125] and testicular[126] tissue and the rate of protein synthesis by suspensions of hepatocytes[81] isolated from 3- to 32-month-old Fischer F344 rats is shown. This strain of rats has a mean survival of 28 to 29 months and a maximum survival of 35 months.[129] An age-related decline in protein synthesis was observed from 3 to 18 months of age in all four tissues. After 18 months of age, the protein synthetic activity of the brain and testes decreased only slightly; however, the protein synthetic activity of kidney tissue decreased 63% from 22 to 31 months of age. The dramatic decrease in kidney protein synthesis during senescence might be due to the age-related increase in the severity of renal disease, which was observed by Coleman et al.[129] in Fischer F344 rats. As noted previously (Figure 1), the rate of protein synthesis by isolated hepatocytes increased from 18 to 30 months of age. It appears that the increased protein synthetic activity of the liver during senescence might be a secondary response to proteinuria, which arises from renal failure. This would explain why — of the four tissues studied — only the liver showed an increased protein synthetic activity from 18 to 30 months of age.

Most of the information currently available on the mechanisms responsible for the age-related change in protein synthesis has come from studies with rodents. Although the decrease in cell-free protein synthesis during aging has been reported to be associated only with the microsomal fraction of liver[60,69] or cardiac tissue,[93] most investigators have found that the ability of the cell sap to support protein synthesis also decreases with age.[61,63-65,126,130] Recently, Moldave et al.[71] measured the activity of the elongation factors of protein synthesis, EF-1 and EF-2, in the cell sap from livers of 3- and 30-month-old rats. Although EF-2 activity did not change with age, the activity of EF-1 was 30 to 40% lower in the cell sap from the old rats compared to the young.

Several investigators[70,131-133] have reported that the aminoacylation of tRNA decreased with increasing age, and this decrease was due to a decrease in the ability of tRNA to accept amino acids. Recently, Mays et al.[133] reported that the age-related decrease in tRNA charging was more pronounced with tRNA isolated from whole liver tissue than with tRNA isolated from the cell sap fraction of liver. They found a defective subfraction of tRNA associated with the ribosomal fraction of liver from old rats. Although the aminoacylation of tRNA appears to decrease with increasing age, no age-related increase in the incidence of errors in the aminoacylation of tRNA has been observed.[70,132]

Because of the importance of nucleoside modification on the biological function of tRNA, it is reasonable to suggest that age-related changes in tRNA modification might be responsible for the decrease in tRNA aminoacylation. Wust and Rosen[131] and Mays et al.[134] reported that the methylation of tRNA decreases with increasing age. However, when Hoffman and McCoy[135] determined the nucleoside composition of tRNA isolated from 12- and 30-month-old mice, no age-related change in the tRNA content of modified nucleosides was found. Because Hoffman and McCoy[135] did a mass analysis of all tRNAs, it is possible that they would not have been able to detect changes in the modification of one or two tRNA species.[136] Although no age-related appearance or disappearance of isoaccepting species of tRNA has been observed,[132,133] Mays et al.[133] have reported that the proportion of isoaccepting species of several tRNAs change as a function of age in rat liver. This observation is consistent with the concept that changes in the modification of the tRNA bases occur during the aging process. (See also "Posttranscriptional Modification of RNA in Aging Organisms".)

Several investigators have studied the effects of aging on ribosomal components of the protein synthetic apparatus. Although Mariotti and Ruscitto[70] reported that the fidelity of polyuridylic acid translation by liver ribosomes decreased from 3 to 12 months of age in rats, no age-related decrease in the fidelity of polyuridylic acid translation was observed by ribosomes isolated from mouse liver[67] or rat brain[119] or kidney.[125] Layman et al.[69] proposed that the age-related decrease in liver cell-free protein synthesis was due to a decrease in the aggregation of ribosomes to mRNA. With increasing age, a shift of ribosomal sedimenting material has been observed in liver,[69,137] skeletal muscle,[88,90,91] lung,[137] and the prostate gland.[137] Comolli and co-workers found that the protein content of 40S ribosomal subunits[138] and the ribosome dissociation factor activity[139] decrease as a function of age. These observations led Comolli[139] to propose that a decrease in the initiation of protein synthesis occurs as an organism ages. An age-related decrease in either the initiation of protein synthesis or the availability of mRNA for protein synthesis could be the basis for the decrease in ribosome aggregation to mRNA that occurs during the aging process.

FIBROBLASTS

The concept that fibroblasts age in vitro originated from the observation that fibroblasts in culture undergo only a limited number of doublings.[140,141] Since this initial

TABLE 6
EFFECT OF IN VITRO AGING ON PROTEIN SYNTHESIS IN CULTURES OF FIBROBLASTS

	Change	Ref.
Human diploid fibroblasts		
MRC-5	89% decrease	143
CF-3	No change	144
WI-38	29—49% decrease	145, 148
HF-J and HF-7	No change	149
Chick embryo fibroblasts	50—62% decrease	146, 147

observation, the use of fibroblasts as a model system to study the aging process has gained wide acceptance.[142] A list of the studies that have reported the effect of in vitro aging on protein synthesis is given in Table 6. In these studies, protein synthesis was determined by measuring the in vivo incorporation of radioactively labeled amino acids into either total acid-insoluble material[143-147] or specific proteins.[148,149] Although Dell'Orco and Guthrie[144] found that [^{3}H]-leucine incorporation was similar for early- and late-passage human fibroblasts, Lewis and Tarrant[143] and Razin et al.[145] observed a decrease in the incorporation of radioactively labeled amino acids by late-passage human fibroblasts compared to early-passage fibroblasts. Lewis and Tarrant[143] reported that the decrease in [^{35}S]-methionine incorporation occurred just before (10 doublings) the onset of cell death. Houck et al.[148] observed that collagen synthesis, measured by the incorporation of [^{3}H]-proline into hydroxyproline, decreased 47% after 33 population doublings. Recently, Engelhardt et al.[149] measured the incorporation of [^{35}S]-methionine into 500 specific polypeptides by both phase 2 and 3 human fibroblasts. Polypeptides from extracts of fibroblasts were separated by SDS-polyacrylamide gel electrophosesis, and the incorporation of [^{35}S]-methionine into the polypeptides was quantified by autoradiography. Although quantification of [^{35}S]-methionine incorporation by this method is only approximate, it appears that no major change in [^{35}S]-methionine incorporation into most polypeptides occurred during aging in vitro.

A decrease in the incorporation of radioactively labeled amino acids into acid-insoluble material was also observed in chick embryo fibroblasts.[146,147] Although amino acid incorporation declined constantly between 5 and 33 doublings (lifespan 35 ± 5 population doublings), the largest decline occurred between the 20th and 25th doubling.

Although most of the studies with fibroblasts demonstrate that the incorporation of radioactively labeled amino acids into protein decreases during in vitro aging, one must be cautious in assuming that these observations indicate that protein synthesis declines during aging in vitro. Birckbichler et al.[150] reported that the transport of leucine and α-aminoisobutyrate was similar for early- and late-passage fibroblasts. However, because the cell volume of fibroblasts increases during senescence in vitro,[151,152] it is possible that changes in the specific activity of the amino acid precursor pool might be responsible for the change in incorporation of radioactively labeled amino acids during aging in vitro.

To this author's knowledge, only one report has been published on the effect of in vitro aging on the protein synthetic apparatus. Goldstein and Varmuza[153] have reported that the initial velocity and specific activity of phenylalanyl-tRNA synthetase was lower in late-passage human fibroblasts than in early-passage fibroblasts. They suggested that the phenylalanyl-tRNA synthetase from late-passage cells was less efficient catalytically.

TABLE 7
EFFECT OF AGING ON WHOLE BODY PROTEIN SYNTHESIS IN HUMANS

Subject	Age (range)	N[a]	Total body protein synthesis (g kg^{-1} day^{-1})	Ref.
Young adult (male and female)	20—23 years	4	3.0 ± 0.2	156
Elderly (male and female)	69—91 years	4	1.9 ± 0.2	156
Young male	20—25 years	4	3.33 ± 0.30	157
Elderly male	65—72 years	4	3.18 ± 0.71	157
Young female	18—23 years	4	2.63 ± 0.20	157
Elderly female	67—91 years	5	2.25 ± 0.37	157

N = number of subjects.

HUMANS

Because the ultimate goal of aging research is to apply basic research to humans, it is of interest to know how aging affects protein synthesis in humans. In an early study, Sharp et al.[154] determined the rates of protein metabolism for 24-year-old and 59- to 70-year-old subjects. Protein turnover was approximately 1.5-fold higher in the old subjects than in the young. Lundholm and Schersten[155] measured the incorporation of [^{14}C]-leucine into acid-insoluble material by muscle fibers obtained from biopsies of subjects younger and older than 60 years of age. The in vitro incorporation of [^{14}C]-leucine by muscle fibers from old subjects was approximately 36% higher than that observed from younger subjects. Because Lindholm and Schersten[155] did not determine the specific activity of the leucine pool in the muscle fibers, it is not possible to determine if the increased [^{14}C]-leucine incorporation was due to an age-related increase in protein synthesis by muscle fibers, or to age-related changes in amino acid transport and the size of the leucine pool.

Recently, Young et al. and Winterer et al. measured the rates of total body protein synthesis in human subjects of various ages,[156,157] the data from these studies are presented in Table 7. Total body protein synthesis was determined by measuring the amount of urinary [^{15}N]-urea when constant [^{15}N] enrichment had been achieved after the administration of [^{15}N]-glycine. Young et al.[156] observed that the rate of total body protein synthesis by 69- to 91-year-old subjects was 37% less than the rate of total body protein synthesis by 20- to 23-year-old subjects. This decrease was statistically significant. More recently, Winterer et al.[157] compared the rates of total body protein synthesis of young and elderly subjects on the basis of sex (Table 7). The rate of total body protein synthesis by female subjects was significantly lower than that by male subjects. Although the rate of total body protein synthesis in elderly males and females was respectively lower than the rate of protein synthesis found in young males and females, this age-related decrease in the rate of total body protein synthesis was not statistically significant.

SUMMARY

The majority of the studies (70 to 75%) described herein indicate that protein synthesis decreases with increasing age in living organisms ranging from fungi[35] to humans.[156] However, a substantial number of investigators (see Tables 1 through 7) have reported that protein synthesis either remains constant or increases during aging. These contradictory observations could be the result of several factors, which will be discussed below.

Differences in the methods used to measure protein synthesis are a likely reason for the discrepancies reported in the literature on the effect of aging on protein synthesis. For example, an age-related decline in protein synthesis was observed in more than 90% of the studies in which a cell-free system was used to measure protein synthesis. On the other hand, in the majority of the studies that used either whole cells, tissue slices, perfused organs, or the whole organism, protein synthesis was reported to either increase or not change during aging. In most of the in vivo studies reported herein, the investigators made no attempt to determine the specific activity of the amino acid precursor pool; only the amount of radioactively labeled amino acid incorporated into protein by organisms of various ages was compared. It is essential that the specific activity of the amino acid precursor pool be measured when studying the effect of aging on protein synthesis because age-related changes in the amino acid precursor pool have been reported to occur during the aging process, e.g., the rate of amino acid turnover decreases in flies,[46,47] and the specific activity of the intracellular leucine pool in perfused heart[94,158] and the specific activity of valyl-tRNA in liver in vivo[73] change as a function of age. Therefore, much of the contradictory information on the effect of aging on protein synthesis apparently occurs because protein synthesis was not measured appropriately.

Protein synthesis can be measured accurately and reproducibly with cell-free systems because an investigator can carefully control experimental conditions; problems that arise from the compartmentalization of amino acids are eliminated. However, the rate of cell-free protein synthesis is only 1% of that observed in vivo.[3,4] Therefore, it is necessary to establish that age-related changes observed in cell-free protein synthesis are representative of the changes that occur in vivo. During the past 4 years, Richardson and co-workers have measured the rate of protein synthesis by liver from rats of various ages using a cell-free system derived from the postmitochondrial supernatant of the liver,[69] isolated hepatocytes,[73] and the liver in vivo.[73] Although the rates of protein synthesis were different in the three systems, protein synthesis was observed to decrease approximately 50% from 1 to 18 months of age in all three systems. Therefore, the relative effect of aging on protein synthesis can be determined using a cell-free system. In fact, until accurate in vivo measurements of protein synthesis are made, the best indication of the effect of aging on protein synthesis comes from cell-free studies.

A few investigators have made an effort to measure the specific activity of the amino acid pool when determining the effect of aging on protein synthesis in vivo. In these studies, a decrease in protein synthesis with increasing age was observed. For example, Baumann and Chen[46] and Levenbook and Krishna[47] measured the specific activities of the free amino acid pools extracted from whole flies to correct for age-related changes in the turnover rate of the amino acid pools. They found that the in vivo rate of protein synthesis by old flies was only 30 to 60% of that observed for young flies. Also, Dwyer and Wasterlain[124] recently measured the rate of in vivo protein synthesis by various brain regions of 3- to 23- month-old rats using "flooding" amounts of an amino acid. After an animal is injected with a large quantity of a radioactively labeled amino acid that is not metabolized, Dunlop et al.[159] found that the specific activity of the intracellular amino acid pool in the brain becomes 80 to 90% of the specific activity of the amino acid injected, and the specific activity of the intracellular amino acid pool in the brain remains constant for at least 2 hours. Using this method, the approximate rate of protein synthesis by the brain in vivo can be determined with some degree of accuracy from the specific activity of the amino acid injected. An age-related decrease in the rate of protein synthesis by the brain in vivo was observed by Dwyer and Wasterlain.[124] To this author's knowledge, only one research group has actually determined the specific activity of the amino acid bound to tRNA (the immediate precursor pool for protein synthesis) when determining the effect of aging on protein synthesis in vivo. Ricca et al.[73] determined the rate of valine incorporation by the liver from the specific activity of the valyl-tRNA. The rate of protein synthesis by the liver of 15-month-old rats was approximately one half of that observed for 3-month-old rats.

In addition, a few investigators have accurately measured protein synthesis in either perfused organs or cell suspensions isolated from animals of various ages. Using perfused heart isolated from 1- to 27-month-old mice, Geary and Florini[94] determined the rate of protein synthesis from the specific activity of the intracellular leucine pool. However, McKee et al.[21] showed that both the intracellular and extracellular phenylalanine pools serve as a source of phenylalanine for protein synthesis in perfused heart. At a low perfusate concentration of phenylalanine (0.01 m*M*), the specific activity of phenylalanyl-tRNA is different from the specific activities of either the extracellular or intracellular phenylalanine pools. By increasing the phenylalanine concentration in the perfusate, the specific activities of the extracellular, intracellular, and tRNA-bound phenylalanine become equivalent. The perfusate concentration of leucine used by Geary and Florini[94] was 0.23 m*M*. Assuming that phenylalanine and leucine would behave similarly in the perfused heart, it would appear from the data of McKee et al.[21] that the specific activity of the intracellular leucine would be similar to the specific activity of the leucyl-tRNA when the perfusate concentration of leucine is 0.23 m*M*. Therefore, the rates of leucine incorporation reported by Geary and Florini[94] would be expected to be a relatively accurate measure of protein synthesis in the perfused heart. In fact, the rates of protein synthesis reported by Geary and Florini[94] are similar to those rates determined by McKee et al.[21] for perfused heart using the specific activity of the aminoacyl-tRNA. Geary and Florini[94] observed that protein synthesis decreased 40% from 8 to 27 months of age in perfused mouse heart.

Recently, Ricca et al.[73] demonstrated that the rate of protein synthesis could be determined accurately in suspensions of hepatocytes from the specific activity of either the intracellular or extracellular valine pool. When hepatocytes were incubated with [^{3}H]-valine, the specific activity of the extracellular and intracellular valine became equal within 5 minutes. Because the tRNA derives its amino acids from both the extracellular and intracellular pools,[18-24] the specific activity of valine bound to tRNA would be identical to the specific activity of either the extracellular or intracellular valine. Using hepatocytes isolated from rats ranging in age from 2.5 to 30 months, Coniglio et al.[81] determined the rate of protein synthesis from the specific activity of the extracellular valine. van Bezooijen et al. and van Bezooijen and Knook[79,80] also compared the protein synthetic activity of hepatocytes isolated from rats of various ages, however, they measured only the incorporation of [^{3}H]-leucine into protein; the specific activity of the leucine pool was not determined. Because saturating concentrations of [^{3}H]-leucine were used when measuring protein synthesis, the rate of [^{3}H]-leucine incorporation reported by van Bezooijen et al. and van Bezooijen and Knook[79,80] would be a relatively accurate indication of the rate of protein synthesis. The studies by van Bezooijen et al.,[79] van Bezooijen and Knook,[80] and Coniglio et al.[81] indicated that protein synthesis by hepatocytes decreased with increasing age from 3 to 24 months. After 24 months of age, an increase in protein synthesis was observed (Figure 1).

Another possible reason for the contradictory observations reported in the literature is the different age-groups studied. Most investigators have studied only two age groups, usually a relatively young organism and an old organism. When such a protocol is used, the investigator assumes that any change in protein synthesis would be linear over the age period studied. However, in the few studies in which protein synthesis was measured at several ages, investigators found that the age-related changes in protein synthesis were nonlinear (Figures 1 and 2). Using perfused mouse heart, Geary and Florini[94] reported that the rate of protein synthesis increased until the animals reached middle-age and then protein synthesis decreased during senescence (Figure 2). On the other hand, van Bezooijen et al.,[79] van Bezooijen and Knook,[80] and Coniglio et al.[81] observed that protein synthesis by suspensions of hepatocytes isolated from rats of various ages decreased constantly during the first two years of life and then increased during the third year of life (Figure 1). If only two age groups are used to study protein synthesis in an organism, investigators might observe no change, an increase, or a decrease in protein synthesis depending on the ages compared. This problem is compounded when research groups use different strains of animals or animal colonies to study the effect of aging on protein synthesis because these animals will probably have different survival characteristics. As a result, contradictory results are to be expected when investigators use only two age groups to study a process that may change in a nonlinear fashion during the life span of an organism. Therefore, an investigator must use several age groups over a wide range of ages to determine how protein synthesis changes during the aging process.

REFERENCES

1. **Finch, C. E.,** Enzyme activities, gene function, and aging in mammals, *Exp. Gerontol.*, 7, 53, 1972.
2. **Schimke, R. T.,** The importance of both synthesis and degradation in the control of arginase levels in rat liver, *J. Biol. Chem.*, 239, 3808, 1964.
3. **Henshaw, E. C., Hirsch, C. A., Morton, B. E., and Hiatt, H. H.,** Control of protein synthesis in mammalian tissues through changes in ribosome activity, *J. Biol. Chem.*, 246, 436, 1971.
4. **Waterlow, J. C.,** Protein turnover in the whole body, *Nature (London)*, 253, 157, 1975.
5. **Neuberger, A. and Richards, F. F.,** Protein biosynthesis in mammalian cells, in *Mammalian Protein Metabolism*, Vol. 1, Monro, H. N. and Allison, J. B., Eds., Academic Press, New York, 1964, 243.
6. **Munro, H. N.,** A general survey of techniques used in studying protein metabolism in whole animals and intact cells, in *Mammalian Protein Metabolism*, Vol. 3, Munro, H. N. and Allison, J. B., Eds., Academic Press, New York, 1969, 237.
7. **Waterlow, J. C.,** The assessment of protein nutrition and metabolism in the whole animal, with special reference to man, in *Mammalian Protein Metabolism*, Vol. 3, Munro, H. N. and Allison, J. B., Eds., Academic Press, New York, 1969, 325.
8. **Rannels, D. E., Li, J. B., Morgan, H. E., and Jefferson, L. S.,** Evaluation of hormone effects on protein turnover in isolated perfused organs, in *Methods in Enzymology*, Vol. 37, O'Malley, B. W. and Hardman, J. G., Eds., Academic Press, New York, 1975, 238.
9. **Loftfield, R. B. and Harris, A.,** Participation of free amino acids in protein synthesis, *J. Biol. Chem.*, 219, 151, 1956.
10. **Kipnis, D. M., Reiss, E., and Helmreich, E.,** Functional heterogeneity of the intracellular amino acid pool in mammalian cells, *Biochim. Biophys. Acta*, 51, 519, 1961.
11. **Manchester, K. L. and Wool, I. G.,** Insulin and incorporation of amino acids into protein of muscle. II. Accumulation and incorporation studies with the perfused rat heart, *Biochem. J.*, 89, 202, 1963.
12. **Rosenberg, L. E., Berman, M., and Segal, S.,** Studies of the kinetics of amino acid transport, incorporation into protein, and oxidation in kidney-cortex slices, *Biochim. Biophys. Acta*, 71, 664, 1963.
13. **Mortimore, G. E., Woodside, K. H., and Henry, J. E.,** Compartmentation of free valine and its relation to protein turnover in perfused rat liver, *J. Biol. Chem.*, 247, 2776, 1972.
14. **Ward, W. F. and Mortimore, G. E.,** Compartmentation of intracellular amino acids in rat liver. I. Evidence for an intralysosomal pool derived from protein degradation, *J. Biol. Chem.*, 253, 3581, 1978.
15. **Hider, R. C., Fern, E. B., and London, D. R.,** Relationship between intracellular amino acids and protein synthesis in the extensor digitorum longus muscle of rats, *Biochem. J.*, 114, 171, 1969.

16. **van Venrooij, W. J., Kuijper-Lenstra, A. H., and Kramer, M. F.,** Interrelationship between amino acid pools and protein synthesis in the rat submandibular gland, *Biochim. Biophys. Acta,* 312, 392, 1973.
17. **van Venrooij, W. J., Moonen, H., and van Loon-Klaassen, L.,** Source of amino acids used for protein synthesis in HeLa cells, *Eur. J. Biochem.,* 50, 297, 1974.
18. **Khairallah, E. A. and Mortimore, G. E.,** Assessment of protein turnover in perfused rat liver. I. Evidence for amino acid compartmentation from differential labeling of free and RNA-bound valine, *J. Biol. Chem.,* 251, 1976.
19. **Airhart, J., Vidrich, A., and Khairallah, E. A.,** Compartmentation of free amino acids for protein synthesis in rat liver, *Biochem. J.,* 140, 539, 1974.
20. **Vidrich, A., Airhart, J., Bruno, M. K., and Khairallah, E. A.,** Compartmentation of free amino acids for protein biosynthesis. I. Influence of diurnal changes in hepatic amino acid concentration on the composition of the precursor pool charging aminoacyl-transfer ribonucleic acid, *Biochem. J.,* 162, 257, 1977.
21. **McKee, E. E., Cheung, J. Y., Rannels, D. E., and Morgan, H. E.,** Measurement of the rate of protein synthesis and compartmentation of heart phenylalanine, *J. Biol. Chem.,* 253, 1030, 1978.
22. **Martin, A. F., Rabinowitz, M., Blough, R., Prior, G., and Zak, R.,** Measurements of half-life of rat cardiac myosin heavy chain with leucyl-tRNA as precursor pool, *J. Biol. Chem.,* 252, 3422, 1977.
23. **Seglen, P. O. and Solheim, A. E.,** Valine uptake and incorporation into protein in isolated hepatocytes. I. Nature of the precursor pool for protein synthesis, *Eur. J. Biochem.,* 85, 15, 1978.
24. **Robertson, J. H. and Wheatley, D. N.,** Pools and protein synthesis in mammalian cells, *Biochem. J.,* 178, 699, 1979.
25. **Shaw, M. and Manocha, M. S.,** Fine structure in detached, senescing wheat leaves, *Can. J. Bot.,* 43, 747, 1965.
26. **Barton, R.,** Fine structure of mesophyll cells in senescing leaves of *Phaseolus, Planta,* 71, 314, 1966.
27. **Butler, R. D.,** The fine structure of senescing cotyledons of cucumber, *J. Exp. Bot.,* 18, 535, 1967.
28. **Srivastava, B. I. S. and Arglebe, C.,** Studies on ribosomes from barley leaves. I. Changes during senescence, *Plant Physiol.,* 42, 1497, 1967.
29. **BeMiller, J. N., Hoffman, M. E., and Pappelis, A. J.,** Relationship of protein metabolism to senescence of corn (*Zea mays* L.) stalk parenchyma, cob parenchyma, and first-developed leaf tissues, *Mech. Ageing Dev.,* 1, 387, 1972/73.
30. **Pillay, D. T. N.,** Protein synthesis in aging soybean cotyledons — loss in translational capacity, *Biochem. Biophys. Res. Commun.,* 79, 796, 1977.
31. **Shugart, L.,** A possible age-related modification of phenylalanine transfer RNA from wheat tissue, *Exp. Gerontol.,* 7, 251, 1972.
32. **Wright, R. D., Pillay, D. T. N., and Cherry, J. H.,** Changes in leucyl-tRNA species of pea leaves during senescence and after zeatin treatment, *Mech. Ageing Dev.,* 1, 403, 1972/73.
33. **Bick, M. D. and Strehler, B. L.,** Leucyl- tRNA synthetase activity in old cotyledons: evidence on repressor accumulation, *Mech. Ageing Dev.,* 1, 33, 1972/73.
34. **BeMiller, J. N., Hoffman, W. E., and Pappelis, A. J.,** Changes in tRNA methylase activity in senescing cob and stalk parenchyma tissue and the first-developed leaf of corn (*Zea mays* L.), *Mech. Ageing Dev.,* 2, 363, 1973.
35. **Gottlieb, D.,** The aging process in the fungus *Rhizoctonia solani, Phytophylactica,* 7, 81, 1975.
36. **Gottlieb, D., Molitoris, H. P., and van Etten, J. L.,** Changes in fungi with age. III. Incorporation of amino acids into cells, *Arch. Microbiol.,* 61, 394, 1968.
37. **Ricciardi, R. P., Holloman, D. W., and Gottlieb, D.,** Age-dependent changes in fungi: ribosomes and protein synthesis in *Rhizoctonia solani* mycelium, *Arch. Microbiol.,* 95, 325, 1974.
38. **Obrig, T. G. and Gottlieb, D.,** In vitro protein synthesis and aging in *Rhizoctonia solani, J. Bacteriol.,* 101, 755, 1970.
39. **Gottlieb, D. and Sharma, V. D.,** Changes in ribonuclease with age in the fungus *Rhizoctonia solani, Mech. Ageing Dev.,* 5, 25, 1976.
40. **Clarke, J. M. and Smith, J. M.,** Increase in the rate of protein synthesis with age in *Drosophila subobscura, Nature (London),* 209, 627, 1966.
41. **Baker G. T.,** Insect flight muscle: maturation and senescence, *Gerontology,* 22, 334, 1976.
42. **Heslop, J. P.,** Effect of age on [^{14}C] valine turnover into locust wing proteins, *Biochem. J.,* 104(Abstr.), 5P, 1967.
43. **Wattiaux, J. M., Libion-Mannaert, M., and Delcour, J.,** Protein turnover and protein synthesis following actinomycin-D injection as a function of age in *Drosophila melanogaster, Gerontologia,* 17, 289, 1971.
44. **Rockstein, M. and Baker, G. T.,** Effects of X-irradiation of pupae on aging of the thoracic flight muscle of the adult house fly *Musca domestica* L., *Mech. Ageing Dev.,* 3, 271, 1974.

45. **Dinamarca, M. L. and Levenbook, L.**, Oxidation, utilization, and incorporation into protein of alanine and lysine during metamorphosis of the blowfly *Phormia regina* (Meigen), *Arch. Biochem. Biophys.*, 117, 110, 1966.
46. **Baumann, D. and Chen, P. S.**, Alterung und proteinsynthesis bei *Drosophila melanogaster, Rev. Suisse Zool.*, 75, 1051, 1969.
47. **Levenbook, L. and Krishna, I.**, Effect of aging on amino acid turnover and rate of protein synthesis in the blowfly *Phormia regina, J. Insect Physiol.*, 17, 9, 1971.
48. **Baker, G. T. and Schmidt, T.**, Changes in 80S ribosomes from *Drosophilia melanogaster* with age, *Experientia*, 32, 1505, 1976.
49. **Hosbach, H. A. and Kubli, E.**, Transfer RNA in aging *Drosophila:* extent of aminoacylation, *Mech. Ageing Dev.*, 10, 131, 1979.
50. **Gershon, D.**, Studies on aging in nematodes. I. The nematode as a model organism for aging research, *Exp. Gerontol.*, 5, 7, 1970.
51. **Prasanna, H. R. and Lane, R. S.**, Impaired protein synthesis in aged *Turbatrix aceti, Fed. Proc.*, 36 (Abstr.), 292, 1977.
52. **Wallach, Z. and Gershon, D.**, Altered ribosomal particles in senescent nematodes, *Mech. Ageing Dev.*, 3, 225, 1974.
53. **Sundararaman, V. and Cummings, D. J.**, Morphological changes in aging cell lines of *Paramecium aurelia.* III. The effects of emetine on polysome formation, *Mech. Ageing Dev.*, 6, 393, 1977.
54. **Bolla, R. and Brot, N.**, Age-dependent changes in enzymes involved in macromolecular synthesis in *Turbatrix aceti, Arch. Biochem. Biophys.*, 169, 227, 1975.
55. **Reitz, M. S. and Sanadi, D. R.**, An aspect of translational control of protein synthesis in aging: changes in the isoaccepting forms of tRNA in *Turbatrix aceti, Exp. Gerontol.*, 7, 119, 1972.
56. **Gibson, D. C., Adelman, R. C., and Finch, C.**, Development of the Rodent as a Model System of Aging, Department of Health, Education and Welfare, Publ. No. (NIH)79-161, U. S. Government Printing Office, Washington, D. C., 1978.
57. **Buetow, D. E., Moudgil, P. G., Eichholz, R. L., and Cook, J. R.**, Protein synthesis in senescent liver, in *Liver and Aging*, Platt, D., Ed., Schattauer Verlag, New York, 1977, 211.
58. **Chen. J. C., Ove, P., and Lansing, A. I.**, In vitro synthesis of microsomal protein and albumin in young and old rats, *Biochim. Biophys. Acta*, 312, 598, 1973.
59. **Beauchene, R. E., Roeder, L. M., and Barrows, C. H.**, The effect of age and ethionine feeding on RNA and protein synthesis of rats, *J. Gerontol.*, 22, 318, 1967.
60. **Mainwaring, W. I. P.**, Effect of age on protein synthesis in mouse liver, *Biochem. J.*, 113, 869, 1969.
61. **Hrachovec, J. P.**, Age changes in amino acid incorporation by rat liver microsomes, *Gerontologia*, 15, 52, 1969.
62. **Hrachovec, J. P.**, The effect of age on tissue protein synthesis. I. Age changes in amino acid incorporation by rat liver purified microsomes, *Gerontologia*, 17, 75, 1971.
63. **Junghahn, I. and Bielka, H.**, Regulation der translation in eukaryotischen zellen. II. Uber die altersbhangige wirkung des zytosols der leber auf die in vitro proteinsynthese in einem polysomesystem, *Acta Biol. Med. Ger.*, 32, 267, 1974.
64. **Buetow, B. E. and Gandhi, P. S.**, Decreased protein synthesis by microsomes isolated from senescent rat liver, *Exp. Gerontol.*, 8, 243, 1973.
65. **Hallthaler, V. G., Reifegerste, D., Köhler, R., and Rotzsch, W.**, Zur molekularbiologie des alterns. VII. Mitteilung: einfluβ der cytosolfraktion auf die aminosäurinkorporation durch rattenlebermikrosomen in abhangigheit vom lebensalter, *Z. Alternsforsch.*, 31, 457, 1976.
66. **Comolli, R.**, Polyamine effects on ^{14}C- leucine transfer to microsomal protein in a rat liver cell-free system during aging, *Exp. Gerontol.*, 8, 307, 1973.
67. **Kurtz, D. I.**, The effect of aging on in vitro fidelity of translation in mouse liver, *Biochim. Biophys. Acta*, 407, 479, 1975.
68. **Kurtz, D. I.**, A decrease in the number of active mouse liver ribosomes during aging, *Exp. Gerontol.*, 13, 397, 1978.
69. **Layman, D. K., Ricca, G. A., and Richardson, A.**, The effect of age on protein synthesis and ribosome aggregation to messenger RNA in rat liver, *Arch. Biochem. Biophys.*, 173, 246, 1976.
70. **Mariotti, D. and Ruscitto, R.**, Age-related changes of accuracy and efficiency of protein synthesis machinery in rat, *Biochim. Biophys. Acta*, 475, 96, 1977.
71. **Moldave, K., Harris, J., Sabo, W., and Sadnik, I.**, Protein synthesis and aging: studies with cell-free mammalian systems, *Fed. Proc.*, 38, 1979, 1979.
72. **Du, J. T., Beyer, T. A., and Lang, C. A.**, Protein biosynthesis in aging mouse tissues, *Exp. Gerontol.*, 12, 181, 1977.
73. **Ricca, G. A., Liu, D. S. H., Coniglio, J. J., and Richardson, A.**, Rates of protein synthesis by hepatocytes isolated from rats of various ages, *J. Cell. Physiol.*, 97, 137, 1978.
74. **Comolli, R., Ferioli, M. E., and Azzola, S.**, Protein turnover of the lysosomal and mitochondrial fractions of rat liver during aging, *Exp. Gerontol.*, 7, 369, 1972.

75. **Beauchene, R. E., Roeder, L. M., and Barrows, C. H.,** The interrelationship of age, tissue protein synthesis, and proteinuria, *J. Gerontol.*, 25, 359, 1970.
76. **Ove, P., Obenrader, M., and Lansing, A.,** Synthesis and degradation of liver proteins in young and old rats, *Biochim. Biophys. Acta*, 277, 211, 1972.
77. **Kanungo, M. S., Koul, O., and Reddy, K. R.,** Concomitant studies on RNA and protein synthesis in tissues of rats of various ages, *Exp. Gerontol.*, 5, 261, 1970.
78. **Knook, D. L.,** Use of isolated parenchymal and nonparenchymal liver cells for studies on the mechanisms of cellular aging, in *Genetic Effects on Aging*, Bergsma, D. and Harrison, D. E., Eds., Alan R. Liss, New York, 1978, 171.
79. **van Bezooijen, C. F. A., Grell, T., and Knook, D.,** The effect of age on protein synthesis by isolated liver parenchymal cells, *Mech. Ageing Dev.*, 6, 293, 1977.
80. **van Bezooijen, C. F. A. and Knook, D. L.,** Aging changes in bromsulfophthalein uptake, albumin, and total protein synthesis in isolated hepatocytes, in *Liver and Aging*, Platt, D., Ed., Schattauer Verlag, New York, 1977, 227.
81. **Coniglio, J. J., Liu, D. S. H., and Richardson, A.,** A comparison of protein synthesis by liver parenchymal cells isolated from Fischer F344 rats of various ages, *Mech. Ageing Dev.*, in press.
82. **van Bezooijen, C. F. A., Grell, T., and Knook, D. L.,** Albumin synthesis by liver parenchymal cells isolated from young, adult, and old rats, *Biochem. Biophys. Res. Commun.*, 71, 513, 1976.
83. **Salatka, K., Kresge, D., Harris, Jr., L., Edelstein, D., and Ove, P.,** Rat serum protein changes with age, *Exp. Gerontol.*, 6, 25, 1971.
84. **Everitt, A. V.,** The urinary excretion of protein, nonprotein nitrogen, and creatinine and uric acid in aging male rats, *Gerontologia*, 2, 33, 1958.
85. **Berg, B. N.,** Spontaneous nephrosis with proteinuria hyperglobulinemia and hypercholesterolemia in the rat, *Proc. Soc. Exp. Biol. Med.*, 119, 417, 1965.
86. **Perry, S. W.,** Proteinuria in the Wistar rat, *J. Pathol. Bacteriol.*, 80, 729, 1965.
87. **Obenrader, M., Chen, J., Ove, P., and Lansing, A. I.,** Etiology of increased albumin synthesis in old rats, *Exp. Gerontol.*, 9, 173, 1974.
88. **Breuer, C. B. and Florini, J. R.,** Amino acid incorporation into protein by cell-free systems from rat skeletal muscle. IV. Effects of animal age, androgens, and anabolic agents on activity of muscle ribosomes, *Biochemistry*, 4, 1544, 1965.
89. **Srivastava, U. and Chaudhary, K. D.,** Effect of age on protein and ribonucleic acid metabolism in mouse skeletal muscle, *Can. J. Biochem.*, 47, 231, 1969.
90. **Srivastava, U.,** Polyribosome concentration of mouse skeletal muscle as a function of age, *Arch. Biochem. Biophys.*, 130, 129, 1969.
91. **Britton, G. W. and Sherman, F. G.,** Altered regulation of protein synthesis during aging as determined by in vitro ribosomal assays, *Exp. Gerontol.*, 10, 67, 1975.
92. **Millward, D. J., Garlick, P. J., Stewart, R. J. C., Nnayelugo, D. O., and Waterlow, J. C.,** Skeletal-muscle growth and protein turnover, *Biochem. J.*, 150, 235, 1975.
93. **Meerson, F. Z., Javich, M. P., and Lerman, M. I.,** Decrease in the rate of RNA and protein synthesis and degradation in the myocardium under long-term compensatory hyperfunction and on aging , *J. Mol. Cell. Cardiol.*, 10, 145, 1978.
94. **Geary, S. and Florini, J. R.,** Effect of age on rate of protein synthesis in isolated perfused mouse hearts, *J. Gerontol.*, 27, 325, 1972.
95. **Florini, J. R., Saito, Y., and Manowitz, E. J.,** Effect of age on thyroxine-induced cardiac hypertrophy in mice, *J. Gerontol.*, 28, 293, 1973.
96. **Johnson, T. C.,** Cell-free protein synthesis by mouse brain during early development, *J. Neurochem.*, 15, 1189, 1968.
97. **Johnson, T. C.,** Aminoacyl-RNA synthetase and transfer RNA binding activity during early mammalian brain development, *J. Neurochem.*, 16, 1125, 1969.
98. **Johnson, T. C. and Belytschko, G.,** Alteration in microsomal protein synthesis during early development of mouse brain, *Proc. Natl. Acad. Sci. U.S.A.*, 62, 844, 1969.
99. **Chou, L., Lerner, M. P., and Johnson, T. C.,** In vitro binding of phenylalanyl-tRNA to neonatal and adult mouse brain ribosomes, *J. Neurochem.*, 18, 2535, 1971.
100. **Lerner, M. P. and Johnson, T. C.,** Regulation of protein synthesis in developing mouse brain tissue, *J. Biol. Chem.*, 245, 1388, 1970.
101. **Gilbert, B. E., Grove, B. K., and Johnson, T. C.,** Characteristics and products of a cell-free polypeptide synthesizing system from neonatal and adult mouse brain, *J. Neurochem.*, 19, 2835, 1972.
102. **Gilbert, B. E. and Johnson, T. C.,** Fetal development: the effects of maturation on in vitro protein synthesis by mouse brain tissue, *J. Neurochem.*, 23, 811, 1974.
103. **Goertz, B.,** Regulation of protein synthesis during postnatal maturation of mouse brain, *Mech. Ageing Dev.*, 10, 261, 1979.
104. **Murthy, M. R. V. and Rappoport, D. A.,** Biochemistry of the developing rat brain. V. Cell-free incorporation of L[1-^{14}C] leucine into microsomal protein, *Biochim. Biophys. Acta*, 95, 121, 1965.

105. **Adams, D. H. and Lin, L.,** Amino acid incorporation by preparations from the developing rat brain, *Biochem. J.*, 99, 261, 1966.
106. **Murthy, M. R. V.,** Protein synthesis in growing rat tissues. II. Polyribosome concentration of brain and liver as a function of age, *Biochim. Biophys. Acta*, 119, 599, 1966.
107. **Yamagami, S., Kritz, R. R., and Rappoport, D. A.,** Biochemistry of the developing rat brain. VII. Changes in the ribosomal system and nuclear RNAs, *Biochim. Biophys. Acta*, 129, 532, 1966.
108. **Yamagami, S. and Mori, K.,** Changes in polysomes in the developing rat brain, *J. Neurochem.*, 17, 721, 1970.
109. **Andrews, T. M. and Tata, J. R.,** Protein synthesis by membrane-bound and free ribosomes of the developing rat cerebral cortex, *Biochem. J.*, 124, 883, 1971.
110. **Roberts, S., Zomzelly, C. E., and Bondy, S. C.,** Development alterations in cerebral ribonucleic acid and protein synthesis, in *Cellular Aspects of Neural Growth and Differentiation*, Pease, D. C., Ed., UCLA Press, Berkeley, 1971, 447.
111. **Barra, H. S., Unates, L. E., Sayavedra, M. S., and Capatto, R.,** Capacities for binding amino acids by tRNAs from rat brain and their changes during development, *J. Neurochem.*, 19, 2289, 1972.
112. **Burnotte, R. E., Gobert, J. G., and Temmerman, J. J.,** Piracetum (2-pyrolidinone acetamide)-induced modifications of the brain: polyribosome pattern in aging rats, *Biochem. Pharmacol.*, 22, 811, 1973.
113. **Fellous, A., Francon, J., Nunez, J., and Sokoloff, L.,** Protein synthesis by highly aggregated and purified polysomes from young and adult rat brain, *J. Neurochem.*, 21, 211, 1974.
114. **Harris, C. L. and Maas, J. W.,** Transfer RNA and the regulation of protein synthesis in rat cerebral cortex during neural development, *J. Neurochem.*, 22, 741, 1974.
115. **Dunlop, D. S., van Elden, W., and Lajtha, A.,** Developmental effects on protein synthesis rates in regions of the CNS in vivo and in vitro, *J. Neurochem.*, 29, 939, 1977.
116. **Dunlop, D. S., van Elden, W., and Lajtha, A.,** Protein degradation rates in regions of the central nervous system in vivo during development, *Biochem. J.*, 170, 637, 1978.
117. **Yang, J. W., Liu, D. S. H., and Richardson, A.,** Biochemical studies of chick brain development and maturation, I. Alteration in macromolecular content and cell-free protein synthesis, *Mech. Ageing Dev.*, 6, 77, 1977.
118. **Yang, J. W., Liu, D. S. H., and Richardson, A.,** Biochemical studies of chick brain development and maturation. II. Alterations in the mechanism of cell-free protein synthesis, *Mech. Ageing Dev.*, 6, 95, 1977.
119. **Ekstrom. R., Liu, D. S. H., and Richardson, A.,** Changes in brain protein synthesis during the life span of male Fischer rats, *Gerontology*, 26, 121, 1980.
120. **McMartin D. N. and Schedlbauer, L. M.,** Incorporation of ^{14}C-leucine into protein and tublin by brain slices from young and old mice. *J. Gerontol.*, 30, 132, 1975.
121. **Orrego, F. and Lipmann, F.,** Protein synthesis in brain slices: effects of electrical stimulation and acidic amino acids, *J. Biol. Chem.*, 242, 665, 1967.
122. **Finch, C. E.,** Catecholamine metabolism in the brains of aging male mice. *Brain Res.*, 52, 261, 1973.
123. **Gordon, S. M. and Finch, C. E.,** An electrophoretic study of protein synthesis in brain regions of senescent male mice, *Exp. Gerontol.*, 9, 269, 1974.
124. **Dwyer, B. E. and Wasterlain, C. G.,** Brain protein synthesis declines with age, *Age*, 1 (Abstr.), 163, 1978.
125. **Hardwick, J., Heish, W. H., Liu, D. S. H., and Richardson, A.,** Cell-free protein synthesis by rat kidney: the effect of age on kidney protein synthesis, *Biochim. Biophys. Acta*, 652, 204, 1981.
126. **Liu, D. S. H., Ekstrom, R., Spicer, J. W., and Richardson, A.,** Age-related changes in protein, RNA, and DNA content and protein synthesis in rat testes, *Exp. Gerontol.*, 13, 197, 1978.
127. **Haining, J. L. and Legan, J. S.,** Catalase turnover in rat liver and kidney as a function of age, *Exp. Gerontol.*, 8, 85, 1973.
128. **Niedermuller, H., Skalicky, M., Hofecker, G., and Kment, A.,** Investigations on the kinetics of collagen-metabolism in young and old rats, *Exp. Gerontol.*, 12, 159, 1977.
129. **Coleman, G. L., Barthold, S. W., Osbaldiston, G. W., Foster, S. J., and Jonas, A. M.,** Pathological changes during aging in barrier-reared Fischer 344 male rats, *J. Gerontol.*, 32, 258, 1977.
130. **Comolli, R., Delpiano, C., and Schubert, A. C.,** Dependency on the source of supernatant factors for optimal ^{14}C-polyphenylalanine synthesis by high-salt wash treated ribosomal subunits in rats of different ages, *Exp. Gerontol.*, 11, 5, 1976.
131. **Wust, C. J. and Rosen, L.,** Aminoacylation and methylation of tRNA as a function of age in the rat, *Exp. Gerontol.*, 7, 331, 1972.
132. **Frazer, J. M. and Yang, W. K.,** Isoaccepting transfer ribonucleic acids in liver and brain of young and old BC3F$_1$ mice, *Arch. Biochem. Biophys.*, 153, 610, 1972.
133. **Mays, L. L., Lawrence, A. E., Ho, R. W., and Ackley, S.,** Age-related changes in function of transfer ribonucleic acid of rat livers, *Fed. Proc.*, 38, 1984, 1979.

134. **Mays L. L., Borek, E., and Rinch, C. E.,** Glycine N-methyl transferase is a regulatory enzyme which increases in ageing animals, *Nature (London),* 243, 411, 1973.

135. **Hoffman, J. L. and McCoy, M. T.,** Stability of the nucleoside composition of tRNA during biological ageing of mice and mosquitoes, *Nature (London),* 249, 558, 1974.

136. **Borek, E.,** tRNA and ageing, *Nature (London),* 251, 260, 1974.

137. **Mainwaring, W. I. P.,** Changes in the ribonucleic acid metabolism of aging mouse tissues with particular reference to the prostate gland, *Biochem. J.,* 110, 79, 1968.

138. **Comolli, R.,** Deficiency in accessory protein of native 40S ribosomal subunits in the liver of aging rats, *Exp. Gerontol.,* 10, 31, 1975.

139. **Comolli, R., Schubert, A. C., and Delpiano, C.,** Dissociation of monomer ribosomes into subunits by liver and hepatoma DF extracts and its relation with age, *Exp. Gerontol.,* 12, 89, 1977.

140. **Hayflick, L. and Moorhead, P. S.,** The serial cultivation of human diploid cell strains, *Exp. Cell Res.,* 25, 585, 1961.

141. **Hayflick, L.,** The limited in vitro lifetime of human diploid cell strains, *Exp. Cell Res.,* 37, 614, 1965.

142. **Hayflick, L.,** Cell biology of aging, *Bioscience,* 25, 629, 1975.

143. **Lewis, C. M. and Tarrant, G. M.,** Error theory and aging in human diploid fibroblasts, *Nature (London),* 239, 316, 1972.

144. **Dell'Orco, R. T. and Guthrie, P. L.,** Altered protein metabolism in arrested populations of aging human diploid fibroblasts, *Mech, Ageing Dev.,* 5, 399, 1976.

145. **Razin, S., Pfendt, E. A., Matsumura, T., and Hayflick, L.,** Comparison by autoradiography of macromolecular biosynthesis in "young" and "old" human diploid fibroblast cultures: a brief note, *Mech. Ageing Dev.,* 6, 379, 1977.

146. **Macieira-Coelho, A. and Lima, L.,** Aging in vitro: incorporation of RNA and protein precursors and acid phosphatase activity during the life span of chick embryo fibroblasts, *Mech. Ageing Dev.,* 2, 13, 1973.

147. **Macieria-Coelho, A., Loria, E., and Berumen, L.,** Relationship between cell kinetic changes and metabolic events during cell senescence in vitro, in *Advances in Experimental Medicine and Biology,* Vol. 53, Cristofalo, V. J. and Holeckova, E., Eds., Plenum Press, New York, 1975, 51.

148. **Houck, J. C., Sharma, V. K., and Hayflick, L.,** Functional failures of cultured human diploid fibroblasts after continued population doublings, *Proc. Soc. Exp. Biol. Med.,* 137, 331, 1971.

149. **Engelhardt, D. L., Lee, G. T-Y., and Moley, J. F.,** Patterns of peptide synthesis in senescent and presenescent human fibroblasts, *J. Cell. Physiol.,* 98, 193, 1979.

150. **Birckbichler, P. J., Whittle, W. L., and Dell'Orco, R. T.,** Amino acid uptake in growing and arrested human diploid cell populations, *Proc. Soc. Exp. Biol. Med.,* 149, 530, 1975.

151. **Simons, J. W. I. M.,** The use of frequency distributions of cell diameters to characterize cell populations in tissue culture, *Exp. Cell Res.,* 45, 336, 1967.

152. **Macieira-Coelho, A. and Ponten, J.,** Analogy in growth between late passage human embryonic and early passage human adult fibroblasts, *J. Cell Biol.,* 43, 374, 1969.

153. **Goldstein, S. and Varmuza, S. L.,** Phenylalanyl synthetase function in cultured fibroblasts from subjects with progeria, *Can. J. Biochem.,* 56, 73, 1978.

154. **Sharp, G. S., Lassen, S., Shankman, S., Hazlet, J. W., and Kendis, M. S.,** Studies of protein retention and turnover using nitrogen-15 as a tag, *J. Nutr.,* 63, 155, 1957.

155. **Lundholm, K. and Schersten, T.,** Leucine incorporation into proteins and cathepsin D activity in human skeletal muscles: the influence of the age of the subject, *Exp. Gerontol.,* 10, 155, 1975.

156. **Young, V. R., Steffee, W. P., Pencharz, P. B., Winterer, J. G., and Scrimshaw, N. W.,** Total human body protein synthesis in relation to protein requirements at various ages, *Nature (London),* 253, 192, 1975.

157. **Winterer, J. C., Steffee, W. P., Davy, W., Perera, A., Uauy, R., Scrimshaw, N. S., and Young, V. R.,** Whole body protein turnover in aging man, *Exp. Gerontol,* 11, 79, 1976.

158. **Florini, J. R.,** Biosynthesis of contractile proteins in normal and aged muscle, in *Aging,* Vol. 6, Kaldor, G. and DiBattista, W. J., Eds., Raven Press, New York, 1978, 49.

159. **Dunlop, D. S., van Elden, W., and Lajtha, A.,** A method for measuring brain protein synthesis rates in young and adult rats, *J. Neurochem.,* 24, 337, 1974.

POSTTRANSLATIONAL ALTERATION OF PROTEINS

Morton Rothstein

ALTERED ENZYMES IN AGED ANIMALS

A number of enzymes have been found to become altered or partly altered in old organisms.[1-11] Characteristically, the altered molecules possess a reduced specific activity. Few other obvious differences in properties between enzymes from young and old organisms have been noted, except for altered sensitivity to heat which usually but not always occurs. Inhibitor effects, behavior during isolation, Km, molecular weight, charge as determined by isoelectric focusing, and electrophoretic patterns typically show insignificant differences. Table 1 lists the enzymes which thus far have been found to be altered in old organisms using the criterion of activity per milligram of pure enzyme or activity per amount of antiserum. Lowered enzyme activity in crude homogenates is not a satisfactory test for the presence of altered enzymes as this measurement may simply reflect the presence of *fewer* enzyme molecules rather than less effective molecules.

The heat-sensitivity patterns thus far observed with "old" enzymes fall into one of three general categories: (1) identical to "young" enzyme, (2) biphasic, consisting of a more heat-sensitive component and a remainder identical with "young" enzyme, (3) biphasic, both components being different from the corresponding "young" enzyme. These findings can be explained as follows: "old" enzyme in (1) consists of normal enzyme molecules and inactive molecules. The latter react with antiserum prepared to the enzyme, and thus increase the antiserum required per unit of activity. On the other hand, being inactive they do not affect the temperature-sensitivity pattern. In the case of (2), "old" enzyme may consist of both altered molecules of low specific activity and normal molecules. The former would yield the heat-sensitive component and account for the increased antibody requirement per unit of activity. "Old" enzyme in (3) would consist entirely of two types of altered molecules, both being more heat-sensitive than normal and having a lowered specific activity.

UNALTERED ENZYMES IN AGED ANIMALS

Though it is clear from Table 1 that altered enzymes may accumulate in old organisms, there are a number of reports of enzymes which have not become altered in aged animals.[12-15] These enzymes are listed in Table 2.

Of the unaltered enzymes reported, pure triosephosphate isomerose[15] from *Turbatrix aceti* and creatine kinase in human muscle homogenates[12] present clear-cut examples in which no change in the respective "young" and "old" enzymes has occurred. Human muscle aldolase[12] from old tissue showed a small (13%) increase in the amount of antibody required per unit of activity; the heat-sensitivity curves are bothersome in that there is considerable variation between age groups. The authors attribute the problem to the effects of deamidation of the enzyme, a process which would be expected to occur during storage of the tissues. Aldolase B from old rat liver shows an increase of 28% in the heat-labile component, but immunotitration indicates that no major amount of cross-reacting material (altered enzyme) is present.[13] The above inconsistencies may reside in use of crude homogenates in the experiments. However, the data showing that "young" and "old" triosephosphate isomerase are identical are indisputable. It is therefore reasonable to conclude that all enzymes do not become altered with age.

Table 1
PROPERTIES OF ALTERED ENZYMES

Enzyme	Source	Preparation	Specific activity[a] (U/mg protein) Young	Specific activity[a] (U/mg protein) Old	Age	Pattern of heat-stability curves Young	Pattern of heat-stability curves Old	Ref.
Isocitrate lyase	*T. aceti*	C.h.[b]	—[c]	—[c]	5 vs. 32 days			1
Aldolase	*T. aceti*	C.h.	—[d]	—[d]	5—60 days	Bi.[e]	Same	2
	T. aceti	Pure	8.0 (0.129)	4.2 (0.072)	7 vs. 35 days	Bi.	Bi.[f]	3
Enolase	*T. aceti*	Pure	1200 (16)	700 (11)	4—6 vs. 22—26 days	Mono.[e]	Bi.[g]	4
Phosphoglycerate kinase	*T. aceti*	Pure	700 (4)	350 (2.2)	6 vs. 27 days	Bi.	Same	5
Isocitrate lyase	*T. aceti*	Pure	210 (11)	83 (3)	6 vs. 27 months	Mono.	Bi.	6
Superoxide dismutase	Rat liver	Pure	2460 (21)	1009 (8.5)	8 vs. 32 months (rat)	Mono.	Bi.	7
	Rat and mouse liver, brain, heart	C.h.	—[h]	—[h]	8 vs. 32 months (rat); 8 vs. 28 months (mouse)			8
Aldolase	Mouse liver	C.h.	(0.058)	(0.029)	3 vs. 31 months			9
	Mouse muscle	C.h.	(0.39)	(0.31)[i]	2.5 vs. 32 months			10
	Mouse muscle	Pure	0.049	0.032	3 vs. 30 months			11
	Mouse heart	Pure	0.044	0.028	3 vs. 30 months			11

[a] Figures in parentheses represent units of enzyme activity per mg of protein in crude homogenates, as defined by the respective authors.
[b] C.h. = crude homogenate.
[c] More antiserum required to precipitate the same amount of activity in "old" preparations.
[d] Reported as a 50% drop in specific activity between 7- and 50-day-old organisms.
[e] Bi. and mono. refer to biphasic and monophasic patterns, respectively.
[f] The "young" enzyme shows more of a heat-labile component.
[g] Both components more heat-labile than the "young" component.
[h] Approximately 2.5-fold increase in the amount of antiserum required to precipitate 50% of the "old" enzyme starting with the same activity.
[i] "Old" enzyme requires more antiserum (30—40% excess) per unit of activity.

Table 2
ENZYMES WHICH APPEAR TO BE UNALTERED IN OLD ANIMALS

Enzyme	Preparation	Source	Procedures	Age	Ref.
Creatine kinase[a]	Crude homogenate	Human muscle	Immunotitration, heat lability	24—47 vs. 64—84 years	12
Aldolase A[a]	Crude homogenate	Human muscle	Immunotitration, heat lability[b]	24—47 vs. 64—84 years	12
Aldolase B	Crude homogenate	Rat liver	Immunotitration, heat lability[c]	3—5 vs. 27—30 months	13
	Crude homogenate	Rat liver	Isotope dilution, immunotitration, activity/mg pure enzyme	2 vs. 24 months	14
Triosephosphate isomerase	Pure	Nematode	Immunotitration, heat lability, activity/mg pure enzyme	6 vs. 27 days	15

[a] Old samples showed about 50% less enzyme present than in young preparations.
[b] Results of heat-stability experiments yielded variable results which did not show an age-related trend.
[c] Heat-stability pattern was biphasic for both ''young'' and ''old'' preparations with about 28% more of a heat-sensitive component for ''old'' enzyme.

Table 3
ALTERED ENZYMES IN CELLS IN TISSUE CULTURE

Cells	Enzyme[b]	Altered enzyme (%)[a] Early passage	Late passage	Increase	Other tests	Ref.
MRC-5	G6PD	5	15—25	10—20		19
	6GP	Near 0	25	25		19
	G6PD	5.8[c]	16.7[c]	11		20
	PGI	0	0	0	Ab titration	21
Mouse embryo	Ald.			0	Ab titration	22
Human skin	G6PD	5	5	0	Ab titration	23
	G6PD	1.1	4.3	3		24
	6GP	0.8	4.9	4		25
	HGPRT	7.7	24.4	17		25
Fetal lung	G6PD	<10	35	25[e]	Ab titration	26
Human liver	Several[d]			0	Ab titration, electrofocusing	27

[a] From heat-lability patterns.
[b] G6PD: glucose-6-phosphate dehydrogenase; 6GP: 6-phosphogluconate dehydrogenase; PGI: phosphoglucose isomerase; Ald.: aldolase; HGPRT:hypoxanthine-guanine phosphoribosyl-transferase.
[c] Mean values.
[d] Phosphoglycerate kinase, pyruvate kinase, PGI, and G6PD.
[e] Altered behavior brought about by components present in "old" homogenates.

In addition to the lack of age-related change in the enzymes reported above, a number of enzymes in human polymorphonuclear leukocytes from old subjects have been reported to be unchanged.[16] Thus, immunological studies of four cytoplasmic enzymes (glucose-6-phosphate dehydrogenase, glucose phosphate isomerase, pyruvate kinase, and lactic dehydrogenase) and two lysosomal enzymes (α-mannosidase and β-glycuronidase) show no age-related changes in the ratio of enzyme activity to immunological reactivity. In addition, superoxide dismutase is not altered in red blood cells from old human subjects,[17] and α-amylase appears to be unchanged in the saliva of old humans.[18] These enzymes differ from those in Tables 1 and 2 in that they are "packaged" in isolated environments.

ALTERED ENZYMES IN TISSUE CULTURE

Late-passage cells in culture have been used extensively for studies on aging. Therefore, a number of investigators have looked for altered enzymes in these cells. The results of these experiments are given in Table 3. From the data, it is obvious that the findings obtained with cells in tissue culture are not consistent. In MRC-5 cells, a substantial fraction of the glucose-6-phosphate dehydrogenase (G6PD) and 6-phosphoglycerate dehydrogenase is reported to be altered in late-passage cells,[19,20] whereas phosphoglucose isomerase is unchanged.[21] In human skin fibroblasts, G6PD and 6-phosphogluconate dehydrogenase[24,25] show small increases, and hypoxanthine-guanine phosphoribosyltransferase[25] shows a substantial degree of alteration in late-passage cells. On the other hand, G6PD is reported to show no change in this respect.[23]

There are a number of possible explanations for these results. The most obvious is that in tissue culture not all enzymes become altered. Thus in MRC-5 cells, G6PD becomes altered and phosphoglucose isomerase does not. Similarly, none of the enzymes examined in late-passage liver cells become altered.[27] The different results obtained with the same enzyme (G6PD) in skin fibroblasts are more difficult to explain unless one assumes that the problem lies either in the tissues sampled or the techniques used in the different laboratories.[23,24] One serious problem may lie in the determination of the heat-sensitivity of an enzyme in crude homogenates where the concentration of proteins or other components may vary from experiment to experiment or with the passage number of the cells. These considerations may affect the stability of the enzyme during the heating process. An example of the difficulties which may arise can be seen in the fact that Zeelon et al.[2] found that aldolase in homogenates prepared from young and old *T. aceti* yielded identical heat-sensitivity patterns. In pure preparations, however, the "old" enzyme was clearly shown to be the more stable of the two.[3] The work of Kahn et al.[26] substantiates this concern. These authors studied G6PD in both human liver and fetal lung fibroblasts and found substantial amounts of heat-sensitive enzyme in late-passage cells. When G6PD was removed from homogenates of early- and late-passage fetal lung cells by a specific antiserum and replaced with pure leukocyte G6PD, enzyme placed in the "old" homogenates developed a substantial heat-labile component. In other words, some agent present in "old" homogenates caused part of the added G6PD to become heat-labile. The causative agent appears to be present in the protein fractions obtained by chromatography with CM Sephadex®.

Taken together, the above results suggest that until the situation becomes clear, caution should be used in interpreting the finding of altered enzymes in late-passage cells in tissue culture.

In addition to the observation made with late-passage cells, substantial amounts of heat-sensitive G6PD,[20,24] 6-phosphogluconate dehydrogenase,[24] and hypoxanthine-guanine phosphoribosyltransferase[25] have been reported in skin fibroblasts obtained from subjects with Werner's syndrome and progeria.[24,28] However, these altered enzymes do not increase with passage number and presumably are not related to cell senescence.

CHANGE IN SEQUENCE VS. POSTSYNTHETIC MODIFICATION

The formation of altered enzymes must result either from a change in sequence or a postsynthetic modification. The idea of age-related errors in the protein synthesizing system originated with Orgel,[29] who proposed that initial errors in proteins involved in protein synthesis would lead in turn to more errors until an "error catastrophe" occurred. In fact, the original experiments of Gershon and Gershon[1] with isocitrate lyase in the free-living nematode, *T. aceti,* and with glucose-6-phosphate dehydrogenase in MRC-5 cells in tissue culture[19] were initiated with the idea that if altered enzymes could indeed be found in old organisms, their existence could be explained by the error theory. In the intervening years, evidence against this hypothesis had mounted. Much information has been uncovered which strongly suggests that the changes observed in proteins are postsynthetic in nature. Militating against the idea of sequence change is the fact that no differences in charge have been noted after isoelectric focusing of several pure enzymes.[4,7,30] The procedure can readily detect the loss of a single amide group in one of four protein chains of aldolase. Thus, if errors in sequence occur in altered enzymes, they must all have the unlikely limitation of exchanges of amino acids resulting in the same net charge. Moreover, errors in the synthesizing system should apply to all proteins. Yet, as previously noted, several enzymes in old animals are unaltered. In the case of an error catastrophe, a variety of molecules with different properties should arise from each enzyme. Many of these would be expected to be lost during purification; however, during purification yields of "young" and "old" enzymes are essentially equal.

A most telling observation is the in vitro conversion of "young" nematode enolase to a product very similar to "old" enolase by repeated passage of the former through an ion-exchanger (DE-52).[31] The thrice-columned "young" enolase reacts more effectively with antiserum prepared to "old" enolase than to "young" enolase.[32] Moreover, some of the "young" enolase is denatured to an inactive form of enolase which is immunologically identical to inactive enolase already present in homogenates of old (but not young) *T. aceti.* Finally, Sharma and Rothstein[31] present strong spectral evidence that the altered properties of "old" enolase result from conformational changes, i.e., a subtle denaturation of the enzyme. (Considerations such as proteolytic changes in SH groups, phosphorylation, deamidation, or acylation have been shown not to be involved.[31]) When the above information is added to the previously mentioned fact that newly synthesized enzymes in old humans are error-free (leukocytic,[16] salivary,[18] and erythrocytic enzymes[17]), then the case for errors in sequence becomes weak indeed.

By contrast, Rothstein and co-workers have hypothesized that the formation of altered enzymes can be explained by a slowing of protein turnover in old animals.[31-35] The resulting increase in the dwell time of cellular proteins would result in some enzymes becoming subtly denatured to new forms (heat-sensitive or heat-stable) possessing a lower specific activity. Those enzymes which are inherently stable would be unaltered. Those enzymes which by their structure had no metastable intermediate forms would, in part, be converted directly to denatured proteins not recognized by antibodies prepared to the pure enzyme. Such enzymes would be found to be unaltered but present in reduced amounts in old organisms (e.g., creatine kinase and triosephosphate isomerase). This theory satisfies all of the experimental results reported so far.

Though experimental results tend to support the idea that protein synthesis and degradation slow with age, this evaluation has not been established unequivocally. In fact, relatively little information is available. There are a few reports that cell-free systems from old animals have a reduced ability to incorporate labeled amino acids into protein, but the studies are not definitive. Menzies and Gold[36] found no differences in the half-lives of mitochondrial proteins from various tissues of 12- vs. 24-month-old rats. Winterer et al. provide suggestive evidence that protein synthesis slows in old humans.[37] In *T. aceti,* the picture seems clear. The rate of enolase synthesis slows dramatically with increasing age,[38] as does the half-life of aldolase.[2] Nonetheless, in higher animals, the precise relationship of protein turnover to aging remains to be determined.

ERRORS AND FIDELITY OF PROTEIN SYNTHESIS

Though they may not represent a situation directly comparable to normal aging,[39] it is interesting to note that late-passage cells fail to demonstrate errors in protein synthesis. In this regard Holland et al.[40] observed that late-passage cells support the normal production of three viruses (polio virus type 1, herpes simplex virus type 1, and vesicular stomatitis virus). In a similar vein, Tomkins et al.[41] infected early- and late-passage WI-38 cells with an RNA-type virus (polio virus) and a DNA-type virus (herpes virus type 1). There were apparently no differences in the viral proteins produced as determined by acrylamide gel electrophoresis. Pitha et al. and Pitha et al. obtained similar results using viral probes.[42,43] Using MRC-5 cells, Linn et al. reported increased errors by semi-purified DNA polymerase from late- compared to early-passage cells.[44] The authors point out that the levels of misincorporation are much greater than expected in vivo. On the other hand, Buchanan and Stevens could not demonstrate with certainty an increase in the misincorporation of methionine in late-passage MRC-5 cells.[45]

Few experiments have been performed in direct attempts to determine the fidelity of protein synthesis in aged animals. Kurz examined microsomes from young and old mouse liver and found that the misincorporation of leucine in a system synthesizing polyphenylalanine decreased with age.[46] Somewhat similar experiments with rat liver by Mariotti and Ruscitto came to the opposite conclusion,[47] though the "young" and "old" animals were 90 and 265 days old, respectively. Ogrodnik et al. claim that there is a general decrease in the ability of old mouse liver preparations to distinguish between methionine and ethionine in the synthesis of ribosomal proteins.[48] However, Medvedev and Medvedeva were unable to find age-related differences in misincorporation of methionine into H1 histone from mouse tissues.[49] No age-related deterioration of the ability to discriminate between normal amino acids and analogs such as ethionine and fluorophenylalanine was found in *Drosophila*.[50]

A number of papers discuss the idea of errors or the error catastrophe hypothesis; several recent examples are cited.[51-53] Of particular interest is the finding that experimentally induced errors in the fidelity of the protein synthesizing system of *E. coli* does not lead to an error catastrophe, but to a stable level of errors which does not affect viability.[54]

On the basis of the results available so far, the idea of an age-related loss of fidelity in the synthesis of proteins is unsubstantiated; particularly at the level of enzymes synthesized by old animals, there is little evidence to support the idea. The eventual sequencing of an altered enzyme and its young counterpart should provide absolute proof one way or the other as to whether or not errors are made in the synthesis of proteins in aged animals.

REFERENCES

1. **Gershon, H. and Gershon, D.**, Detection of inactive molecules in ageing organisms, *Nature (London)*, 227, 144, 1970.
2. **Zeelon, P., Gershon, H., and Gershon, D.**, Inactive enzyme molecules in aging organisms: nematode fructose-1, 6-dephosphate aldolase, *Biochemistry*, 12, 1743, 1973.
3. **Reznick, A. Z. and Gershon, D.**, Age-related alterations in purified fructose-1,6-diphosphate aldolase from the nematode, *Turbatrix aceti, Mech. Ageing Dev.*, 6, 345, 1977.
4. **Sharma, H. K., Gupta, S. K., and Rothstein, M.**, Age-related alteration of enolase in the free-living nematode *Turbatrix aceti, Arch. Biochem. Biophys.*, 174, 324, 1976.
5. **Gupta, S. K. and Rothstein, M.**, Phosphoglycerate kinase from young and old *Turbatrix aceti, Biochim. Biophys. Acta*, 445, 632, 1976.
6. **Reiss, U. and Rothstein, M.**, Age-related changes in isocitrate lyase from the free-living nematode, *Turbatrix aceti, J. Biol. Chem.*, 250, 826, 1975.
7. **Reiss, U. and Gershon, D.**, Rat liver superoxide dismutase: purification and age-related modifications, *Eur. J. Biochem.*, 63, 617, 1976.
8. **Reiss, U. and Gershon, D.**, Comparison of cytoplasmic superoxide dismutase in liver, heart, and brain of aging rats and mice, *Biochem. Biophys. Res. Commun.*, 73, 255, 1976.
9. **Gershon, H. and Gershon, D.**, Inactive enzyme molecules in aging mice: liver aldolase, *Proc. Natl. Acad. Sci. U.S.A.*, 70, 909, 1973.
10. **Gershon, H. and Gershon, D.**, Altered enzyme molecules in senescent organisms: mouse muscle aldolase, *Mech. Ageing Dev.*, 2, 33, 1973.
11. **Chetsanga, C. J. and Liskiwskyi, M.**, Decrease in specific activity of heart and muscle activity in old mice, *Int. J. Biochem.*, 8, 753, 1977.
12. **Steinhagen-Thiessen, E. and Hilz, M.**, The age-dependent decrease in creatine kinase and aldolase activities in human striated muscle is not caused by an accumulation of faulty proteins, *Mech. Ageing Dev.*, 5, 447, 1976.
13. **Weber, A., Gregori, C., and Schapira, F.**, Aldolase B in the liver of senescent rats, *Biochim. Biophys. Acta*, 444, 810, 1976.
14. **Anderson, P. J.**, The specific activity of aldolase in the livers of old rats, *Can. J. Biochem.*, 54, 194, 1976.

15. **Gupta, S. K. and Rothstein, M.**, Triosephosphate isomerase from young and old *Turbatrix aceti*, *Arch. Biochem. Biophys.*, 174, 333, 1976.
16. **Rubinson, H., Kahn, A., Boivin, P., Schapira, F., Gregori, C., and Dreyfus, J. C.**, Aging and accuracy of protein synthesis in man: search for inactive enzymatic cross-reacting material in granulocytes of aged people, *Gerontology*, 22, 438, 1976.
17. **Stevens, C., Goldblatt, M. J., and Freedman, J. C.**, Lack of erythrocyte superoxide dismutase change during human senescence, *Mech. Ageing Dev.*, 4, 415, 1975.
18. **Helfman, P. M. and Price, P. A.**, Human parotid α-amylase — a test of the error theory of aging, *Exp. Gerontol.*, 9, 209, 1974.
19. **Holliday, R. and Tarrant, G. M.**, Altered enzymes in ageing human fibroblasts, *Nature (London)*, 238, 26, 1972.
20. **Holliday, R., Porterfield, J. S., and Gibbs, D. D.**, Premature ageing and occurrence of altered enzyme in Werner's syndrome fibroblasts, *Nature (London)*, 248, 762, 1974.
21. **Shakespeare, V. and Buchanan, J. H.**, Studies on phosphoglucose isomerase from cultured human fibroblasts: absence of detectable aging effects on the enzyme, *J. Cell. Physiol.*, 94, 105, 1978.
22. **Danot, J. and Gershon, D.**, The lack of altered enzyme molecules in "senescent" mouse embryo fibroblasts in culture, *Mech. Ageing Dev.*, 4, 289, 1975.
23. **Pendergrass, W. R., Martin, G. M., and Bornstein, P.**, Evidence contrary to the protein error hypothesis for *in vitro* senescence, *J. Cell. Physiol.*, 87, 3, 1976.
24. **Goldstein, S. and Moerman, E. J.**, Defective proteins in normal and abnormal human fibroblasts during aging *in vitro*, *Interdiscip. Top. Gerontol.*, 10, 24, 1976.
25. **Goldstein, S. and Moerman, E. J.**, Heat-labile enzymes in Werner's syndrome fibroblasts, *Nature (London)*, 255, 159, 1975.
26. **Kahn, A., Guillouzo, A., Leibovitch, M. P., Cottreau, D., Bourel, M., and Dreyfus, J. C.**, Heat lability of glucose-6-phosphate dehydrogenase in some senescent human cultured cells: evidence for its postsynthetic nature, *Biochem. Biophys. Res. Commun.*, 77, 760, 1977.
27. **Kahn, A., Guillouzo, A., Cottreau, D., Marie, J., Bourel, M., Boivin, P., and Dreyfus, J. C.**, Accuracy of protein synthesis and *in vitro* aging, *Gerontology*, 23, 174, 1977.
28. **Goldstein, S. and Moerman, E.**, Heat-labile enzymes in skin fibroblasts from subjects with progeria, *New Eng. J. Med.*, 292, 1306, 1975.
29. **Orgel, L.**, The maintenance of the accuracy of protein synthesis and its relevancy to aging, *Proc. Natl. Acad. Sci. U.S.A.*, 49, 517, 1963.
30. **Goren, P., Reznick, A. Z., Reiss, U., and Gershon, D.**, Isoelectric properties of nematode aldolase and rat liver superoxide dismutase from young and old animals, *FEBS Lett.*, 84, 83, 1977.
31. **Sharma, H. K. and Rothstein, M.**, Age-related changes in the properties of enolase from *Turbatrix aceti*, *Biochemistry*, 17, 2869, 1978.
32. **Sharma, H. K. and Rothstein, M.**, Serological evidence for the alteration of enolase during aging, *Mech. Ageing Dev.*, 8, 341, 1978.
33. **Reiss, U. and Rothstein, M.**, Heat-labile isozymes of isocitrate lyase from aging *Turbatrix aceti*, *Biochem. Biophys. Res. Comm.*, 61, 1012, 1974.
34. **Rothstein, M.**, Recent developments in the age-related alteration of enzymes: a review, *Mech. Ageing Dev.*, 6, 241, 1977.
35. **Rothstein, M.**, The formation of altered enzymes in aging animals, *Mech. Ageing Dev.*, 9. 197, 1979.
36. **Menzies, R. A. and Gold, P. H.**, The turnover of mitochondria in a variety of tissues of young adult and aged rats, *J. Biol. Chem.*, 246, 2425, 1971.
37. **Winterer, J. C., Steffee, W. P., Davy, W., Perera, A., Uauy, R., Scrimshaw, N. S., and Young, V. R.**, Whole body protein turnover in aging man, *Exp. Gerontol.*, 11, 79, 1976.
38. **Sharma, H. K., Prasanna, H. R., Rothstein, M., and Lane, R. S.**, Age-related reduction in the synthesis of enolase in the free-living nematode, *Turbatrix aceti*, *Fed. Proc.*, 37, 1334, 1978.
39. **Schneider, E. L. and Mitsu, Y.**, The relationship between *in vitro* cellular aging and *in vivo* human age, *Proc. Natl. Acad. Sci., U.S.A.*, 73, 3584, 1976.
40. **Holland, J. J., Kohne, D., and Doyle, M. V.**, Analysis of virus replication in ageing human fibroblast cultures, *Nature (London)*, 245, 316, 1973.
41. **Tomkins, G. A., Stanbridge, E. J., and Hayflick, L.**, Viral probes of aging in the human diploid cell strain W1-38 (38110), *Proc. Soc. Exp. Biol. Med.*, 146, 385, 1974.
42. **Pitha, J., Adams, R., and Pitha, P. M.**, Viral probe into events of cellular *(in vitro)* aging, *J. Cell. Physiol.*, 83, 211, 1974.
43. **Pitha, J., Stork, E., and Wimmer, E.**, Protein synthesis during aging of human cells in culture, *Exp. Cell Res.*, 94, 310, 1975.
44. **Linn, S., Kairis, M., and Holliday, R.**, Decreased fidelity of DNA polymerase activity isolated from aging human fibroblasts, *Proc. Natl. Acad. Sci. U.S.A.*, 73, 2818, 1976.

45. **Buchanan, J. H. and Stevens, A.,** Fidelity of histone synthesis in cultured human fibroblasts, *Mech. Ageing Dev.*, 7, 321, 1978.
46. **Kurz, D. I.,** The effects of ageing on in vitro fidelity of translation in mouse liver, *Biochim. Biophys. Acta*, 407, 479, 1975.
47. **Mariotti, D. and Ruscitto, R.,** Age-related changes of accuracy and efficiency of protein synthesis machinery in rat, *Biochim. Biophys. Acta*, 475, 96, 1977.
48. **Ogrodnik, J. P., Wulf, J. H., and Cutler, R. G.,** Altered protein hypothesis of mammalian aging processes. II. Discrimination ratio of methionine vs. ethionine in the synthesis of ribosomal protein and RNA of C57BL/6J mouse liver, *Exp. Gerontol.*, 10, 119, 1975.
49. **Medvedev, Z. A. and Medvedeva, M. N.,** Use of H1 histone to test the fidelity of protein biosynthesis, *Biochem. Soc. Trans.*, 6, 610, 1978.
50. **Reis, R. J. S.,** Enzyme fidelity and metazoan aging, *Interdiscip. Top. Gerontol.*, 10, 11, 1976.
51. **Gershon, D. and Gershon, H.,** An evaluation of the "error catastrophe" theory of ageing in the light of recent experimental results, *Gerontology*, 22, 212, 1976.
52. **Menninger, J. R.,** Ribosome editing and the error catastrophe hypothesis of cellular aging, *Mech. Ageing Dev.*, 6, 131, 1977.
53. **Dreyfus, J. C., Rubinson, H., Schapira, F., Weber, A., Marie, J., and Kahn, A.,** Possible molecular mechanisms of ageing, *Gerontology*, 23, 211, 1977.
54. **Edelman, P. and Gallant, J.,** On the translational error theory of aging, *Proc. Natl. Acad. Sci. U.S.A.*, 74, 3396, 1977.

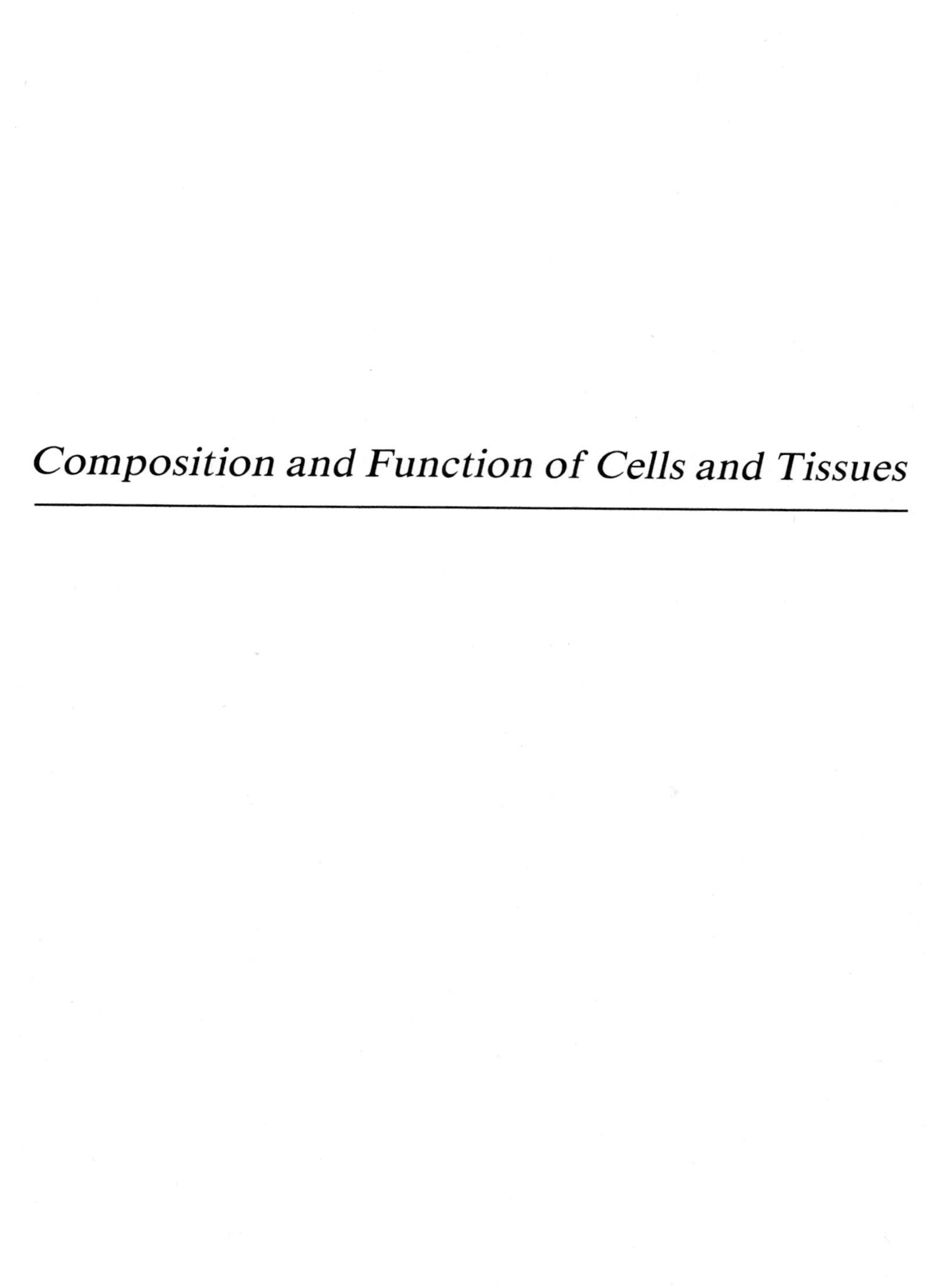

Composition and Function of Cells and Tissues

EFFECT OF AGE ON THE DNA, RNA, AND PROTEIN CONTENT OF TISSUES

Charles H. Barrows, Jr. and Gertrude C. Kokkonen

INTRODUCTION

Age related changes in biochemical systems have been expressed most frequently on the basis of protein or DNA content of the preparation. However, there does exist data on age changes in the tissue contents of these important biochemical compounds. In addition, recent biochemical findings have designed the relationships among DNA, RNA, and protein in genetic informational transfer. Thus far little information is found in the gerontological literature regarding the effects of age on these relationships. It is the purpose of this presentation to review available data so that they may serve as general indicators of approximate levels to be expected in working with new systems.

NORMAL ANIMALS

DNA

Early studies have employed the DNA content of tissues primarily as an estimate of cell number. This estimate is based on the constancy with age of (1) the DNA content of nuclei and (2) the cellular populations in tissues. In an effort to establish these criteria, Falzone et al. isolated nuclei from the livers of rats and determined the mean DNA per nucleus, as well as the distribution of nuclei according to size classes.[1] These data (Table 1) indicate that neither the mean DNA per nucleus, nor the percentage of different types of nuclei isolated from liver change with age during adulthood.

In order to establish the validity of the mean DNA of suspensions containing tetraploid as well as diploid cells, Falzone et al. also used continuous density gradients to separate rat liver nuclei into two distinct sedimentation velocity classes[2] (summarized in Table 2). The observed mean DNA per nucleus and differential counts on fractions 2 and 4 were used in simultaneous equations to calculate the mean DNA per nucleus for hypothetical preparations containing 100% small or large nuclei. The value of 6.7 pg and 15.1 pg were obtained for small and large nuclei, respectively, and compare well with values obtained by other investigators using these as well as other techniques. More recent studies by Knook have separated various types of liver cells.[3] Unfortunately, the yields have only approximated 50% of the cells in the liver. Therefore, at present it is not possible to evaluate the effect of age on changes in cell populations in liver.

Franks et al. have reported that the mean DNA of nuclei of brains of C57BL/Icrf/a' mice did not vary significantly between the ages of 4 and 144 weeks.[4] Therefore, on the basis of data presently available, the DNA content of tissue may serve as a reasonable index of the numbers of cells in tissue preparations. The reported DNA content of various tissues is presented in Tables 3 through 10 and Figures 1 through 5.

RNA

Early studies on aging measured the RNA content of tissues in the apparent hope that RNA would ultimately prove to be biochemically important. Further stimulus to study the effect of age on the RNA content of tissues resulted from a better understanding of the role RNA plays in genetic informational transfer, and the possibility proposed by Wulff that compensatory RNA synthesis may occur due to age-associated errors in transcription.[32] The reported RNA content of various tissues is summarized in Tables 11 through 13 and Figures 5 through 8.

Protein

The protein content of tissue has traditionally been used as a basis for the expression of various biochemical variables. It is difficult to infer the intent of various investigators as to whether the protein represented an index of cell number, of selectivity of synthesis of various proteins, or a measure of protein synthesis. The protein content of tissue is generally used as the basis for biochemical activities, therefore, it is frequently not reported per se. Although a mean value for protein content can frequently be calculated from such data, such values are not presented here since estimates of variance are not obtainable. The protein content reported for various tissues is presented in Tables 14 through 18 and Figures 9 through 12.

Summary

There is no evidence for consistent age-associated changes during adulthood in the DNA, RNA, or protein content of tissues. The inconsistencies in the values obtained may be attributed to the differences in species, strains, or assay methods employed. Nevertheless, the data presented here should be useful to investigators calculating expected concentrations, necessary dilutions, etc. when starting work on new systems.

DIETARILY RESTRICTED ANIMALS

It is well known that dietary restriction increases the life span of a variety of species;[41] a number of investigators have reported a relationship between life span and nutritional manipulations. For this reason, studies on the effects of dietary restriction on tissue DNA and protein content have been included in this report. Ross reported that dietary restriction is accompanied by a decrease in the number of hepatocytes per liver, an increase in the number of hepatocytes per gram of liver, and a decrease in the size of the hepatocytes.[42] In addition, these data suggested that these changes were accompanied by a decrease in total hepatic nitrogen, as well as a reduced nitrogen content of hepatocytes.[42] If DNA is taken as an index of cell number, then the reduction in the number of hepatocytes per liver is confirmed by the data on the animals fed the 4%-protein diet (Table 19).[44] The increase in the DNA per unit wet weight suggests an increase in the number of cells per unit wet weight, as well as a decrease in cellular size. If it may be assumed, as reported by Ross, that hepatic nitrogen is a measure of the protein content of the tissue, then these data indicate that total hepatic protein is decreased with the *ad libitum* feeding of a low-protein diet.[42] In addition, the decrease in protein per unit DNA agrees with the decrease in nitrogen per hepatocyte reported by Ross.[42] However, another method of dietary restriction which has been reported to increase life span, i.e., intermittent feeding, failed to bring about changes similar to those caused by the *ad libitum* feeding of a low-protein diet.[46,47] The mean values of the intermittent-fed and intermittent-fasted animals were essentially the same as those of the 24% protein *ad libitum*-fed controls. During fasting period, the biochemical changes were the same as those fed the low-protein diet. During refeeding, they returned to, or exceeded, those found in the 24% protein *ad libitum*-fed controls. Essentially the same results were obtained when the kidney was examined (Table 20).[44] Therefore, these data suggest that dietary restriction sufficient to increase life span causes a reduction in the number, size, and protein content of hepatic and renal cells.

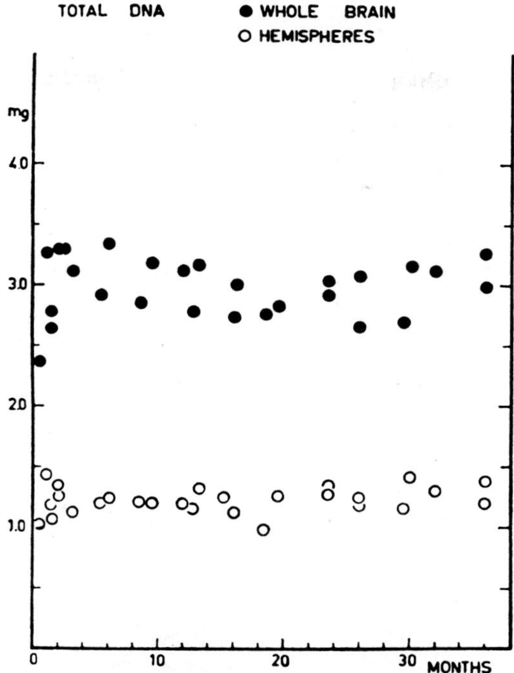

FIGURE 1. Total DNA in brain during the life span of the male Wistar rat.[26] DNA determined by the method of Burton.[27]

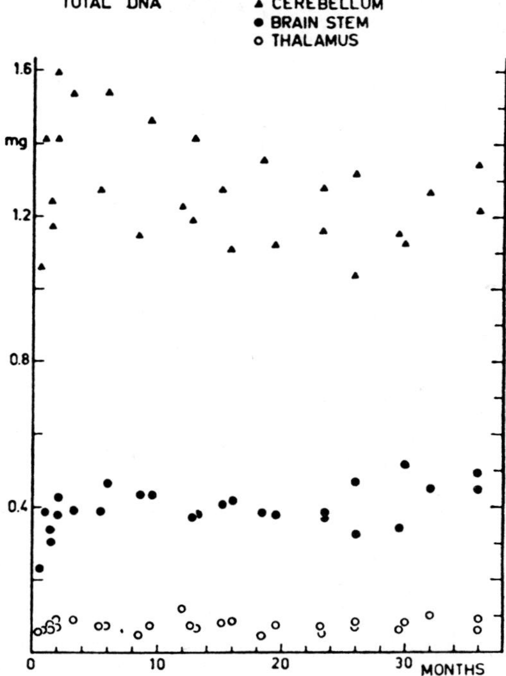

FIGURE 2. Total DNA in parts of the brain during the life span of the male Wistar rat.[26] DNA determined by the method of Burton[27]

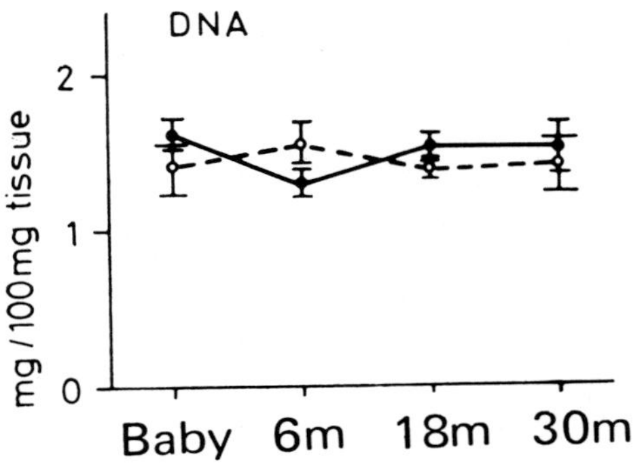

FIGURE 3. Total DNA in male (●) and female (○) C57BL/Icrf/a[t] mouse kidneys of different ages.[28] DNA was determined by the method of Kissane and Robins.[15]

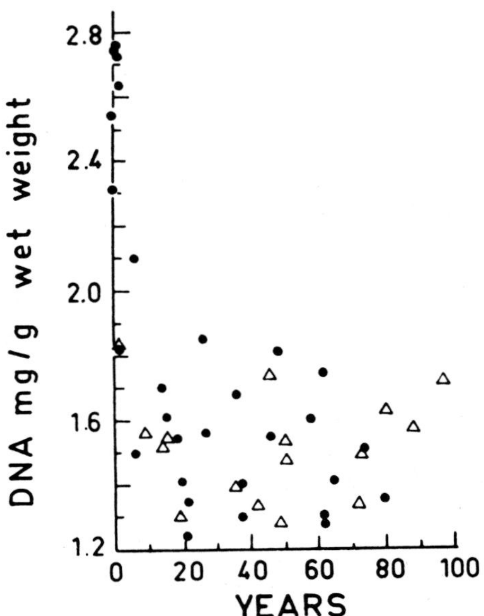

FIGURE 4. Effect of age on the DNA content of normal human aorta (male = ●; female = △).[29] DNA estimated by the method of Schneider.[30]

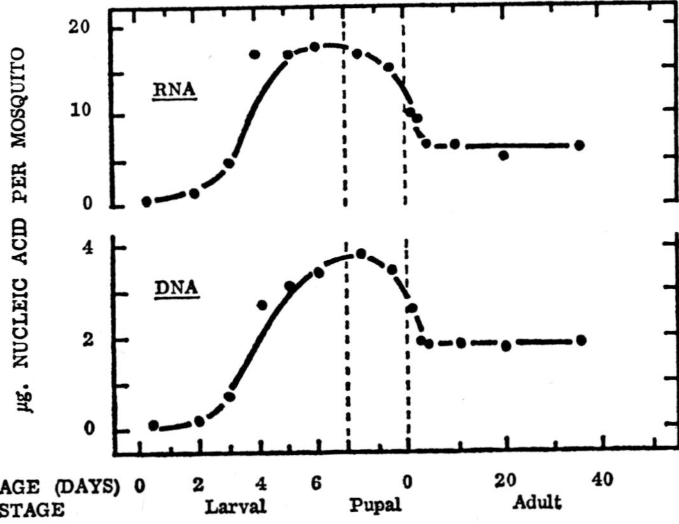

FIGURE 5. Nucleic acid content of the mosquito during its life span.[31] DNA estimated by the method of Burton.[27] RNA estimated by the method of Schneider.[30]

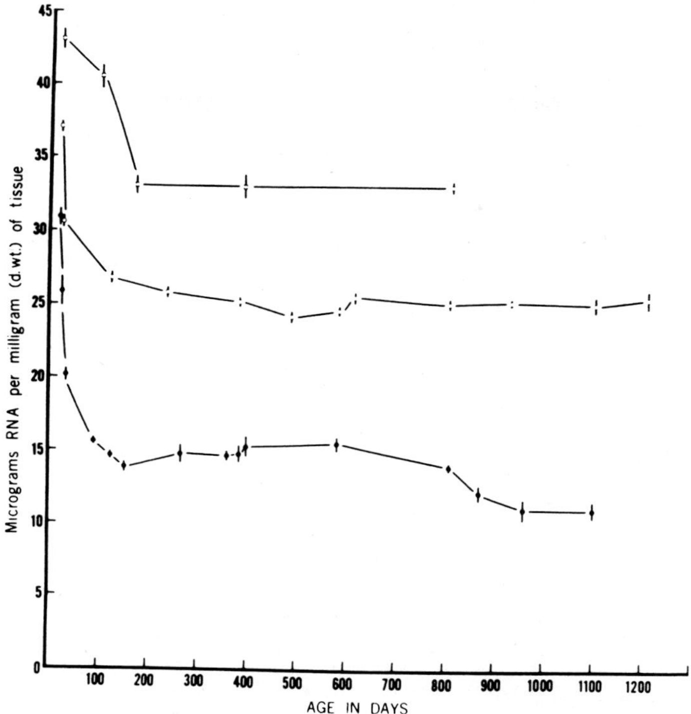

FIGURE 6. The relationship between age and RNA extracted with ribonuclease from spinal ganglia (□), ventricular muscle (○), and folia of the cerebellum (●) of Carworth CFN rats. Each point represents the mean of three to eight experiments (six samples per experiment), and the vertical bars drawn through each point represents the standard error of the mean.[35]

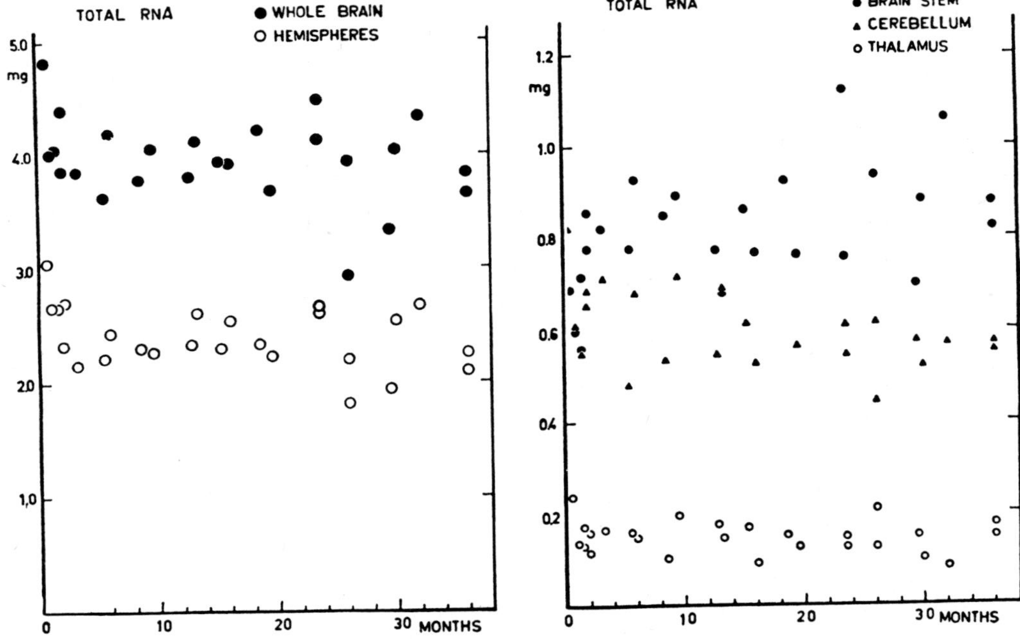

FIGURE 7. Total RNA in brain during the life span of the male Wistar rat.[26] RNA was measured by the method of Schneider.[36]

FIGURE 8. Total RNA in parts of the brain during the life span of the male Wistar rat.[26] RNA was measured by the method of Schneider.[36]

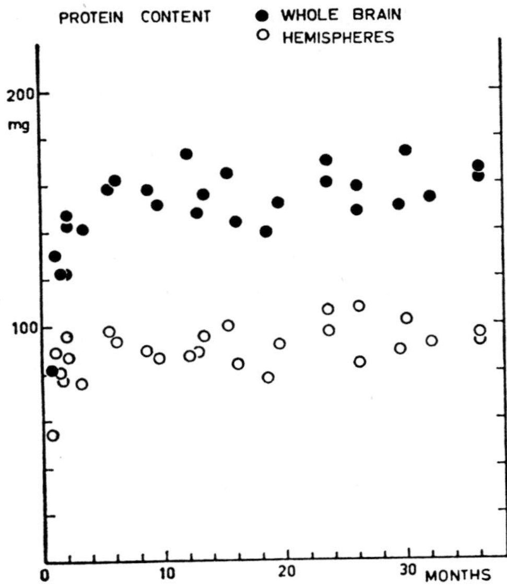

FIGURE 9. Total protein in brain during the life span of the male Wistar rat.[26] Protein was measured by the method of Hiller et al.[38]

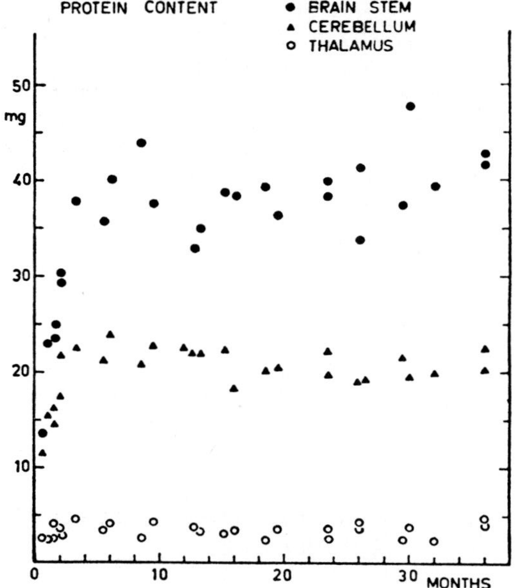

FIGURE 10. Total protein in parts of the brain during the life span of the male Wistar rat.[26] Protein was measured by the method of Hiller et al.[38]

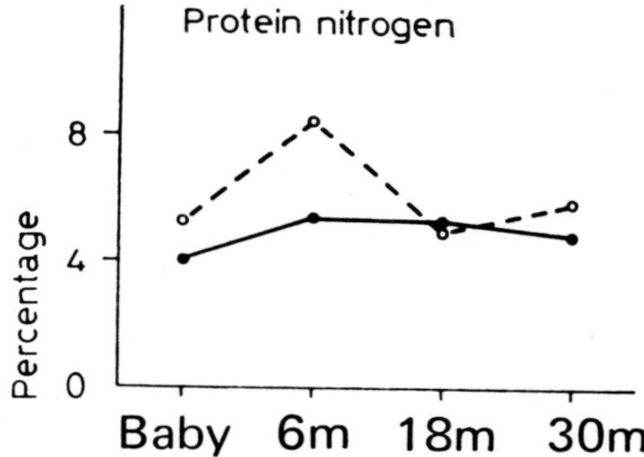

FIGURE 11. Total protein nitrogen in male (●) and female (○) C57BL/Icrf/a[t] mouse kidneys of different ages.[28] Protein was measured by the method of Hiraoka and Glick.[39]

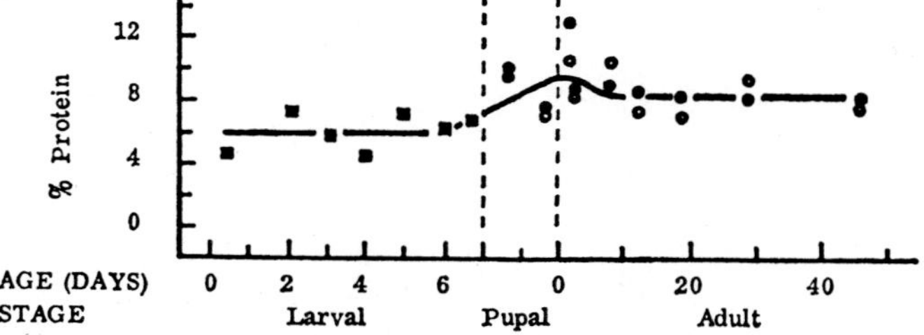

FIGURE 12. The protein content of the mosquito during its life span both sexes (■); female (○); and male (●).[31] Protein was measured by the method of Lowry et al.[37]

Table 1
EFFECT OF AGE ON NUMBER AND DNA CONTENT OF NUCLEI FROM RAT LIVERS[1]

N	Age (months)	Sex	Mean DNA[a] nucleus (pg)	Large nuclei (%) (minor axis > 6.5 μ)	Small nuclei (%)[a] (minor axis < 6.5 μ)
9	12—14	F	11.8 ± 0.4	72.4 ± 1.2	26.7 ± 1.1
10	24—27	F	12.6 ± 0.4	68.3 ± 1.6	30.6 ± 1.5
9	12—14	M	11.9 ± 0.4	72.7 ± 0.6	26.4 ± 0.5
10	24—27	M	11.9 ± 0.5	71.5 ± 0.9	27.4 ± 0.9

[a] By this criterion, the small class of nuclei is derived mainly from stromal elements, but also contains a small proportion of probable diploid hepatic nuclei.

Table 2
DNA CONTENT OF NUCLEI ISOLATED FROM RAT LIVER CELLS

Parameter	Unfractionated nuclei	Density gradient fraction 2	Density gradient fraction 4
N	8	12	11
Large nuclei (%)[a]	64.8 ± 2.26	6.69 ± 1.11	90.5 ± 0.72
DNA per nucleus[b]	11.2 ± 0.50	7.32 ± 0.22	14.3 ± 0.45

[a] See Table 1.
[b] Values are mean pg DNA/nucleus ± SEM.

From Falzone, J. A., Barrows, C. H., and Yiengst, M. J., *Exp. Cell Res.*, 26, 552, 1962. With permission.

Table 3
EFFECT OF AGE ON DNA CONTENT OF RAT LIVER

Strain	Sex	N	Age (months)	μg DNA per 100 mg wet weight	Method	Ref.
McCollum	F	10	12—14	325 ± 9	5	6
	F	10	24—27	306 ± 6		
	M	10	12—14	301 ± 15	5	6
	M	10	24—27	308 ± 8		
	F	13	12—14	342 ± 8	5	7
	F	11	24—27	347 ± 5		
	M	10	12—14	292 ± 12	5	7
	M	13	24—27	311 ± 13		
Sprague-	F	10	1	323 ± 7	5	8
Dawley	F	10	4	378 ± 11		
	F	10	12	392 ± 15		
	F	10	24	368 ± 3		
	M	8	12—14	375 ± 10	5	9
	M	8	27—28	396 ± 12		
Wistar	F	10	12—14	351 ± 8	5	9
	F	9	24—31	345 ± 10		
	F	10	10—11	378 ± 14	5	9
	F	9	26—28	364 ± 9		
	M	8	12—14	351 ± 9	5	9
	M	8	24—26	341 ± 10		
	M	11	11—14	308 ± 10	5	10
	M	13	23—28	358 ± 6		
Rattus	F	6	14	369 ± 21	5	11
norwegicus	F	8	33—35	391 ± 16		

Table 4
EFFECT OF AGE ON DNA CONTENT OF MOUSE LIVER

Strain	Sex	N	Age (months)	μg DNA per 100 mg wet weight	Method	Ref.
C57BL/6J	F	10	10	524 ± 16	12	13
	F	10	29	598 ± 35		
	F	10	1	482 ± 16	12	14
	F	10	3	438 ± 13		
	F	10	7	401 ± 22		
	F	10	14	403 ± 13		
	F	10	24	452 ± 13		
	F	4	28	403 ± 24		
	F	9	3—4	299 ± 10	5	9
	F	6	27—28	338 ± 11		
C57BL/Icrf/a^t	M	4	0.25	9070	15	16
	M	4	6	8150		
	M	4	18	10400		
	M	4	30	9430		
	F	4	0.25	8730	15	16
	F	4	6	6860		
	F	4	18	9360		
	F	4	30	9010		

Table 5
EFFECT OF AGE ON DNA CONTENT OF RAT KIDNEY

Strain	Sex	N	Age (months)	μg DNA per 100 mg wet weight	Method	Ref.
McCollum	F	8	12—14	383 ± 13	5	6
	F	8	24—27	397 ± 11		
	M	7	12—14	365 ± 16	5	6
	M	8	24—27	360 ± 12		
	F	10	12—14	395 ± 6	5	6
	F	10	24—27	366 ± 6		
	M	10	12—14	362 ± 7	5	6
	M	10	24—27	358 ± 6		
	F	13	12—14	366 ± 6	5	7
	F	11	24—27	356 ± 8		
	M	10	12—14	355 ± 8	5	7
	M	13	24—27	359 ± 6		
Sprague-Dawley	F	13	2—4	394 ± 11	5	17
	F	13	12—15	382 ± 7		
	F	14	26—33	361 ± 7		
	F	10	1	544 ± 21	5	8
	F	10	4	424 ± 26		
	F	10	12	439 ± 11		
	F	10	24	394 ± 14		
	F	13	12	422 ± 10	5	18
	F	11	21	400 ± 11		
Rattus norwegicus	F	6	14	377 ± 17	5	11
	F	8	33—35	343 ± 16		

Table 6
EFFECT OF AGE ON KIDNEY DNA CONTENT OF FEMALE C57BL/6J MICE

N	Age (months)	μg DNA per 100 mg wet weight	Method	Ref.
10	10	686 ± 13	12	13
	29	704 ± 25		
	1	711 ± 17	12	14
	3	719 ± 13		
	7	683 ± 30		
	14	601 ± 23		
	24	608 ± 30		
4	28	577 ± 39		

Table 7
EFFECT OF AGE ON DNA CONTENT OF WISTAR RAT BRAINS

Area	Sex	N	Age (months)	μg DNA per 100 mg wet weight	Method	Ref.
Prosencephalon	F	10	3	141 ± 7	15	19
	F	10	6	137 ± 8		
	F	10	12	138 ± 7		
	F	10	24	139 ± 7		
Cortex	F	10	3	120 ± 8	15	19
	F	10	6	117 ± 7		
	F	10	12	120 ± 8		
	F	10	24	126 ± 7		
Prosencephalon	F	10	10—12	131 ± 8	15	19
	F	10	26—32	123 ± 5		
Cerebellum	F	10	10—12	577 ± 52	15	19
	F	10	26—32	599 ± 53		
Brain stem	F	10	10—12	123 ± 6	15	19
	F	10	26—32	114 ± 6		

Table 8
EFFECT OF AGE ON DNA CONTENT OF MOUSE BRAIN

Strain	Area	Sex	N	Age (months)	μg DNA per 100 mg wet weight	Method	Ref.
C57BL/6J	Whole brain	F	10	4	166 ± 44	15	19
		F	8	28—29	176 ± 6		
		M	10	4	153 ± 6	15	19
		M	9	28—29	159 ± 5		
	Cerebellum—	—	6—10	1	10.9 ± 0.3[a]	20	21
	molecular	—	6—10	8	7.5 ± 0.8[a]		
		—	6—10	30	8.4 ± 0.6[a]		
	Granular	—	6—10	1	85.5 ± 3.0[a]	20	21
		—	6—10	8	84.0 ± 3.3[a]		
		—	6—10	30	88.5 ± 4.2[a]		
	White	—	6—10	1	6.8 ± 6[a]	20	21
		—	6—10	8	3.0 ± 2[a]		
		—	6—10	30	4.0 ± 4[a]		
C57BL/10	Whole brain	F	8	4	106	22	23
	— left half	F	8	8	117		
		F	8	16	103		
		F	8	24	113		
		M	8	4	111	22	23
		M	8	8	110		
		M	8	16	101		
		M	8	24	102		

[a] μg DNA per mg dry wt.

Table 9
EFFECT OF AGE ON DNA CONTENT OF RODENT HEARTS

Strain	Sex	N	Age (months)	μg DNA per 100 mg wet weight	Method	Ref.
			Rats			
McCollum	F	10	12—14	112 ± 3	5	6
	F	10	24—27	108 ± 3		
	M	10	12—14	106 ± 4	5	6
	M	10	24—27	106 ± 3		
			Mice			
C57BL/6J	F	10	10	282 ± 8	12	13
	F	10	21	296 ± 16		
	F	10	1	328 ± 8	12	14
	F	10	3	284 ± 8		
	F	10	7	300 ± 23		
	F	10	14	262 ± 10		
	F	10	24	275 ± 9		
	F	4	28	293 ± 16		

Table 10
EFFECT OF AGE ON DNA CONTENT OF RODENT TISSUES

Sex	N	Age (months)	μg DNA per 100 mg wet weight	Method	Ref.
		C57 Mice — Ventral Prostate			
F	4	9	173.2 ± 10.5	15	24
	4	18	166.0 ± 3.9		
	4	24	171.6 ± 8.0		
	4	30	175.7 ± 4.3		
		C57BL/Icrf/a' Mice — Lung			
M	4	0.25	8400	15	16
	4	6	8530		
	4	18	9900		
	4	30	9200		
F	4	0.25	7120		
	4	6	7130		
	4	18	8730		
	4	30	9120		
		Guinea Pigs — Articular Cartilage			
F	—	2 weeks	5.130 ± 0.750	15	25
	—	12 weeks	6.210 ± 1.380		
	—	1 year	0.625 ± 0.056		
	—	2.5 years	0.695 ± 0.078		
	—	5.75 years	0.466 ± 0.020		

Table 11
EFFECT OF AGE ON RNA CONTENT OF RAT LIVER

Strain	Sex	N	Age (months)	μg RNA per 100 mg wet weight	Method	Ref.
McCollum	F	9	12	987 ± 21	33	11
	F	9	24—27	1095 ± 52		
	F	10	12	1014 ± 32	33	11
	F	10	24—27	1016 ± 27		
	F	12	12	954 ± 21	33	11
	F	11	24—27	995 ± 19		
Wistar	M	11	11—14	902 ± 14	33	10
	M	13	23—28	988 ± 17		
Rattus	F	6	14	852 ± 25	33	11
norwegicus	F	8	33—35	949 ± 12		

Table 12
EFFECT OF AGE ON RNA CONTENT OF RAT KIDNEY

Strain	Sex	N	Age (months)	μg RNA per 100 mg wet weight	Method	Ref.
McCollum	F	9	12	549 ± 14	33	11
	F	9	24—27	509 ± 12		
	F	10	12	540 ± 7	33	11
	F	10	24—27	494 ± 13		
	F	12	12	513 ± 9	33	11
	F	11	24—27	493 ± 11		
Rattus	F	6	14	475± 14	33	11
norwegicus	F	8	33—35	427 ± 10		
Sprague-	F	12	12	505 ± 8	33	18
Dawley	F	11	21	487 ± 14		

Table 13
EFFECT OF AGE ON RNA CONTENT OF MOUSE TISSUES

Strain	Sex	N	Age (months)	μg RNA per 100 mg wet weight	Method	Ref.
			Whole Brain			
C57BL/6J	F	10	4	386 ± 11	33	19
	F	8	28—29	389 ± 15		
	M	10	4	420 ± 38	33	19
	M	9	28—29	476 ± 22		
C57BL/10	F	8	4	471	22	23
	F	8	8	507		
	F	8	16	487		
	F	8	24	541		
	M	8	4	449	22	23
	M	8	8	494		
	M	8	16	455		
	M	8	24	570		
			Ventral Prostate Gland			
C57	M	4	9	172 ± 24	34	24
	M	4	18	164 ± 10		
	M	4	24	150 ± 14		
	M	4	30	163 ± 12		

Table 14
EFFECT OF AGE ON THE PROTEIN CONTENT OF RODENT LIVERS

Strain	Sex	N	Age (months)	mg protein per 100 mg wet weight	Method	Ref.
			Rats			
Wistar	M	11	11—14	18.4 ± 0.5	37	10
	M	13	23—28	17.9 ± 0.4		
	F	10	12—14	16.2 ± 0.5	37	9
	F	9	24—31	16.5 ± 1.0		
	F	10	10—11	16.5 ± 0.7	37	9
	F	9	26—28	16.6 ± 0.4		
	M	8	12—14	17.8 ± 0.3	37	9
	M	8	24—26	17.0 ± 0.3		
Sprague-Dawley	M	8	12—14	16.7 ± 0.4	37	9
	M	8	27—28	16.4 ± 0.4		
McCollum	F	10	12—14	2.92 ± 0.05[a]	38	6
	F	10	24—27	2.88 ± 0.04[a]		
	M	10	12—14	2.97 ± 0.08[a]	38	6
	M	10	24—27	2.88 ± 0.03[a]		
	F	13	12—14	2.83 ± 0.04[a]	38	7
	F	11	24—27	2.82 ± 0.02[a]		
	M	10	12—14	2.77 ± 0.05[a]	38	7
	M	13	24—27	2.86 ± 0.05[a]		
			Mice			
C57BL/6J	F	9	3-4	16.4 ± 0.6	37	9
	F	6	27-28	16.9 ± 0.5		
C57BL/Icrf/a[t]	F	4	0.25	3.04	39.	16
	F	4	6	1.95		
	F	4	18	3.36		
	F	4	30	6.10		
	M	4	0.25	8.64	39	16
	M	4	6	4.44		
	M	4	18	4.26		
	M	4	30	4.14		

[a] mg protein nitrogen per 100 mg wet weight.

Table 15
EFFECT OF AGE ON THE PROTEIN CONTENT OF RODENT KIDNEYS

Strain	Sex	N	Age (months)	mg protein nitrogen per 100 mg wet weight	Method	Ref.
			Rats			
McCollum	F	10	12—14	2.68 ± 0.03[a]	38	6
	F	10	24—27	2.55 ± 0.04[a]		
	M	10	12—14	2.80 ± 0.05[a]	38	6
	M	10	24—27	2.66 ± 0.04[a]		
	F	13	12—14	2.52 ± 0.02[a]	38	7
	F	11	24—27	2.44 ± 0.04[a]		
	M	10	12—14	2.57 ± 0.04[a]	38	7
	M	13	24—27	2.47 ± 0.04[a]		
Sprague-Dawley	F	13	12	2.20 ± 0.03[a]	38	18
	F	11	21	2.14 ± 0.02		
			Mice			
C57BL/6	F		6	19.9 ± 0.8	37	40
	F		23	19.6 ± 0.4		
	M		6	18.9 ± 0.5	37	40
	M		23	19.4 ± 0.5		

[a] mg protein nitrogen per 100 mg wet weight.

Table 16
EFFECT OF AGE ON THE BRAIN PROTEIN CONTENT OF FEMALE WISTAR RATS

Area	N	Age (months)	mg protein per 100 mg wet weight	Method	Ref.
Prosencephalon	10	3	12.4 ± 4.8	37	19
	10	6	13.0 ± 4.9		
	10	12	12.5 ± 5.3		
	10	24	12.7 ± 4.3		
Cortex	10	3	13.3 ± 6.8	37	19
	10	6	12.9 ± 4.8		
	10	12	13.2 ± 4.4		
	10	24	12.2 ± 2.3		
Prosencephalon	10	10—12	10.7 ± 3.5	37	19
	10	26—32	10.4 ± 3.5		
Cerebellum	10	10—12	11.2 ± 6.8	37	19
	10	26—32	10.0 ± 4.2		
Brain stem	10	10—12	9.5 ± 4.7	37	19
	10	26—32	9.5 ± 3.5		

Table 17
EFFECT OF AGE ON THE PROTEIN CONTENT OF MOUSE BRAINS

Strain	Area	Sex	N	Age (months)	mg protein per 100 mg wet weight	Method	Ref.
C57BL/6J	Whole brain	F	10	4	14.5 ± 1.3	37	19
		F	8	28—29	11.2 ± 1.3		
C57BL/10	Whole brain— left half	F	8	4	10.6	22	23
		F	8	8	11.7		
		F	8	16	10.3		
		F	8	24	11.3		
		M	8	4	11.1	22	23
		M	8	8	11.0		
		M	8	16	10.1		
		M	8	24	10.2		

Table 18
EFFECT OF AGE ON THE PROTEIN CONTENT OF VARIOUS RODENT TISSUES

Strain	Sex	N	Age (months)	mg protein per 100 mg wet weight	Method	Ref.
			Rats — Heart			
McCollum	F	10	12—14	2.95 ± 0.05[a]	38	6
	F	10	24—27	2.86 ± 0.09[a]		
	M	10	12—14	2.85 ± 0.06[a]	38	6
	M	10	24—27	2.76 ± 0.02[a]		
			Mice—Ventral Prostate			
C57	M	4	9	3.18 ± 0.48	37,39	24
	M	4	18	3.26 ± 0.17		
	M	4	24	3.15 ± 0.27		
	M	4	30	2.35 ± 0.22		
			Mice—Lung			
C57BL/Icrf/a[t]	F	4	0.25	6.12	39	16
	F	4	6	5.84		
	F	4	18	6.08		
	F	4	30	7.36		
	M	4	0.25	6.76	39	16
	M	4	6	8.96		
	M	4	18	5.52		
	M	4	30	6.12		
			Guinea Pigs—Articular Cartilage			
	F	—	2 weeks	100 ± 7[b]	37	25
	F	—	12 weeks	173 ± 16[b]		
	F	—	1 yr	175 ± 19[b]		
	F	—	2.5 yr	178 ± 28[b]		
	F	—	5.75 yr	236 ± 17[b]		

[a] mg protein nitrogen per 100 mg wet weight.

[b] mg noncollagen protein per g dry weight.

Table 19
CONCENTRATION OF DNA AND PROTEIN IN THE LIVERS OF FEMALE MICE FED DIFFERENT DIETARY REGIMES[44]

Age (months)	24% Protein	4% Protein	Intermittent[a] fed	Intermittent[b] fasted
		DNA Concentration[c]		
(γ/mg tissue)				
2[d]	3.52 ± 0.08[e]	4.04 ± 0.07[f]	3.19 ± 0.09[f]	4.16 ± 0.19[f]
7[d]	4.13 ± 0.19	4.55 ± 0.17	3.49 ± 0.11[f]	5.24 ± 0.18[f]
22[g]	3.64 ± 0.16	4.43 ± 0.16	3.35 ± 0.13	
(mg/total liver)				
2	4.39 ± 0.14	3.16 ± 0.12[f]	4.28 ± 0.28	4.38 ± 0.19
7	6.56 ± 0.17	3.28 ± 0.25[f]	5.56 ± 0.14[f]	5.37± 0.24[f]
22	6.20 ± 0.25	5.69 ± 0.30	5.26 ± 0.62	
		Protein Concentration[c]		
(mg/g tissue)				
2	191.3 ± 3.3	166.1 ± 4.4[f]	203.5 ± 6.2	212.1 ± 5.0
7	191.7 ± 6.1	157.2 ± 3.5[f]	190.0 ± 4.2	206.3 ± 8.0
22	182.1 ± 4.3	158.2 ± 5.3[f]	191.0 ± 9.3	
(mg/mg DNA)				
2	54.7 ± 1.7	41.1 ± 0.8[f]	63.8 ± 0.6[f]	51.6 ± 1.6
7	46.7 ± 0.9	34.8 ± 1.1[f]	54.8 ± 1.8[f]	39.6 ± 1.9[f]
22	51.0 ± 2.9	36.2 ± 1.8[f]	57.8 ± 4.6	
(mg/total liver)				
2	238.4 ± 5.5	129.0 ± 5.1[f]	272.7 ± 16.7	231.3 ± 6.0
7	305.6 ± 7.4	115.1 ± 10.2[f]	302.7 ± 6.1	212.9 ± 15.0[f]
22	314.9 ± 20.2	203.0 ± 7.8[f]	293.4 ± 25.5	

[a] Fed *ad libitum* a 24% protein diet on Monday, Wednesday, and Friday; sacrificed on Tuesday or Thursday.
[b] Fed *ad libitum* a 24% protein diet on Monday, Wednesday, and Friday; sacrificed on Wednesday or Friday.
[c] DNA assayed according to Ceriotti.[12] Protein assayed according to Miller.[45]
[d] C57BL/6J mice fed dietary regimes from weaning (N = 10).
[e] Mean ± SEM.
[f] $P<0.05$ when compared to values obtained for animals fed the 24%-protein diet.
[g] CBA mice fed dietary regimes from 17 months of age (N = 6 to 10).

Table 20
CONCENTRATION OF DNA AND PROTEIN IN THE KIDNEYS OF FEMALE MICE FED DIFFERENT DIETARY REGIMES[44]

Age (months)	24% Protein	4% Protein	Intermittent[a] fed	Intermittent[b] fasted
		DNA Concentration[c]		
(γ/g tissue)				
2[d]	6.46 ± 0.33[e]	8.08 ± 0.13[f]	5.89 ± 0.11[f]	6.45 ± 0.15
7[d]	6.63 ± 0.18	8.82 ± 0.18[f]	6.00 ± 0.11[f]	7.36 ± 0.18[f]
22[g]	6.34 ± 0.18	6.97 ± 0.25[f]	5.41 ± 0.07[f]	
(mg/total kidney)				
2	1.81 ± 0.11	1.40 ± 0.05[f]	1.49 ± 0.05[f]	1.60 ± 0.06
7	2.31 ± 0.07	1.59 ± 0.05[f]	1.85 ± 0.05[f]	1.90 ± 0.03[f]
22	2.76 ± 0.10	2.15 ± 0.08[f]	2.44 ± 0.06[f]	
		Protein Concentration[c]		
(mg/g tissue)				
2	173.0 ± 6.3	178.8 ± 5.6	193.4 ± 3.3[f]	173.1 ± 3.7
7	172.6 ± 3.8	179.7 ± 3.7	163.5 ± 2.9	171.4 ± 5.0
22	163.4 ± 2.9	156.4 ± 3.8	159.6 ± 3.0	
(mg/mg DNA)				
2	27.4 ± 1.7	22.1 ± 0.5[f]	33.0 ± 1.0[f]	26.8 ± 0.6
7	26.2 ± 0.8	20.4 ± 0.6[f]	27.3 ± 0.5	23.4 ± 0.9[f]
22	25.9 ± 0.8	22.5 ± 0.5[f]	29.5 ± 0.4[f]	
(mg/total kidney)				
2	48.33 ± 1.67	31.36 ± 1.44[f]	49.41 ± 1.29	42.94 ± 1.43[f]
7	60.10 ± 1.18	32.68 ± 1.57[f]	50.46 ± 1.29[f]	44.48 ± 1.68[f]
22	71.09 ± 2.15	48.24 ± 1.74[f]	72.14 ± 1.90	

[a] Fed *ad libitum* a 24% protein diet on Monday, Wednesday, and Friday; sacrificed on Tuesday or Thursday.
[b] Fed *ad libitum* a 24% protein diet on Monday, Wednesday, and Friday; sacrificed on Wednesday or Friday.
[c] DNA assayed according to Ceriotti.[12] Protein assayed according to Miller.[45]
[d] C57BL/6J mice fed dietary regimes from weaning (N = 10).
[e] Mean ± SEM.
[f] $P<0.05$ when compared to values obtained for animals fed the 24%-protein diet.
[g] CBA mice fed dietary regimes from 17 months of age (N = 6 to 10).

REFERENCES

1. **Falzone, J. A., Barrows, C. H., and Shock, N. W.,** Age and polyploidy of rat liver nuclei as measured by volume and DNA content, *J. Gerontol.,* 14, 2, 1959.
2. **Falzone, J. A., Barrows, C. H., and Yiengst, M. J.,** Fractionation of rat liver nuclei into diploid and tetraploid DNA classes by continuous density gradient sedimentation, *Exp. Cell Res.,* 26, 552, 1962.
3. **Knook, D. L.,** Use of isolated parenchymal and nonparenchymal liver cells for studies on the mechanisms of cellular aging, *Birth Defects,* 14, 171, 1978.
4. **Franks, L., Wilson, P., and Whelan, R.,** The effects of age on total DNA and cell number in the mouse brain, *Gerontologia,* 20, 21, 1974.
5. **Stumpf, P. K.,** A colorimetric method for the determination of desoxyribosenucleic acid, *J. Biol. Chem.,* 169, 367, 1947.
6. **Barrows, C. H., Yiengst, M. J., and Shock, N. W.,** Senescence and the metabolism of various tissues of rats, *J. Gerontol.,* 13, 351, 1959.
7. **Barrows, C. H., Falzone, J. A., and Shock, N. W.,** Age differences in the succinoxidase activity of homogenates and mitochondria from the livers and kidneys of rats, *J. Gerontol.,* 15, 130, 1960.
8. **Barrows, C. H. and Roeder, L. M.,** Effect of age on protein synthesis in rats, *J. Gerontol.,* 16, 321, 1961.
9. **Beauchene, R. E., Roeder, L. M., and Barrows, C. H.,** The effect of age and of ethionine feeding on the ribonucleic acid and protein synthesis of rats, *J. Gerontol.,* 22, 318, 1967.
10. **Beauchene, R. E., Roeder, L. M., and Barrows, C. H.,** The interrelationships of age, tissue protein synthesis, and proteinuria, *J. Gerontol.,* 25, 359, 1970.
11. **Barrows, C. H., Roeder, L. M., and Falzone, J. A.,** Effect of age on the activities of enzymes and the concentration of nucleic acids in the tissues of female wild rats, *J. Gerontol.,* 17, 144, 1962.
12. **Ceriotti, G. J.,** A microchemical determination of desoxyribonucleic acid, *J. Biol. Chem.,* 198, 297, 1952.
13. **Leto, S., Kokkonen, G. C., and Barrows, C. H.,** Age changes in various biological measurements of C57BL/6J female mice, *J. Gerontol.,* 26, 24, 1971.
14. **Leto, S., Kokkonen, G. C., and Barrows, C. H.** Dietary protein, life span, and biochemical variables in female mice, *J. Gerontol.,* 31, 144, 1976.
15. **Kissane, J. M. and Robins, E.,** The fluorimetric measurement of deoxyribonucleic acid in animal tissues with special reference to the central nervous system, *J. Biol Chem.,* 233, 184, 1958.
16. **Wilson, P. D.,** Enzyme patterns in young and old mouse livers and lungs, *Gerontologia,* 18, 36, 1972.
17. **Adams, J. R. and Barrows, C. H.,** Effect of age on PAH accumulation by kidney slices of female rats, *J. Gerontol.,* 18, 37, 1963.
18. **Barrows, C. H., Roeder, L. M., and Olewine, D. A.,** Effect of age in renal compensatory hypertrophy following unilateral nephrectomy in the rat, *J. Gerontol.,* 17, 148, 1962.
19. **Hollander, J. and Barrows, C. H.,** Enzymatic studies in senescent rodent brains, *J. Gerontol.,* 23, 174, 1968.
20. **Hess, H. H. and Thalheimer, C.,** Microassay of biochemical structural components in nervous tissues. I. Extraction and partition of lipids and assay of nucleic acids, *J. Neurochem.,* 12, 193, 1965.
21. **Maker, H. S., Lehrer, M., and Weiss, C.,** DNA content of mouse cerebellar layers, *Brain Res.,* 50, 226, 1973.
22. **Wannemacher, R. M., Banks, W. L., and Wunner, H. H.,** Use of a single tissue extract to determine cellular protein and nucleic acid concentrations and rate of amino acid incorporation, *Anal. Biochem.,* 11, 320, 1965.
23. **Ordy, J. M. and Schjeide, O. A.,** Univariate and multivariate models for evaluating long-term changes in neurobiological development, maturity, and aging, *Prog. Brain Res.,* 40, 25, 1973.
24. **Mainwaring, W. I. P.,** The aging process in the mouse ventral prostate gland: A preliminary biochemical survey, *Gerontologia,* 13, 177, 1967.
25. **Silberberg, R., Stamp, W. G., Lesker, P. A., and Hasler, M.,** Aging changes in ultrastructure and enzymatic activity of articular cartilage of guinea pigs, *J. Gerontol.,* 25, 184, 1970.
26. **Von Hahn, H. P.,** Distribution of DNA and RNA in brain during the life-span of the albino rat, *Gerontologia,* 12, 18, 1966.
27. **Burton, K.,** A study of the conditions and mechanism of diphenylamine reaction for the colorimetric estimation of DNA, *Biochem. J.,* 62, 315, 1956.
28. **Wilson, P. D. and Franks, L. M.,** Enzyme patterns in young and old mouse kidneys, *Gerontologia,* 17, 16, 1971.

29. **Eisenberg, S., Stein, Y., and Stein, O.,** Phospholipases in arterial tissue. IV. The role of phosphatide acyl hydrolase, lysophosphatide acyl hydrolase, and sphingomyelin choline phosphohydrolase in the regulation of phospholipid composition in the normal human aorta with age, *J. Clin. Invest.*, 48, 2320, 1969.
30. **Schneider, W. C.,** Determination of nucleic acids in tissues by pentose analysis, in *Methods of Enzymology*, Vol. 3, Colowick, S. P. and Kaplan, N. O., Eds., Academic Press, New York, 1957, 680.
31. **Lang, C. A.,** Macromolecular changes during the life span of the mosquito, *J. Gerontol.*, 22, 53, 1967.
32. **Wulff, V. J., Quastler, H., and Sherman, F. G.,** An hypothesis concerning RNA metabolism and aging, *Proc. Natl. Acad. Sci. U.S.A.*, 48, 1373, 1962.
33. **Volkin, E. and Cohn, W. E.,** Estimation of nucleic acids, in *Methods of Biochemical Analysis*, Vol. 1, Glick, D., Ed., Interscience, New York, 1954, 298.
34. **Fleck, A. and Begg, D.,** The estimation of ribonucleic acid using ultraviolet absorption measurements, *Biochim. Biophys. Acta*, 108, 333, 1965.
35. **Wulff, V. J.,** Piekielniak, M., and Wayner, M. J., The ribonucleic acid content of tissues of rats of different ages, *J. Gerontol.*, 18, 322, 1963.
36. **Schneider, W. C.,** Phosphorus compounds in animal tissues. I. Extraction and estimation of desoxypentose nucleic acid and of pentose nucleic acid, *J. Biol. Chem.*, 161, 293, 1945.
37. **Lowry, O. H., Rosebrough, N. J., Farr, L. A., and Randall, R. J.,** Protein measurement with folin phenol agent, *J. Biol. Chem.*, 193, 265, 1951.
38. **Hiller, A., Plazin, J., and Van Slyke, D. D.,** A study of conditions for kjeldahl determination of nitrogen in proteins: description of methods with mercury as catalyst and titrimetric and gasometric measurements of the ammonia formed, *J. Biol. Chem.*, 176, 1401, 1948.
39. **Hiraoka, T. and Glick, D.,** Studies in histochemistry. LXXI. Measurement of protein in millimicrogram amounts by quenching of dye fluorescence, *Anal. Biochem.*, 5, 497, 1963.
40. **Zorzoli, A. and Li, J. B.,** Gluconeogenesis in mouse kidney cortex: effect of age and fasting on glucose production and enzyme activities, *J. Gerontol.*, 22, 151, 1967.
41. **Barrows, C. H. and Kokkonen, G. C.,** Relationship between nutrition and aging, in *Advances in Nutritional Research*, Draper, H. H., Ed., Plenum Press, New York, 1977, 253.
42. **Ross, M.,** Aging, nutrition, and hepatic enzyme activity patterns in the rat, *J. Nutr.*, 97, 565, 1969.
43. **Ma, T. S. and Zuazaga, G.,** Micro-Kjeldahl determination of nitrogen: a new indicator and improved rapid method, *Ind. Eng. Chem.*, 14, 280, 1942.
44. **Barrows, C. H. and Kokkonen, G.,** The effect of various dietary restricted regimes on biochemical variables in the mouse, *Growth*, 42, 71, 1978.
45. **Miller, G. L.,** Protein determination for large numbers of samples, *Anal. Chem.*, 31, 964, 1959.
46. **Carlson, A. J. and Hoelzel, F.,** Apparent prolongation of the life span of rats by intermittent fasting, *J. Nutr.*, 31, 363, 1946.
47. **Tucker, S. M., Mason, R. L., and Beauchene, R. E.,** Influence of diet and feed restriction on kidney function of aging male rats, *J. Gerontol.*, 31, 364, 1976.

Organelles and Enzymes

ENERGY METABOLISM

Richard G. Hansford

INTRODUCTION

This section describes age-linked changes in the energy-metabolism of mammals. For this purpose, direct measurements of the flux through energy-yielding and energy-utilizing pathways would be most informative as, presumably, it is these fluxes which relate most closely to the physiology of the animal. Some such results obtained with intact tissues are presented in Table 1. However, it is difficult to stimulate metabolism maximally in intact tissues (or enforce any known degree of stimulation), and this has given rise to a large volume of work with homogenates and isolated mitochondria (Table 2A). These preparations can be stimulated, typically, by addition of ADP, and give access to substrates (see footnote to Table 2A), yet necessarily introduce artefacts of preparation.

The other approach to the definition of flux through pathways (and possible changes with age) is to measure the activities of enzymes known to catalyse nonequilibrium reactions (Table 3).[1] This is a powerful tool in comparing potential maximal activities between tissues or age groups, but has not been widely used in aging research.[2] Emphasis on flux and nonequilibrium reactions dictates measurement of the activities of enzymes which are frequently complex, comprising several subunits, and which are sensitive to various types of control. By contrast, the object of discriminating between the various theories of the mechanism of aging by searching for altered proteins may very reasonably lead to the measurement of activities such as aldolase or lactate dehydrogenase, which catalyse near-equilibrium reactions. There are many such measurements in the aging literature; they have been omitted from these tables to allow for a more detailed description of changes in overall fluxes or rate-limiting enzymes. Unfortunately this leads to the omission of excellent work, for instance that done on lactate dehydrogenase.[3] However, information on many enzymes catalysing near-equilibrium reactions is available from Wilson's contribution to this volume. The major portion of this review (Tables 1, 2, and 3) is concerned with pathways which provide ATP; however, a limited attempt is also made to include enzymes which hydrolyse ATP in the performance of cellular work (Table 4). Finally, the tabulation has been restricted to work on mammals. This does not imply that work on flies or nematodes, for instance, is not relevant, but that time and space are limited.

Table 1
DETERMINATION OF FLUX THROUGH ENERGY-YIELDING PATHWAYS AND OF STEADY-STATE CONCENTRATIONS OF "HIGH-ENERGY" COMPOUNDS IN INTACT ORGANS AND TISSUE SLICES

Tissue and preparation	Animal, (age range), sex	Activity or content measured	Assay method	Change with increasing age	Comments	Ref.
Arterial tissue						
Slices	Man, (1 day—17 years, 21—73 years)	Succinate oxidation	Manometric determination of O_2 uptake at 37° with succinate as substrate	Decrease; arch (56%), thoracic (57%), abdominal (26%)	Activity in the vena cava was unchanged with age	29
		Cytochrome *c* oxidase	Manometric determination of O_2 uptake at 37° with p-phenylendiamine as substrate	Decrease; arch (44%), thoracic (58%), abdominal (45%)	Activity in the vena cava was unchanged with age; the time course of the change within the adult group is not known	29
Brain						
Slices of cerebral cortex	Rat, CD, (3 months, 1 year, 2 years) M	Glucose oxidation	$^{14}CO_2$ release from [U-^{14}C] glucose	Decrease (25%) from 1 to 2 years	The decrease was statistically significant for both glucose and 3-hydroxybutyrate oxidation	30
		3-Hydroxybutyrate oxidation	$^{14}CO_2$ release from D,L-3-hydroxy [3-^{14}C] butyrate	Decrease (27%) from 1 to 2 years	3-Hydroxybutyrate dehydrogenase, 3-oxo acid CoA transferase and acetoacetyl CoA thiolase were all decreased in activity from 3 months to 2 years, but the decrement was mainly from 3 months to 1 year, i.e., out of synchrony with the flux changes above	30

Elastic cartilage						
Slices	Rat, Wistar, (12, 45, 65 weeks)	O_2 uptake with glucose or galactose as substrate	Manometric determination of O_2 uptake	Decrease	O_2 uptake declines from 34 to 45 weeks with glucose and from 12 to 65 weeks with galactose; glucose uptake declines significantly from 12 to 45 weeks	31
		Glucose uptake	Disappearance of glucose	Decrease		31
Heart muscle						
Whole organ	Rat, Sprague-Dawley, (6—9, 18—24, 24—30 months)	Creatine-phosphate content	The heart was removed, weighed, and then extracted in trichloroacetic acid	Decrease (43%) from 6—9 to 18—24 months	The decrease in creatine phosphate content in senescence was significant; there was no significant difference in hexosephosphate, inorganic phosphate, or ATP content between these age groups; absolute levels of creatine phosphate are low and levels of inorganic phosphate high compared to more recent work, questioning the rate of quenching of metabolism	32
Slices	Rat, McCollum, (12—14, 24—27 months), M and F	Succinate oxidation	Manometric determination of O_2 uptake at 37° with succinate as substrate	Decrease (9%, M; 8%, F)	Decrease is significant on a wet weight or DNA basis	33
	Rat, White, (8—12, 28—32 months)	ATP/ADP ratio	The heart was labeled in vivo with ^{32}Pi, removed and extracted with trichloracetic acid; adenine nucleotides separated by chromatography	Decrease from 0.86 to 0.52	The absolute magnitude of this ratio is low compared to more recent work, questioning the rate of quenching of metabolism	7

Table 1 (continued)
DETERMINATION OF FLUX THROUGH ENERGY-YIELDING PATHWAYS AND OF STEADY-STATE CONCENTRATIONS OF "HIGH-ENERGY" COMPOUNDS IN INTACT ORGANS AND TISSUE SLICES

Tissue and preparation	Animal, (age range), sex	Activity or content measured	Assay method	Change with increasing age	Comments	Ref.
		$\frac{NAD^+ + NADP^+}{NADH + NADPH}$ ratio		Decrease	No statistical evaluation of this change was given; this paper also reported a decreased glycogen and increased lactate content of hearts from 28—32 month animals	7
Sections	Rat, Wistar, (6—8, 24—25 months)	Oxidation of endogenous substrate	Manometrics determination of O_2 uptake at 37°, with no added substrate	Decrease (49%)	O_2 uptake with succinate as substrate is also decreased with age; the statistical significance of the increase in glycolytic flux is not clear; added glycogen is not likely to permeate the muscle; the paper also presented results obtained under conditions of hypodynamia	34
		Glycolysis	Measurement of lactate produced with and without added glycogen	Increase		34
Perfused heart	Rat, Fisher 344, (5 to 28 months)	O_2 uptake with glucose and palmitate	Polarographic determination	Decrease (from 5 to 24 months)	Age-linked decrements were seen on a per gram dry weight basis; on a "per heart" basis, activities were unchanged with age; efficiency was also essentially unchanged with age at both low and high pressure development	28
		Palmitate utilization (presence of glucose)	Measurement of $^{14}CO_2$ release from [U-^{14}C] palmitate	Decrease (from 5 to 24 months)		28
		Glycolytic flux (presence of glucose and palmitate)	Measurement of ^3H_2O formation from [5-^{3}H] glucose	Increase	Increment in glycolytic rate was not statistically significant	28

Kidney						
Slices	Rat, McCollum, (12—14, 24—27 months), M and F	O_2 uptake with endogenous substrate	Manometric determination at 37°	Decrease (9% F; 7% M)	Decrease is statistically significant but could reflect changed availability of endogenous oxidizable substrate	33
Liver						
Slices	Rat, McCollum, (12—14, 24—27 months), M and F	Oxidation of endogenous substrate	Manometric determination of O_2 uptake at 37°	No change (M and F)	Tissue DNA content was also unchanged with age on a wet weight basis	33
		Succinate oxidation	As above, with succinate as substrate	No change (M and F)		33
		Glycolysis	Manometric determination of CO_2 production from a bicarbonate buffer at 37°	No change (M and F)		33
Skin						
Slices	Rat, Wistar, (4 to 65 weeks), M and F	O_2 uptake with glucose or galactose as substrate	Manometric determination of O_2 uptake at 37°	Decrease	O_2 uptake declines significantly from 12 to 65 weeks	35
		Glucose uptake	Disappearance of glucose	Decrease	(both M, F); over this period there was no change in DNA per tissue dry weight; glucose uptake declines significantly from 12 to 65 weeks (M)	35
Striated muscle						
Sections of M. quadriceps femoris	Rat, Wistar, (6—8, 24—25 months)	Oxidation of endogenous substrates	Manometric determination of O_2 uptake at 37°, with no added substrate	Decrease (20%)	The decreased oxidation activity is statistically significant; an increased glycolytic	34
		Oxidation of succinate	Manometric determination of O_2 uptake with succinate at 37°	Decrease (19%)	activity is found at 24—25 months compared to 6—8 months but the statistical significance is not clear	34

Table 1 (continued)
DETERMINATION OF FLUX THROUGH ENERGY-YIELDING PATHWAYS AND OF STEADY-STATE CONCENTRATIONS OF "HIGH-ENERGY" COMPOUNDS IN INTACT ORGANS AND TISSUE SLICES

Tissue and preparation	Animal, (age range), sex	Activity or content measured	Assay method	Change with increasing age	Comments	Ref.
White muscles (M. rectus femoris and peripheral M. gluteus maximus)	Rat, Wistar, (7—9, 17, 25—33 months), M, F	$\frac{[\text{Creatinephosphate}] \times 100}{[\text{Creatine}] + [\text{Creatinephosphate}]}$	Muscles were dissected from the animal in the cold, frozen and extracted in trichloroacetic acid	Decrease (7—9 months, 50%: 17 months, 40%: 25—37 months, 18%)	Resting [creatinephosphate] × 100/[creatine] + [creatinephosphate] is higher in young animals in both groups of muscles; after exercise, this ratio returns to its resting value within 10 min for animals of each age group; changes due to exercise may be minimized by the relatively slow quenching technique	36
Red muscles (M. piriformis, M. intermedius, and central M. gluteus maximus)		$\frac{[\text{Creatinephosphate}] \times 100}{[\text{Creatine}] + [\text{Creatinephosphate}]}$	Muscles were dissected from the animal in the cold, frozen and extracted in trichloracetic acid	Decrease (7—9 months, 24%: 17 months, 23%: 25—33 months, 13%)		36

White muscles of the thigh	Rat, Wistar, (6, 26—30 months) M, F	$\frac{[\text{Creatinephosphate}] \times 100}{[\text{Creatine}] + [\text{Creatinephosphate}]}$	Muscles were dissected from the animal in the cold, frozen and extracted in trichloroacetic acid	—	This paper corroborates the work presented above (see Ref. 36) and extends it to show that if the old rats are fed glucose for 7 days prior to the experiment (work followed by rest) they regain [creatinephosphate] × 100/ [creatine] + [creatinephosphate] ratios similar to those of the young animals; glucose feeding elevated the ratio in young animals also, but to a lesser extent; the reviewer raises the possibility that larger glycogen stores owing to glucose feeding allow increased glycolysis, and the consequent maintenance of high [creatinephosphate] during the removal and preparation of this muscle	37
White muscles (M. rectus femoris: M. gluteus maximus, periphery)	Rat, Wistar, (5—6, 15—30 months), M, F	ATP/ADP Ratio	Muscles were dissected from the animal in the cold, frozen and extracted in trichloroacetic acid	Decrease from 6.7 (5—6 months) to 2.2 (15—30 months) at rest	This paper also corroborates results above (see Ref. 36) in a lower [creatinephosphate] at rest in the old animal; the quenching technique used may not be fast enough to preserve in vivo patterns of adenine nucleotides, creatine, and creatinephosphate	36

Table 1 (continued)
DETERMINATION OF FLUX THROUGH ENERGY-YIELDING PATHWAYS AND OF STEADY-STATE CONCENTRATIONS OF "HIGH-ENERGY" COMPOUNDS IN INTACT ORGANS AND TISSUE SLICES

Tissue and preparation	Animal, (age range), sex	Activity or content measured	Assay method	Change with increasing age	Comments	Ref.

Note: This table presents results of studies in which the flux through metabolic pathways has been measured by the consumption of substrate or the appearance of product. Unlike those presented in Table 2A, these studies have used relatively intact tissue in the form of isolated organs or tissue slices. This preserves the cellular environment to a greater degree but can raise problems in that access of substrates or O_2 to the cells may be limited. This problem may perhaps be overcome by perfusion of larger organs or by use of thin slices of material. Although flux measurements through a metabolic pathway are probably the best way of determining whether the capacity of that pathway is altered in senscence (see Introduction), this is really only true if the pathway is maximally activated (e.g., by the availability of ADP for many energy-yielding pathways). Thus, a drawback of many of the studies using organ slices which are presented above is that the metabolic status of the tissue is unknown but usually tends toward resting. A greater degree of tissue damage to the preparation may, for instance, result in a greater ATP-ase at both the mitochondrial and plasma membrane level by dissipation of ion gradients and, thus, activate glycolysis and respiration. Under these circumstances, comparison of preparations from young adult and senscent animals becomes difficult. A preparation which appears to avoid these difficulties is the isolated, perfused working heart.[28] Here, a given degree of physical work, and hence activation of energy-yielding pathways, can be enforced and any difference in the efficiency of energy-coupling (in the broadest sense) between young and old tissues might be expected to emerge. This table also presents data on the steady-state tissue contents of adenylates and other compounds involved in mediating energy transfer, as these are often available in the flux studies. It is emphasized that although mechanisms of metabolic control can be identified by comparison of Kequ. and mass-action ratio for enzymic reactions under conditions of known flux,[2] inferences of flux changes from changes in steady-state intermediate contents alone are not valid, but are common in the aging literature. Thus, changes in ATP/ADP ratio cannot be permissibly interpreted in terms of a changed rate of phosphorylation alone, for this ignores dephosphorylation. These criticisms do not apply to statements on flux based on depletion of, for instance, glycogen, which may not be replenished significantly in the isolated tissue.

Table 2A
OXIDATIVE PROPERTIES OF HOMOGENATES AND MITOCHONDRIAL FRACTIONS FROM THE TISSUES OF ADULT AND SENESCENT MAMMALS

Tissue and preparation	Animal, age range (months), sex[a]	Activity measured	Assay method	Change with increasing age	Comments	Ref.
Brain						
Mitochondria	Rat, Sprague-Dawley, (3—4, 24)	Succinate oxidation	Manometric determination of O_2 uptake at 30°	No change	P/O ratio was also unchanged with age; ATPase was unchanged, but showed unusually little uncoupler sensitivity	5
Heart muscle	Rat, Wistar, (12—14, 24—27)	3-Hydroxybutyrate oxidation	Polarographic determination of O_2 uptake at 26°	No change	No statistically significant change in the rate of O_2 uptake on the basis of protein or cytochrome *c* oxidase content; RC ratios were high and unchanged with age; the mitochondrial preparation involved tissue digestion with collagenase	6
Mitochondria	Rat, White, (8—12, 28—32)	Succinate oxidation	Manometric determination of O_2 uptake at 26° in the presence of cytochrome *c*, $CaCl_2$, $AlCl_3$	Increase (60%)		7
		Cytochrome *c* oxidase	Manometric determination of O_2 uptake at 26° with cytochrome *c* and paraphenylene diamine as substrate	No change	Rates were slightly diminished when cytochrome *c* was not added	7
		Succinate oxidation	Manometric determination of O_2 uptake at 26° with ADP and hexokinase plus glucose as phosphate acceptor	No change	Lack of change of ADP-stimulated O_2 uptake with age seems to be inconsistent with the increase in succinate oxidation, above; P/O ratio was increased with both succinate and 2-oxoglutarate in preparations from senescent compared to young adult (8—12 months) rats; low absolute values for this ratio for the latter age group raise the question of artefactual mitochondrial damage	7
		2-Oxoglutarate oxidation	Manometric determination of O_2 uptake at 26° with ADP and hexokinase plus glucose as phosphate acceptor	Decrease (23%)		7

Table 2A (continued)
OXIDATIVE PROPERTIES OF HOMOGENATES AND MITOCHONDRIAL FRACTIONS FROM THE TISSUES OF ADULT AND SENESCENT MAMMALS

Tissue and preparation	Animal, age range (months), sex[a]	Activity measured	Assay method	Change with increasing age	Comments	Ref.
Homogenate		Endogenous respiration	Manometric determination of O_2 uptake at 37° with no added substrate	Decrease (55%)	Possibly reflects decreased substrate availability to mitochondria	7
Mitochondria	Rat, Sprague-Dawley, (6, 24), M	Succinate-cytochrome *c* reductase	Spectrophotometric determination of reduced cytochrome *c*	No change	Assay possibly limited by access of the exogenous cytochrome *c*, through this may have been improved by freeze-thawing	8
	Rat, Fisher 344, (3 to 28), M	Malate *plus* glutamate oxidation	Polarographic determination of O_2 uptake at 25°	Decrease (20%) from 12 to 28 months	Decreases in activity were statistically significant; investigations at multiple age points between immaturity and senescense allow evaluation of the development of the changes shown; there was no generalized decrease in the efficiency of oxidative phosphorylation, as P/O and RC ratios were unchanged with age; instead, highly substrate-specific changes in state 3 rates focus attention on dehydrogenases and ancillary enzymes (transaminases, carnitine acyltransferases) as loci of age changes; omission of malate might have limited full expression of oxidative activity with palmitoylcarnitine and palmitoyl-CoA *plus* carnitine as substrate	9
		Palmitoylcarnitine oxidation	Polarographic determination of O_2 uptake at 25°	Decrease (20%) from 12 to 28 months		
		Glutamate *plus* pyruvate oxidation	Polarographic determination of O_2 uptake at 25°	Decrease (30%) from 8 to 24 months		
		3-Hydroxybutyrate oxidation	Polarographic determination of O_2 uptake at 25°	Decrease (30%) from 8 to 24 months		
		Succinate, ascorbate *plus* cytochrome *c*, pyruvate *plus* malate, 2-oxoglutarate and palmitoyl-CoA *plus* L-carnitine oxidations (measured separately)	Polarographic determination of O_2 uptake at 25°	No change		

	Rat, Sprague-Dawley, (7, 24—31)	Cytochrome *c* oxidase	Polarographic determination of O_2 uptake at 25° with N,N,N',,N'-tetra-methyl-p-phenylenediamine *plus* ascorbate as substrate	Decrease (27%)	Activity was maximized by solubilizing the mitochondria with deoxycholate	10
Homogenate		Cytochrome *c* oxidase	Polarographic determination of O_2 uptake at 25° with N,N,N',N'-tetramethyl-p-phenylenediamine *plus* ascorbate as substrate	Decrease (28%)	Activity was maximized by using deoxycholate; activity cited on a wet weight basis; comparison of specific activity in homogenates and mitochondrial fractions shows no change with age in the mitochondrial content of the tissue	10
Mitochondria and homogenate	Rat, Wistar, normal and Okamoto (spontaneously hypertensive) strain, (2 to 17), M	Cytochrome *c* oxidase	Polarographic determination of O_2 uptake at 30° with cytochrome *c* and ascorbate as substrate	—	Comparison of specific activity in homogenates and mitochondrial fractions shows a 20% decrease in mitochondrial content from 6 to 17 months in normotensive rats and a 28% decrease in hypertensive rats, on a heart protein basis	11

Table 2A (continued)
OXIDATIVE PROPERTIES OF HOMOGENATES AND MITOCHONDRIAL FRACTIONS FROM THE TISSUES OF ADULT AND SENESCENT MAMMALS

Tissue and preparation	Animal, age range (months), sex[a]	Activity measured	Assay method	Change with increasing age	Comments	Ref.
Mitochondria	Rat, Wistar, (6, 24), M	Palmitoyl-L-carnitine *plus* malate oxidation	Polarographic determination of O_2 uptake at 25° and 37°	Decrease (25—30%)	Decreases in activity shown are statistically significant; lack of a change with age of pyruvate *plus* malate oxidation makes the decrease with other substrates less likely to be an artefact of preparation; this paper also presents the activities of mitochondrial enzymes involved in fatty acid oxidation; there is evidence for a decline with senescence in the activities of acyl-CoA synthetase, carnitine acetyltransferase and 3-hydroxyacyl-CoA dehydrogenase, but no change in the activity of carnitine palmitoyltransferase or acyl-CoA dehydrogenase; carnitineylcarnitine exchange across the mitochondrial membrane was shown to be impaired with age; the mitochondrial preparation involved tissue digestion with Nagarse	12
		Palmitoyl-CoA *plus* malate *plus* D, L-carnitine oxidation	Polarographic determination of O_2 uptake at 25° and 37°	Decrease (12%) at 37°		
		Octanoate *plus* malate oxidation	Polarographic determination of O_2 uptake at 25° and 37°	Decrease (37-44%)		
		Acetyl-L-carnitine *plus* malate oxidation	Polarographic determination of O_2 uptake at 25° and 37°	Decrease (20%)		
		Pyruvate oxidation in the presence of malonate and D,L-carnitine	Polarographic determination of O_2 uptake at 25° and 37°	Decrease (22%)		
		Pyruvate *plus* malate and glutamate *plus* malate oxidations (measured separately)	Polarographic determination of O_2 uptake at 25° and 37°	No change		
Kidney						
Mitochondria	Rat, McCollum, (12—14, 24—27), M and F	Succinate oxidation	Manometric determination of O_2 uptake at 37°	No change	Tissue fractions were derived from the cortex; comparison of specific activities of succinate oxidation in	13

Homogenate		Succinate oxidation	Manometric determination of O_2 uptake at 37°	Decrease (11% in F, 11% in M)	mitochondrial and homogenate preparations indicates a diminished cortex content of mitochondria with age; DNA content and phosphorylation with succinate as oxidative substrate were undiminished with age in homogenates	
	Rat, wild *(Rattus norvegicus)*, (14, 33—35), F	Succinate oxidation	Manometric determination of O_2 uptake	Decrease (19%)	This decrease is significantly greater than the decrease in tissue DNA	14
Mitochondria	Rat, Wistar, (12—14, 24—27)	3-Hydroxybutyrate oxidation	Polarographic determination of O_2 uptake at 26°	No change	Activity unchanged with age on the basis of either mitochondrial protein or cytochrome *c* oxidase content	6
Homogenate	Mouse, C57/BL, (18, 30), M and F	Succinate dehydrogenase	Spectrophotometric determination of methylene blue reduction in the presence of cyanide	Decrease in M and F	Activities of succinate dehydrogenase and cytochrome *c* oxidase are expressed on the basis of tissue DNA; statistical significance of the changes cannot be evaluated; measurement of cytochrome *c* oxidase depends upon mitochondrial swelling in the M/30 phosphate buffer removing the outer membrane	15
		Cytochrome *c* oxidase	Spectrophotometric determination of the oxidation of prereduced cytochrome *c*	Increase in M		
Mitochondria	Rat, Sprague-Dawley, (16, 24), M	Succinate-cytochrome *c* reductase	Spectrophotometric determination of reduced cytochrome *c*	Decrease (31%)	Km for cytochrome *c* was found to be increased at 24 months, but caution is needed in interpretation because of possibly poor access of exogenous cytochrome *c*	8
Liver						
Mitochondria	Rat, Sprague-Dawley, (3—4, 24)	3-Hydroxybutyrate oxidation	Measurement of acetoacetate formation at 30°	Decrease (38%)	The decreased state 3 rate of O_2 uptake was specific for 3-hydroxybutyrate, of the substrates tested; P/O ratios were undiminished with age; the composition of the mitochondrial incubation medium was very different from that of more recent studies and precludes comparison; the paper also identifies an increased fragility of mitochondria from the old animals (not the cause of the decreased oxidation of 3-hydroxybutyrate)	5
		Succinate, 2-oxoglutarate, glutamate and malate oxidations (measured separately)	Manometric determination of O_2 uptake at 30°	No change		

Table 2A (continued)
OXIDATIVE PROPERTIES OF HOMOGENATES AND MITOCHONDRIAL FRACTIONS FROM THE TISSUES OF ADULT AND SENESCENT MAMMALS

Tissue and preparation	Animal, age range (months), sex[a]	Activity measured	Assay method	Change with increasing age	Comments	Ref.
	Rat, McCollum, (12—14, 24—27), M and F	Succinate oxidation	Manometric determination of O_2 uptake at 37°	No change in M or F	The medium used was hypotonic, though this may not be crucial for measurement of O_2 uptake with succinate	13
Homogenate		Succinate oxidation	Manometric determination of O_2 uptake at 37°	No change in M or F	There was no change in activity with age on either a protein or DNA basis. ADP-phosphorylation by the homogenate was also unchanged with age	13
	Rat, wild *(Rattus norwegicus)*, (14, 33—35), F	Succinate oxidation	Manometric determination of O_2 uptake at 37°	No change		14
Homogenate		Succinate oxidation	Manometric determination at O_2 uptake at 37°	No change	Homogenate succinate oxidation was unchanged on either a wet weight or DNA basis	14
Mitochondria	Rat, Wistar, (12—14, 24—27)	3-Hydroxybutyrate oxidation	Polarographic determination at O_2 uptake at 26°	No change	No statistically significant change in rate on the basis of protein or cytochrome *c* oxidase content; no change with age in P/O or RC ratio	6
	Rat, Sprague-Dawley, (6, 24), M	Succinate — cytochrome *c* reductase	Spectrophotometric determination of reduced cytochrome *c*	Increase	Statistical significance not clear	8
Homogenate	Mouse, C57/BL, (18, 30), M and F	Succinate dehydrogenase	Spectrophotometric determination of methylene blue reduction in the presence of cyanide	Decrease (90% in M and 52% in F)	There is a sharp maximum in acitvity at 18 months; statistical significance is not given	16
		Cytochrome *c* oxidase	Spectrophotometric determination of the oxidation of prereduced cytochrome *c*	Decrease (48% in M and 67% in F)	This method depends upon accessibility to the exogenous cytochrome *c*, which could be limiting despite the hypotonic buffer (M/30 phosphate) used	16

		NADH dehydrogenase	Spectrophotometric determination of 2, 6-dichlorophenolindophenol reduction by NADH	Decrease (91% in M and 27% in F)	Evaluation must be tentative, as exogenous NADH has no access to the active site of NADH dehydrogenase in intact mitochondria	16
Mitochondria	Mouse, C57/BL, (6, 30), M	Succinate oxidation	Polarographic determination of O_2 uptake at 30°	No change	RC ratios were very low for both age groups	17
		Cytochrome *c* oxidase	Spectrophotometric determination of the oxidation of prereduced cytochrome *c*	No change	See comments above concerning assay (cf. Ref. 16)	17
Homogenate		Cytochrome *c* oxidase	Spectrophotometric determination of the oxidation of prereduced cytochrome *c*	No change	There is an 18% decrease in activity in the 30 months, but the difference is probably not statistically significant; cf. results cited above (Ref. 16)	17
Striated muscle						
Mitochondria	Rat, Wistar, (5, 15—30), M, F	Succinate dehydrogenase	Spectrophotometric determination of reduced neotetrazolium chloride at 38°		The determination involved isolated mitochondria but differs from measurements of succinate oxidation cited elsewhere in this table in that an artificial electron acceptor replaced the respiratory chain	18
White muscle (M. rectus femoris; M. gluteus maximus, periphery)				Decrease (35%)		18
Red muscle (M. vastus lateralis; M. intermedius and M. gluteus maximus, center)				Decrease (53%)		18

Table 2A (continued)
OXIDATIVE PROPERTIES OF HOMOGENATES AND MITOCHONDRIAL FRACTIONS FROM THE TISSUES OF ADULT AND SENESCENT MAMMALS

Tissue and preparation	Animal, age range (months), sex[a]	Activity measured	Assay method	Change with increasing age	Comments	Ref.
Mitochondria (M. quadratus femoris and M. adductor brevis)	Rat, Fisher, 344 (3 to 28), M	Malate, *plus* glutamate oxidation	Polarographic determination of O_2 uptake at 25°	Decrease (19%) from 12 to 28 months	P/O ratios and state 4 rates were unchanged with age and indicate preparations with a high degree of intactness; the absolute activity of palmitoylcarnitine and palmitoyl-CoA *plus* carnitine oxidation is low and possibly limited by the lack of added malate	9
		Succinate, ascorbate *plus* cytochrome *c*, palmitoylcarnitine and palmitoyl-CoA *plus* carnitine oxidations (measured separately)	Polarographic determination of O_2 uptake at 25°	No change		
Prostate gland	Mouse, C57, (9, 30), M	Succinate dehydrogenase	Spectrophotometric determination of p-iodo nitrotetrazolium violet reduction at 37°	Decrease (62%)	This decrease is based upon DNA content — decrease based on protein is similar; most of the decrement occurs between 24 and 30 months	19
Homogenate		Cytochrome *c* oxidase	Spectrophotometric determination of the oxidation of prereduced cytochrome *c*	Decrease (35%)	Decrease only significant on the basis of DNA	19

Note: Rates of substrate oxidation referred to are state 3 rates unless a note is made to the contrary; i.e., electron transfer is fully activated by the presence of ADP and phosphate as substrates for phosphorylation.[4] As such, state 3 reveals the maximum potential activity of the pathways involved and is probably best suited to the demonstration of changes in enzyme activity with age. ADP-stimulated substrate oxidation involves a complex sequence of enzymic reactions and the reaction(s) limiting flux through the pathway is (are) not always easily identified. Adenine nucleotide and substrate translocation across the mitochondrial inner membrane and specific dehydrogenases are likely candidates (the former can be bypassed by the use of uncoupling agents to stimulate respiration). In a few cases, segments of the overall pathway have been presented, e.g., the reduction of cytochrome *c* or artificial electron acceptors by succinate, though there has been no attempt systematically to present succinate dehydrogenase results. There is no necessity for the rates obtained to be the same as those achieved in state 3 succinate oxidation (involving the reactions of phosphorylation and of the terminal portion of the respiratory chain), nor in the measurement of succinate dehydrogenase in disaggregated mitochondria (in which succinate permeation is not a factor). In some of the studies cited, the phosphorylation accompanying state 3 respiration is also measured allowing the derivation of a P/O ratio. This is a criterion of the efficiency of oxidative phosphorylation and is discussed, if available, in the Comments column. Some of these studies also include the measurement of state 4 respiration, i.e., resting or controlled respiration occurring in the absence of ADP.[4] If so, this is mentioned indirectly under Comments by allusion to the RC (or respiratory control) ratio, which is the state 3 rate divided by the state 4 rate achieved after the completion of ADP phosphorylation. This is probably the best criterion of the integrity of a mitochondrial preparation. The RC ratio is high for a well-coupled preparation, and is diminished by increased permeability of the inner membrane to ions (in a noncharge-compensated fashion), general disintegration of mitochondrial membrane structure, or the presence in the preparation of extramitochondrial ATPases. It is the reviewer's contention that there is not yet any proof that mitochondria from senescent animals are less well-coupled (lower P/O, RC ratios) than those from young adults, though this has been alleged. The development of optimal conditions for assaying mitochondrial activities involves consideration of mitochondrial permeability properties and this has been lacking in many studies. For instance, nicotinamide nucleotides do not penetrate the inner membrane and added cytochrome *c* may not have ready access to cytochrome *c* oxidase unless the outer membrane is removed. Most intramitochondrial enzyme activities are revealed reliably by using low concentrations of nonionic detergents (e.g., 0.1% Triton X-100). These remarks also apply to the measurement of mitochondrial activities in homogenates, especially where the homogenization medium used will tend to preserve mitochondrial structure (e.g., 0.25 *M* sucrose).

[a] M and F indicates that results for male and female animals were presented separately; M, F indicates that animals of both sexes were used but no discrimination was made.

Table 2B
MITOCHONDRIAL ULTRASTRUCTURE IN SENESCENCE[a]

Tissue	Animal, age (months), sex	Findings and comments	Ref.
Brain	Mouse, C57BL/10, (8, 26)	The number of mitochondria per 100 axons was found to be significantly decreased with age (18%); the neurons studied were motor neurons of the pyramidal tracts	21
Heart muscle	Rat, Sprague-Dawley, (5, 20—21)	The number of mitochondria per unit of cell area was significantly increased with age; the individual sectional area of mitochondria decreased with age; the total percentage of the sectional area of the cell occupied by mitochondria was not found to be changed significantly with age	22
	Rat, Wistar, (6 to 33), M	In a study of left ventricular myocardium, there were statistically significant increases in the number of residual bodies in the mitochondrial cones at the nuclear poles (18 to 33 months) and in the mitochondrial rows between myofilaments (12 to 33 months); in addition, there were significant increases in the number of primary lysosomes in the nuclear pole zones and in the mitochondrial rows between myofilaments; a role of primary lysosomes in the degradation of mitochondria to residual bodies is suggested; it is probably not correct to infer rates from steady-state concentrations (or numbers of organelles), but it is possible that the rate of mitochondrial degradation is increased with senescence	23
	Mouse, C57BL/6J, (8, 30, 43—44), M, F	The proportion of the cellular volume occupied by mitochondria decreased by 16% from 8 months to 43—44 months, reflecting a decreased number of mitochondria per unit cellular volume, with no change in the volume of the average mitochondrion	24
	Mouse, C57BL/6J, (9, 18, 36), M	Corroborates the above finding of decreased number of mitochondria per unit cellular volume with age (9 to 36 months); because of this, the area of the mitochondrial cristael (inner) membrane decreases on a cytosol volume basis (by 35% over this age range); cristael area per volume of mitochondria is unchanged with age; cristael area is probably closely correlated with the capacity for energy transduction	25
Kidney	Mouse, C57BL, (6, 18, 30)	Histochemical determination of succinate dehydrogenase showed no obvious difference with age in the distribution of enzyme activity along the tubule	15
Liver	Rat, Sprague-Dawley, (5, 20—24), M, F	The number of mitochondria per unit of cell area was significantly increased with age; the mean sectional area of individual mitochondria was significantly decreased with age; the percentage of the sectional area of the cell occupied by mitochondria was not found to be changed significantly with age	26
	Man, M, F	The number of mitochondria per unit of cell area was found to decline significantly after age 60 (compared to the under 49 group); over the same age range, mean mitochondrial size, measured by area and circumference, increased significantly; in addition, increased numbers of giant mitochondria and mitochondrial inclusions (osmiophilic granules, myelin-like figures, and fibrillar or crystalline structures) were seen in old age	27

Table 2B (continued)
MITOCHONDRIAL ULTRASTRUCTURE IN SENESCENCE[a]

Tissue	Animal, age (months), sex	Findings and comments	Ref.
	Mouse, C57/BL, (6, 30), M	Mitochondria fixed *in situ* showed a 60% increase in mean size (sectional area) with increased age and a wider distribution of sizes; in addition, in the tissue from the old animals, mitochondria tended to be less elongated and have a less dense matrix and granules than in young animals; after isolation, the morphology of mitochondria from young and old animals was more similar: there was evidence for a loss of the very large mitochondria from the tissue of the old animals during the preparation	20
	Mouse, C57/BL, (3—6, 30—32), M	Histochemical determination of cytochrome *c* oxidase activity in isolated mitochondria suggested a less even distribution of activity in mitochondria from the old animals, with some organelles showing very little activity; there is no statistical evaluation	17
	Mouse, C57BL/6J, (8, 30, 43—44), M, F	The proportion of the cellular volume occupied by mitochondria decreased by 35% from 8 months to 43—44 months, reflecting a decreased number of mitochondria per unit cellular volume, with no change in the mean volume per mitochondrion; there was no significant change from 8 to 30 months	24
	Mouse, C57BL/6J, (9, 18, 36), M	Area of the cristael (inner) mitochondrial membrane was found to be decreased by 35% from 9 to 36 months, on the basis of cytosol volume: this reflects both a decrease in number of mitochondria and a decrease in cristael membrane area per volume of mitochondria (cf. heart)	25

Note: Presented are results on mitochondrial size and the proportion of tissue occupied by mitochondria in liver and heart as a function of age. These results complement biochemical data presented in Table 2A in which the functional tissue content of mitochondria was derived by a comparison of the specific activity of exclusively mitochondrial enzymes in mitochondrial preparations and in tissue homogenates. Microscopy has the added ability to discriminate changes in morphology occurring within a fraction of a mitochondrial population, which mitochondrial isolation, followed by biochemical analysis, does not.[20] Further, microscopic analysis *in situ* may reveal an aberrant fraction of mitochondria which may be selectively lost during tissue homogenization and mitochondrial isolation. Histochemistry may extend this ability to discriminate differences within the mitochondrial population of a tissue (i.e., between cell types or similar cells occupying different positions in the organ) to the level of enzymic activity. However, results are semiquantitative.

Table 3
EFFECT OF AGE UPON THE ACTIVITY OF SOME POTENTIALLY RATE-LIMITING ENZYMES OF GLYCOLYSIS, GLYCOGENOLYSIS, AND THE TRICARBOXYLATE CYCLE

Tissue	Animal	Enzyme	Change with increasing age	Comments	Ref.
Arterial	Man	Hexokinase	No change (10—83 years)	Tissue was from the aorta and pulmonary artery; activities measured may be less than maximal owing to possible substrate (ATP) depletion and endproduct (glucose-6-phosphate) accumulation over 30 min.[1]	39
Aorta	Man	Glycogen phosphorylase	Decrease (on wet weight basis)	The method measures the reverse of the physiological reaction, though there is probably no objection to this for comparative purposes; AMP was present as an activator	40
Pulmonary artery		Glycogen phosphorylase	No significant change		40
Coronary artery		Glycogen phosphorylase	Decrease (on both wet weight and N basis)		40
	Man	Phosphofructokinase	No change (20—87 years)	There was no statistically significant change in aorta, coronary artery, pulmonary artery, or vena cava; measured specific activities are very low, e.g., less than 1% of the activity of heart[1]	41
Brain	Man	Hexokinase	No change (19—91 years)		42
		Phosphofructokinase	No change (19—91 years)		42
	Rat	Hexokinase	No change (20—120 weeks)		42
		Phosphofructokinase	No change (20—120 weeks)		42
	Rat, CD, (3 months, 1 year, 2 years) M	Citrate synthase	No change		30

		NAD-isocitrate dehydrogenase	Decrease (57% from 3 months to 2 years)	Much of the decrease in NAD-isocitrate dehydrogenase occurs between 3 months and 1 year and may reflect maturation: however, a 31% decrease in the 1-yr activity occurs by 2 years; the statistical significance of the latter change is not clear	30
Heart muscle	Rat, White	Glycogen phosphorylase	Decrease (10% from 8—12 to 28—32 months)	This slight decrement is in total phosphorylase (sum of a + b) activity	7
		Hexokinase	Decrease (ca. 50% from 8—12 to 28—32 months)	Thus, overall, this study showed no consistent pattern of change of 3 potentially rate-limiting enzymes in glycogen and glucose metabolism	7
		Phosphofructokinase	Slight increase (from 8—12 to 28—32 months)		7
Liver	Rat, Wistar, M	Hexokinase	Decrease (39% from 3 to 18 months)	Activities are computed on the basis of protein in the soluble fraction of a tissue homogenate	43
	Rat, F	Phosphofructokinase	No change (20—400 days)	Activity is expressed on a wet weight basis	44
		Pyruvate kinase	See Comments	Pyruvate kinase activity decreases from 60 to 180 days then increases to 400 days; activity is increased by sucrose feeding; it is difficult to evaluate whether the animals used in this study were senescent at 400 days	44
Striated muscle	Rat, Wistar, (3, 28—36 months) M			There is a shift with senescence towards a more oxidative enzyme pattern in the EDL, with triosephosphate dehydrogenase activity (a near-equilibrium glycolytic enzyme) decreasing relative to citrate synthase and malate dehydrogenase	45
M. extensor digitorum longum (EDL)		Hexokinase	No change		
		Citrate synthase	No change		
M. soleus		Hexokinase	Decrease (30%)	In the soleus, there is a trend towards a less oxidative pattern with decreased citrate synthase and much-decreased malate dehydrogenase activity; thus, both of these muscles tend to dedifferentiate with age	
		Citrate synthase	Decrease (30%)		
Diaphragm		Hexokinase	No change		
		Citrate synthase	No change		

Table 3 (continued)
EFFECT OF AGE UPON THE ACTIVITY OF SOME POTENTIALLY RATE-LIMITING ENZYMES OF GLYCOLYSIS, GLYCOGENOLYSIS, AND THE TRICARBOXYLATE CYCLE

Tissue	Animal	Enzyme	Change with increasing age	Comments	Ref.

Note: Measurement of the activity of enzymes which catalyze reactions known to be far displaced from equilibrium in living tissues provides a convenient way of comparing the potential activity of a metabolic pathway in different tissues or in tissue derived from animals of different ages. For the glycolytic pathway, the appropriate enzymes are hexokinase, phosphofructokinase, and pyruvate kinase: for glycogenolysis, the enzyme is glycogen phosphorylase. For the tricarboxylate cycle, information on the activity of citrate synthetase, NAD-isocitrate dehydrogenase, and 2-oxoglutarate dehydrogenase would be most useful but very little is available. It is emphasized that the measured activities of enzymes catalyzing nonequilibrium reactions need not give an absolute value for the maximum potential flux through a pathway because of the uncertainty of reproducing in vivo conditions in vitro. However, they are informative in a comparative sense, and a decrement in enzyme activity (e.g., with senescence) can reasonably be expected to be translated into a proportional decrease in flux. By contrast, this is not true of the enzymes catalyzing near-equilibrium reactions, e.g., aldolase and succinate dehydrogenase, where a large decrement could be tolerated without a large change in flux.

Table 4
EFFECT OF AGE UPON ACTOMYOSIN AND Na^+/K^+-ATP-ASE ACTIVITY

Tissue	Animal	Activity	Change with increasing age	Comments	Ref.
Brain					
Prosencephalon	Rat, Wistar, F	Na^+/K^+-ATP-ase	No change	The activity was defined as the activity inhibited by ouabain in the presence of Na^+ and K^+; the lack of change was true on both a wet weight and DNA basis	46
Cerebellum		Na^+/K^+-ATP-ase	No change		46
Brain stem		Na^+/K^+-ATP-ase	No change (10 to 12 26—32 months)		46
Erythrocyte	Human	Na^+/K^+-ATP-ase	No change	Age refers to the age of the cell: cells were separated according to age on the basis of density	47
Heart muscle	Rat, Fischer, M	Actomyosin ATP-ase	Decrease (20%) from 1 to 16 months, then no change through 27 months)	The activity is the specific activity of extracted actomyosin; actomyosin protein content is unchanged with age per gram of tissue	48

Kidney	Rat, Wistar	Na^+/K^+-ATP-ase	Decrease (24%) from 12—14 to 24—28 months)	The activity is that in the presence of Na^+ *plus* K^+, minus that in the presence of Na^+ only; the decrease was only seen in homogenates prepared from inner kidney slices	49
Striated muscle					
Mm. glutaei and M. quadriceps femoris	Rat, Wistar	Myofibrillar ATP-ase	No change (3—10 to 20—31 months)	There was no change in the specific activity of Ca^{2+}-ATP-ase or Mg^{2+}-ATP-ase of a myofibrillar preparation or in EGTA-sensitivity of Mg^{2+}-ATP-ase	50
M. extensor digitorum longus (EDL)	Rat, Wistar, M	Myosin ATP-ase	Decrease (14%) from 3 to 28—33 months)	The decrease in Ca^{2+}-myosin ATP-ase with senesence in the (fast) EDL matches an increased latency period, contraction and relaxation time	51
M. soleus		Myosin ATP-ase	Increase (40% from 3 to 28—33 months)	The increase in Ca^{2+}-myosin ATP-ase with senescence in the (slow) soleus matches a decreased latency period, contraction and relaxation time; a dedifferentiation thus occurs with senescence in respect to these parameters	51
Red muscle	Rat	Myofibrillar ATP-ase	No change	There was no statistically significant change from 4—6 months to >20 months in Ca^{2+}, Mg^{2+}-ATP-ase from any of these muscles	52
White muscle		Myofibrillar ATP-ase	No change		52
Diaphragm		Myofibrillar ATP-ase	No change		52
Heart muscle		Myofibrillar ATP-ase	No change		52
M. extensor digitorum longus (EDL)	Rat, Wistar (3, 28—36 months) M	Myofibrillar ATP-ase (histochemistry)	Change in pattern	There is a decrease in the fibers with high ATP-ase (type II) with senescence in the EDL	45
M. soleus		Myofibrillar ATP-ase (histochemistry)	Change in pattern	There is a decrease in the ATP-ase activity of the few type II fibers found in the soleus; thus both these muscles lose heterogeneous, "mosaic" appearance with senescence	45
Diaphragm		Myofibrillar ATP-ase (histochemistry)	No change	Heterogeneous fiber pattern is maintained with age in the diaphragm	45

Table 4 (continued)
EFFECT OF AGE UPON ACTOMYOSIN AND Na^+/K^+-ATP-ASE ACTIVITY

Tissue	Animal	Activity	Change with increasing age	Comments	Ref.
Muscle not stated	Rat, CD Fischer	Myosin ATP-ase	No change (6 and 28 months)	This is the specific activity of purified myosin A measured in the presence of Ca^{2+}; myosin A has a decreased -SH content with senescence	53
		Actomyosin ATP-ase	Decrease (40%) from 6 to 28 months	This is the specific activity of purified actomyosin in the presence of Mg^{2+}; actomyosin from the senescent animals is more inhibited (relative to the young adult) by Ca^{2+}-chelation	53

Note: This table presents the variation with age in the activities of two enzymes which consume large amounts of ATP in the performance of work. Both have well-defined physiological functions within the cell. The Mg^{2+}-stimulated ATP-ase of tissue homogenates is not included as its function is less clear and may represent a mixture of activities, including that due to damaged mitochondria. The mitochondrial (oligomycin-sensitive) ATP-ase is also omitted as its physiological function is ATP synthesis, not hydrolysis. The Ca^{2+}-ATP-ase of the sarcoplasmic reticulum is relevant, but not included for lack of information. Numerous biosynthetic processes also consume ATP, but are beyond the scope of this summary.

REFERENCES

1. **Crabtree, B. and Newsholme, E. A.,** The activities of phosphorylase, hexokinase, phosphofructokinase, lactate dehydrogenase, and the glycerol 3-phosphate dehydrogenases in muscles from vertebrates and invertebrates, *Biochem. J.*, 126, 49, 1972.
2. **Hansford, R. G.,** A comparison of energy-yielding reactions in the flight muscle of young adult and senescent blowflies, *Comp. Biochem. Physiol.*, 59B, 37, 1978.
3. **Singh, S. N. and Kanungo, M. S.,** Alterations in lactate dehydrogenase of the brain, heart, skeletal muscle, and liver of rats of various ages, *J. Biol. Chem.*, 243, 4526, 1968.
4. **Chance, B. and Williams, G. R.,** The respiratory chain and oxidative phosphorylation, *Adv. Enzymol.*, 17, 65, 1956.
5. **Weinbach, E. C. and Garbus, J.,** Oxidative phosphorylation in mitochondria from aged rats, *J. Biol. Chem.*, 234, 412, 1959.
6. **Gold, P. H., Gee, M. V., and Strehler, B. L.,** Effect of age on oxidative phosphorylation in the rat, *J. Gerontol.*, 23, 509, 1968.
7. **Frolkis, V. V. and Bogatskaya, L. N.,** The energy metabolism of myocardium and its regulation in animals of various age, *Exp. Gerontol.*, 3, 199, 1968.
8. **Grinna, L. S. and Barber, A. A.,** Age-related changes in membrane lipid content and enzyme activities, *Biochim. Biophys. Acta*, 288, 347, 1972.
9. **Chen, J. C., Warshaw, J. B., and Sanadi, D. R.,** Regulation of mitochondrial respiration in senescence, *J. Cell. Physiol.*, 80, 141, 1972.
10. **Abu-Erreish, G. M., Wohlrab, H., and Sanadi, D. R.,** *In vitro* and *in vivo* changes of mitochondria from hearts of senescent rats, *Fed. Proc.*, 33, 1518, 1974.
11. **Farmer, B. B., Harris, R. A., Jolly, W. W., and Vail, W. J.,** Studies on the cardiomegaly of the spontaneously hypertensive rat, *Circ. Res.*, 35, 102, 1974.
12. **Hansford, R. G.,** Lipid oxidation by heart mitochondria from young adult and senescent rats, *Biochem. J.*, 170, 285, 1978.
13. **Barrows, C. H., Jr., Falzone, J. A., Jr., and Shock, N. W.,** Age differences in the succinoxidase activity of homogenates and mitochondria from the livers and kidneys of rats, *J. Gerontol.*, 15, 130, 1960.
14. **Barrows, C. H., Jr., Roeder, L. M., and Falzone, J. A.,** Effect of age on the activities of enzymes and the concentrations of nucleic acids in the tissues of female wild rats, *J. Gerontol.*, 17, 144, 1962.
15. **Wilson, P. D. and Franks, L. M.,** Enzyme patterns in young and old mouse kidneys, *Gerontologia*, 17, 16, 1971.
16. **Wilson, P. D.,** Enzyme patterns in young and old mouse livers and lungs, *Gerontologia*, 18, 36, 1972.
17. **Wilson, P. D., Hill, B. T., and Franks, L. M.,** The effect of age on mitochondrial enzymes and respiration, *Gerontologia*, 21, 95, 1975.
18. **Ermini, M., Szelényi, I., Moser, P., and Verzár, F.,** The aging of skeletal (striated) muscle by changes of recovery metabolism, *Gerontologia*, 17, 300, 1971.
19. **Mainwaring, W. I. P.,** The aging process in the mouse ventral prostate gland; a preliminary biochemical survey, *Gerontologia*, 13, 177, 1967.
20. **Wilson, P. D. and Franks, L. M.,** The effect of age on mitochondrial ultrastructure, *Gerontologia*, 21, 81, 1975.
21. **Samorajski, T., Friede, R. L., and Ordy, J. M.,** Age differences in the ultrastructure of axons in the pyramidal tract of the mouse, *J. Gerontol.*, 26, 542, 1971.
22. **Kment, Von A., Leibetseder, J. and Burger, H.,** Gerontologische Untersuchungen an Rattenherzmitochondrien, *Gerontologia*, 12, 193, 1966.
23. **Travis, D. F. and Travis, A.,** Ultrastructural changes in the left ventricular rat myocardial cells with age, *J. Ultrastruct. Res.*, 39, 124, 1972.
24. **Herbener, G. H.,** A morphometric study of age-dependent changes in mitochondrial population of mouse liver and heart, *J. Gerontol.*, 31, 8, 1976.
25. **Tate, E. L. and Herbener, G. H.,** A morphometric study of the density of mitochondrial cristae in heart and liver of aging mice, *J. Gerontol.*, 31, 129, 1976.
26. **Kment, Von A., Leibetseder, J., and Adamiker, D.,** Gerontologische Untersuchungen an Rattenlebermitochondrien, *Z. Alternsforsch.*, 19, 241, 1966.
27. **Tauchi, H. and Sato, T.,** Age changes in size and number of mitochondria of human hepatic cells, *J. Gerontol.*, 23, 454, 1968.
28. **Abu-Erreish, G. M., Neely, J. R., Whitmer, J. T., Whitman, V., and Sanadi, D. R.,** Fatty acid oxidation by isolated perfused working hearts of aged rats, *Am. J. Physiol.*, 232, E258, 1977.
29. **Maier, N. and Haimovici, H.,** Metabolism of arterial tissue: oxidative capacity of intact arterial tissue, *Proc. Soc. Exp. Biol. Med.*, 95, 425, 1957.

30. **Patel, M. S.,** Age-dependent changes in the oxidative metabolism in rat brain, *J. Gerontol.*, 32, 643, 1977.
31. **Patnaik, B. K.,** Effect of age on the oxygen consumption and glucose uptake by the elastic cartilage of rat, *Gerontologia*, 13, 173, 1967.
32. **Casten, G. G.,** Effects of aging process on acid-soluble phosphorus compounds in myocardium of rats, *Am. Heart J.*, 39, 353, 1950.
33. **Barrows, C. H., Jr., Yiengst, M. J., and Shock, N. W.,** Senescence and the metabolism of various tissues of rats, *J. Gerontol.*, 13, 351, 1958.
34. **Angelova-Gateva, P.,** Tissue respiration and glycolysis in quadriceps femoris and heart of rats of different ages during hypodynamia, *Exp. Gerontol.*, 4, 177, 1969.
35. **Patnaik, B. K. and Kanungo, M. S.,** Metabolic changes in the skin of rats of various ages: oxygen consumption and uptake of glucose, *Biochem. J.*, 98, 374, 1966.
36. **Ermini, M.,** Das Altern der Skelettmuskulatur. Die Restitution des Kreatinphosphates der Skelettmuskulatur nach Arbeit bei Ratten verschiedenen Alters, *Gerontologia*, 16, 65, 1970.
37. **Verzár, F. and Ermini, M.,** Decrease of creatine-phosphate restitution of muscle in old age and the influence of glucose, *Gerontologia*, 16, 223, 1970.
38. **Ermini, M., Szelényi, I., Moser, P., and Verzár, R.,** The aging of skeletal (striated) muscle by changes of recovery mechanism, *Gerontologia*, 17, 300, 1971.
39. **Brandstrup, N., Kirk, J. E., and Bruni, C.,** The hexokinase and phosphoglucoisomerase activities of aortic and pulmonary artery tissue in individuals of various ages, *J. Gerontol.*, 12, 166, 1957.
40. **Kirk, J. E.,** The glycogen phosphorylase activity of arterial tissue in individuals of various ages, *J. Gerontol.*, 17, 154, 1962.
41. **Ritz, E. and Kirk, J. E.,** The phosphofructokinase and sorbitol dehydrogenase activities of arterial tissue in individuals of various ages, *J. Gerontol.*, 22, 433, 1967.
42. **Iwangoff, P., Armbruster, R. and Enz, A.,** The influence of aging on glycolytic enzymes in human and rat brain, *Experientia*, 33, 794, 1977.
43. **Bartoc, R., Bruhis, S., Klein, R., Moldoveanu, E., Oeriv, I., and Oeriv, S.,** Effect of age and -SH active groups on the activity of some enzymes involved in the carbohydrate metabolism, *Exp. Gerontol.*, 10, 161, 1975.
44. **Webb, J. and Bailey, E.,** Changes in activities of some enzymes associated with hepatic lipogenesis in the rat from weaning to old age and the effect of sucrose feeding, *Int. J. Biochem.*, 6, 813, 1975.
45. **Bass, A., Gutmann, E., and Hanzlíková, V.,** Biochemical and histochemical changes in energy supply-enzyme pattern of muscles of the rat during old age, *Gerontologia*, 21, 31, 1975.
46. **Hollander, J. and Barrows, C. H., Jr.,** Enzymatic studies in senescent rodent brains, *J. Gerontol.*, 23, 174, 1968.
47. **Kadlubowski, M. and Agutter, P. S.,** Changes in the activities of some membrane-associated enzymes during *in vivo* aging of the normal human erythrocyte, *Br. J. Haematol.*, 37, 111, 1977.
48. **Chesky, J. A. and Rockstein, M.,** Reduced myocardial actomyosin adenosine triphosphatase activity in the aging male Fischer rat, *Cardiovasc. Res.*, 11, 242, 1977.
49. **Beauchene, R. E., Fanestil, D. D., and Barrows, C. H., Jr.,** The effect of age on active transport and sodium-potassium-activated ATPase activity in renal tissue of rats, *J. Gerontol.*, 20, 306, 1965.
50. **Ermini, M.,** Das Altern der Skelettmuskulatur. Untersuchungen an der Myofibrillen-Adenosin-5'-Triphosphatase bei verschieden alten Ratten, *Gerontologia*, 16, 72, 1970.
51. **Gutmann, E. and Syrový, I.,** Contraction properties and myosin-ATPase activity of fast and slow senile muscles of the rat, *Gerontologia*, 20, 239, 1974.
52. **Honorati, M. C. and Ermini, M.,** Myofibrillar and mitochondrial ATPase activity of red, white, diaphragmatic, and cardiac muscle of young and old rats, *Experientia*, 30, 215, 1974.
53. **Kaldor, G. and Min, B. K.,** Enzymatic studies on the skeletal myosin A and actomyosin of aging rats, *Fed. Proc.*, 34, 191, 1975.

ENZYME LEVELS IN ANIMALS OF VARIOUS AGES

Patricia D. Wilson*

Published data for enzyme levels in various animal organs at different ages are summarized in the table following this discussion. The enzyme levels in young adults, middle-aged, and senescent animals have been included while changes during the developmental stages have been excluded.

It is apparent that a wide variety of enzymes have been studied in many mammals. However, the data are confusing and often conflicting. This may be due to strain and species differences and the difficulty in assessing physiological age. Much of the early work was carried out on animal colonies without reference to colony survival data. More recent studies on long-lived strains of mice[1] and rats[2] show that the onset of functional decline and death occurs at approximately 24 months and animals of 30 months and over can confidently be called senescent. However, it may well be that in selecting such an animal one is dealing with the "physiological elite", i.e., an exceptional animal able to survive to such an age.

Another problem in assessing age is that not only do individuals age at different rates, but so do organs, tissues, and cells. Some tissues such as muscle and nerve are postmitotic and age at the same rate as the individual; others such as blood cells have a very short life span. Most organs undergo continual cell replacement and so contain cells of different ages. Also, different cell types may have different turnover rates within a single organ.

There are a number of problems associated with the correct interpretation of biochemical enzyme assay data. The conditions used in the assay media are those which are optimal for the enzyme being measured. This is rarely, if ever, the case in vivo. In measuring enzyme-specific activity, a reference base line such as protein, wet weight, tissue nitrogen, or DNA is used. However, it is not always the case that this base line remains constant during the aging of an organ. For instance it has been shown that total protein levels increase with age in mouse and rat livers[3,161]

The preparation of the tissue before assay may influence the results obtained. Most of the early work was carried out on whole homogenates which may or may not contain interfering molecules such as inhibitors, activators, or cofactors. Membrane-bound enzyme activities may be masked by insufficient membrane disruption. In recent studies cellular fractions have been used; however, then one cannot rule out the danger of the loss of altered organelles from old tissues during the fractionation procedure. In one study it was shown that there was a selective loss of "abnormal" mitochondria (which are characteristic of old mouse liver tissue) during the differential centrifugation preparation process.[4,5] The most valid studies are probably those using purified enzyme extracts, although differential loss from young and old tissues is still possible.

A criticism of all biochemical assays carried out to date is that only an overall average of enzyme-specific activity within an organ can be determined. There can be no indication of any focal change in enzyme activity or differential change within different cell types. By contrast, histochemical techniques have revealed focal changes in alkaline phosphatase in old mouse liver, but these techniques cannot be used for reliable quantitative studies. The combined use of biochemical assay and histochemical techniques should provide maximum information. When studying the liver it is now possible to compare such in vivo studies with similar studies carried out on isolated cells. Using pure preparations of parenchymal, Kupffer, and endothelial cells it has been

* Present address: Physiologisches Institut der Universität München, München, West Germany.

possible to show that while the lysosomal enzyme cathepsin D is significantly increased in parenchymal cells from old rat livers, it is unchanged in the sinus-lining cells.[6]

The data presented in Table 1 show the reported changes in enzyme levels in mammalian tissues from young adulthood, through middle age, and into senescence. It can be seen that in many instances the data are incomplete for the whole life span. There are many inconsistencies and even contradictions of directions of change in particular enzyme levels with age; no universal trend could be determined. Although many enzymes showed decreased specific activity levels in senescence, this was by no means the rule. Neither was there a universal increase in hydrolytic degradative enzymes with age. In a number of instances there was a trend towards increased enzyme activity from adulthood into middle age, followed by a decline.[7] Some discrepancies may be explained by the use of different base lines for expressing the specific activity measurements and different methods of tissue preparation. Also, it is desirable to study several stages throughout the life span.

Some organs and tissues such as the arteries, brain, and liver have been studied in detail. Others such as the endocrine and reproductive organs and the digestive tract have been surprisingly neglected. The postmitotic tissues of muscle and nerves are attracting increasing interest and are quite suitable for aging studies.

Additional information is available from histochemical studies of enzyme distribution in some organs during aging. Although these types of enzyme studies do not provide reliable quantitative data, they are invaluable for qualitative information which may have significant bearing on the interpretation of quantitative data obtained using biochemical methods. Many enzymes are not uniformly distributed throughout an organ. Light microscope histochemical studies have been carried out during the aging of the brain,[8,9] arteries,[10,11] heart,[12] kidney,[12-14] liver,[3,12,15,16] lungs,[3] stomach,[17] intestine,[18] salivary gland,[19] muscle,[12,20] testis,[21] bone,[22] and cartilage.[23] Electron microscope localization of enzymes during aging has been studied in kidney,[13] brain,[24] liver,[3] and lungs.[16]

Although many enzymes do show a decreased specific activity in senescent tissues which would be consistent with the error catastrophe theory, there are also many instances in which enzyme-specific activity levels are either increased or remain unchanged with age. Similarly conflicting results have been reported for the occurrence of altered enzyme molecules with respect to heat lability and immunological reactivity.

An increased thermolability of glucose-6-phosphate dehydrogenase (G6PD) was first shown in vitro in late-passage human foetal fibroblasts[25] and fibroblasts from patients with Werner's syndrome,[26] but no altered G6PD properties were found in liver cells from old mice.[27] Other enzymes have been reported to be more heat labile in old tissues in vivo; among these are aldolase in mouse liver,[28] glucose-6-phosphatase,[29] and superoxide dismutase in rat liver.[30] By contrast, rat liver adenosine triphosphatase[31] and rat kidney glucose-6-phosphatase[32] decreased in thermolability with age. No immunological modifications have been found in four enzymes studied in senescent human liver cells in vitro.[33] or in seven enzymes in vivo in human granulocytes from individuals of over 80 years of age.[34]

Table 1

Organ or tissue	Function of enzyme	Enzyme	Species	Ages studied	Basis of specific activity measurements	Preparation of tissue	Effect of age	Ref.
Adipose	Hormone action	Adenyl cyclase	Rat	6, 12, 24 months	Protein; cell number	Plasma membrane ghosts	Decrease	35
Adrenal gland	Ion transport	Alkaline phosphatase	Mouse	4, 8, 12, 16, 20, 24 months	Wet weight	Homogenate 15,000 rpm supernatant	Increase to 8 months, then decrease	36
	Steroidogenesis	5–3 Hydroxysteroid dehydrogenase	Rat	4, 6, 12, 18, 24 months	Protein	Unspecified	Decrease to 12 months, then constant	37
		5–3 Hydroxysteroid dehydrogenase	Mouse	3, 13 months	Protein	Homogenate	Decrease	38
Cardiovascular system								
Heart	Carbohydrate metabolism	Lactic dehydrogenase	Rat	2, 24 months	Wet weight	Homogenate; 12,000 g supernatant	Decrease	39
		Lactic dehydrogenase	Rat	4, 18 months	Protein	Homogenate; 10,000 g supernatant	Decrease	40
	Citric acid cycle	Malate dehydrogenase	Rat	5, 24 months	Wet weight	Cytoplasmic fraction	Decrease	41
		Malate dehydrogenase	Rat	5, 24 months	Wet weight	Mitochondrial fraction	Decrease	41
	Respiratory	Succinic dehydrogenase	Horse	18 months, 2—12 years	Dry weight	Unspecified	No change	42
		Succinoxidase	Horse	18 months, 2—12 years	Dry weight	Unspecified	No change	42
		Succinoxidase	Rat	27 months	Wet weight		Decrease	43
		Cytochrome oxidase	Horse	18 months, 2—12 years	Dry weight	Unspecified	No change	42
		Cytochrome oxidase	Rat	13, 26 months			No change	44
		ATPase	Rat	5, 20 months	Protein	Homogenate	No change	45

Table 1 (continued)

Organ or tissue	Function of enzyme	Enzyme	Species	Ages studied	Basis of specific activity measurements	Preparation of tissue	Effect of age	Ref.
	Lipid metabolism	NADH cytochrome *c* reductase	Rat	6, 24 months	Protein	Microsomal fraction	Increase	46
		NADPH cytochrome *c* reductase	Rat	6, 24 months	Protein	Microsomal fraction	No change	46
		Succinate cytochrome *c* reductase	Rat	6, 24 months	Protein	Mitochondrial fraction	No change	46
		β-Hydroxy butyrate dehydrogenase	Rat	6, 24 months	Protein	Mitochondrial fraction	Increase	46
	Hydrolytic degradation	Cathepsin	Rat	3, 12, 24 months	Wet weight	Homogenate	Increase	47
	Neurotransmitter regulation	Guanyl cyclase	Rat	2, 10 months	Protein	Homogenate	Decrease	48
		c-GMP phosphodiesterase	Rat	2, 10 months	Protein	Homogenate	Decrease	48
		Adenyl cyclase	Rat	2, 10 months	Protein	Homogenate	Decrease	48
		DOPA decarboxylase	Rat	4, 24 months	Protein	Homogenate	Increase	49
		Catechol-o-methyltransferase	Rat	4, 24 months	Protein	Homogenate	No change	49
		Monoamine oxidase	Rat	4, 24 months	Protein	Homogenate	Increase	49
		Monoamine oxidase	Rat	2, 24 months	Protein			
	Muscular contraction	ATPase	Rat	5, 20 months	Protein	Homogenate	No change	45
		ATPase	Rat	4, 6, 8, 10, 13, 17, 20, 23, 27 months	Protein	Myocardium actomyosin	Decrease to 16 months, then constant	51
	Anticytotoxic	Superoxide dismutase	Rat	8, 32 months	Protein	Homogenate; 13,000 g supernatant	Decrease	52
		Superoxide dismutase	Mouse	8, 28 months	Protein	Homogenate; 13,000 g supernatant	Decrease	52

Arteries	Carbohydrate metabolism							
	Glycolysis	Aldolase	Man	20—87 years	Wet weight; Nitrogen	Homogenate	Increase to 50 years, then decrease	53, 54
		Phosphoglucoisomerase	Man	20—87 years	Wet weight; Nitrogen	Homogenate	No change	53, 55
		Hexokinase	Man	20—87 years	Wet weight; Nitrogen	Homogenate	No change	53, 55
		Enolase	Man	20—79 years	Wet weight; Nitrogen	Homogenate	No change	56
		Phosphofructokinase	Man	20—87 years	Wet weight; Nitrogen	Homogenate	Increase	57
		Lactic dehydrogenase	Man	20—87 years		Homogenate	Increase to 50 years, then decrease	54, 55
		Glyceraldehyde-3 phosphate DH	Man	20—87 years	Wet weight	Homogenate	Decrease	58
		Phosphoglyceric acid mutase	Man	20—87 years	Wet weight; Nitrogen	Homogenate	Decrease	59
		Phosphomannose isomerase	Man	20—87 years	Wet weight; Nitrogen	Homogenate	Decrease	59
	Hexose monophosphate shunt	Glucose-6-phosphate DH	Man	20—85 years	Wet weight; Nitrogen	Homogenate	Decrease	53
		Glucose-6-phosphate DH	Man	20—85 years	Wet weight; Nitrogen	Homogenate	No change	53
		6-Phosphogluconate DH	Man	20—85 years	Wet weight; Nitrogen	Homogenate	Decrease	60
		6-Phosphogluconate DH	Man	20—85 years	Wet weight; Nitrogen	Homogenate	No change	53
		Ribose-5-phosphate isomerase	Man	20—85 years	Wet weight; Nitrogen	Homogenate	Increase to 50 years then decrease	54

Table 1 (continued)

Organ or tissue	Function of enzyme	Enzyme	Species	Ages studied	Basis of specific activity measurements	Preparation of tissue	Effect of age	Ref.
	Glycogenolysis	Glycogen phosphorylase	Man	20—85 years	Wet weight; Nitrogen	Homogenate	Decrease	54, 61
		Phosphoglucomutase	Man	20—87 years	Wet weight; Nitrogen	Homogenate	Decrease	59
	Citric acid cycle	Fumarase	Man	20—85 years	Wet weight	Homogenate	Decrease	53—55
		Malic dehydrogenase	Man	20—83 years	Wet weight; Nitrogen	Homogenate	No change	53, 55
		Isocitric dehydrogenase	Man	20—85 years	Wet weight; Nitrogen	Homogenate	No change	62
		Aconitase	Man	20—85 years	Wet weight; Nitrogen	Homogenate	No change	63
	Intermediary metabolism	Glutamic dehydrogenase	Man	20—88 years	Wet weight; Nitrogen	Homogenate	Decrease	64
		Malic enzyme	Man	20—85 years	Wet weight; Nitrogen	Homogenate	Decrease	65
	Respiratory	Glyoxalase I	Man	20—88 years	Wet weight; Nitrogen	Homogenate	Decrease	66
		Succinic dehydrogenase	Man	20—85 years	Wet weight	Homogenate	Decrease	53
		Succinoxidase	Man	1 day—17 years; 21—73 years	Dry weight	Slices	Decrease	67
		Cytochrome oxidase	Man	1 day—17 years; 21—73 years	Dry weight	Slices	Decrease	67
		Cytochrome oxidase	Man	20—85 years	Wet weight	Homogenate	Decrease	53, 59
		Cytochrome C reductase	Man	20—87 years	Wet weight; Nitrogen	Homogenate	Decrease	59
		Creatine phosphokinase	Man	20—87 years	Wet weight; Nitrogen	Homogenate	Decrease	59
		ATPase	Man	20—85 years	Wet weight; Nitrogen	Homogenate	No cbange	53
		NAD diaphorase	Man	20—87 years	Wet weight; Nitrogen	Homogenate	No change	68

Protein metabolism	Leucine amino peptidase	Man	20—79 years	Wet weight	Homogenate	Decrease	65
Fat metabolism	α-Glycerophosphate dehydrogenase	Man	20—87 years	Wet weight; Nitrogen	Homogenate	Decrease	58
	Sphingomyelinase	Man	0—19, 20—44, 45—70, 71—97 years	DNA	Homogenate	Decrease	69
	Lecithinase	Man	0—19, 20—44, 45—70, 71—97 years	DNA	Homogenate	Increase	69
	TPN-malic enzyme	Man	20—87 years	Wet weight; Nitrogen	Homogenate	No change	62
	Sorbitol dehydrogenase	Man	90 years	Wet weight; Nitrogen	Homogenate	Decrease	57
Nucleic acid metabolism	Purine nucleoside phosphorylase	Man	20—87 years	Wet weight; Nitrogen	Homogenate	No change	70
Hydrolytic degradation	β-Acetyl glucosaminidase	Man	1—30, 31—60, 60 years	Units	Homogenate	No change	71
	β-Glucuronidase	Man	1—30, 31—60, 60 years	Units	Homogenate	No change	71
	β-Glucuronidase	Man	20—85 years	Wet weight; Nitrogen	Homogenate	Increase to 60 years, then decrease	54
	Cathepsin	Man	20—87 years	Wet weight; Nitrogen	Homogenate	Increase	61
	Purine nucleosidase	Man	20—87 years	Wet weight; Nitrogen	Homogenate	Increase	70
	Acid phosphomonoesterase	Man	20—85 years	Wet weight; Nitrogen	Homogenate	Decrease	72
	Phenol sulfatase	Man	20—85 years	Wet weight; Nitrogen	Homogenate	Decrease	53, 54
	Adenyl pyrophosphatase	Man	20—85 years	Wet weight; Nitrogen	Homogenate	Decrease	72
	β-Glucuronidase	Rat	1, 3, 18 months	Protein	Lysosomal fractions	Decrease	73
	N-acetyl-hexosaminidase	Rat	1, 3, 18 months	Protein	Lysosomal fractions	Decrease	73
	Acid phosphatase	Rat	1, 3, 18 months	Protein	Lysosomal fractions	No change	73

Table 1 (continued)

Organ or tissue	Function of enzyme	Enzyme	Species	Ages studied	Basis of specific activity measurements	Preparation of tissue	Effect of age	Ref.
	Ion transport	Inorganic pyrophosphatase	Man	20—85 years	Wet weight; Nitrogen	Homogenate	Decrease	72
		5′-Nucleotidase	Man	20—85 years	Wet weight; Nitrogen	Homogenate	Increase to 40 years, then decrease	54, 60
	Neurotransmitter regulation	Monoamine oxidase	Rat	2, 24 months	Protein	Homogenate	Decrease	50
Blood cells								
Erythrocytes	Carbohydrate metabolism	Transketolase	Man	15, 25, 35, 45, 55, 65, 75, 85, 95 years	Units	Cells	Decrease	74
	Plasma membrane function	Na^+/K^+-ATPase	Man	18—35 years	Protein	Plasma membrane ghosts	No change	75
		Glyceraldehyde-3-phosphate DH	Man	18—35 years	Protein	Plasma membrane ghosts	No change	75
		NADH-ferricyanide reductase	Man	18—35 years	Protein	Plasma membrane ghosts	No change	75
		Alkaline phosphatase	Man	18—35 years	Protein	Plasma membrane ghosts	Decrease	75
		Mg^{2+}—ATPase	Man	18—35 years	Protein	Plasma membrane ghosts	Decrease	75
		Phosphoglycerate kinase	Man	18—35 years	Protein	Plasma membrane ghosts	Decrease	75
		Purine nucleoside phosphorylase	Man	18—35 years	Protein	Plasma membrane ghosts	Decrease	75
		Adenylate kinase	Man	18—35 years	Protein	Plasma membrane ghosts	Decrease	75
		Acetylcholinesterase	Man	18—35 years	Protein	Plasma membrane ghosts	Decrease	75
		Cholinesterase	Man	20, 30, 40, 50, 60 years	Units	Cells	No change	76

Leucocytes	Protein metabolism	Peptidase	Man	19—32, 67—90 years	Manometric	Cells	Increase	77
Serum	Carbohydrate metabolism	Diastase	Man	12—60, 61—96 years	Units		Decrease	78
		Amylase	Man	12—60, 61—96 years	Units		Decrease	78
		Lactic dehydrogenase	Man	20—80 years	Units		Increase	79
	Protein metabolism	Pepsin	Man	12—60, 61—96 years	Units		Decrease	78
		Trypsin	Man	12—60, 61—96 years	Units		Decrease	78
		Glutamic-pyruvic transaminase	Man	20—80 years	Units		Decrease	79
		Glutamic-oxaloacetic transaminase	Man	20—80 years	Units		Decrease	79
		Ornithine transcarbamylase	Man	21—72 years	Units		Increase	80
	Fat metabolism	Lipase	Man	12—60, 61—96 years	Units		Decrease	78
	Nucleic acid metabolism	Dimethyl-p-phenylenediamine oxidase	Man	20—39, 40—59, 60 years	Units		Increase	81
		Phenylenediamine oxidase	Rat	2—24 months	Units		Increase	82
	Intermediary metabolism	Monoamine oxidase	Man	25, 35, 45, 55, 65, 70 years	Protein		Increase	83
	Hydrolytic degradation	Acid phosphatase	Man	25, 35, 45, 55, 65, 70 years	Units		Decrease	84
	Ion transport	Alkaline phosphatase	Man	25—50, 50—60, 80—92 years	Units		Decrease	85
		Alkaline phosphatase	Man	25—50, 50—60, 80—92 years	Units		Increase	85
		Alkaline phosphatase	Mouse	4, 8, 12, 16, 20, 24 months	Wet weight		No change	36
	Neurotransmitter regulation	Pseudo cholinesterase	Man		Units		Decrease	86
		Cholinesterase	Man	20—90 years	Units		Decrease	87
		Cholinesterase	Rat	13, 26 months	Units		Decrease	87
		Dopamine hydroxylase	Man	16—20, 21—40, 41—60 years	Units		Increase	88
	Detoxification	Paraxonase	Man	18—48, 70—96 years	Units		No change	89

Table 1 (continued)

Organ or tissue	Function of enzyme	Enzyme	Species	Ages studied	Basis of specific activity measurements	Preparation of tissue	Effect of age	Ref.
	Neutrophil turnover	Lysozyme	Man	25, 35, 45, 55, 75 years	Units		Increase	90
Cartilage	Carbohydrate metabolism	Hexokinase	Guinea pig	3 months—5 3/4 years	DNA	Slices	Increase	91
	Glycolytic	Aldolase	Guinea pig	3 months—5 3/4 years	DNA	Slices	Increase	91
		Phosphofructo kinase	Guinea pig	3 months—5 3/4 years	DNA	Slices	Increase	91
		Lactate dehydrogenase	Guinea pig	3 months—5 3/4 years	DNA	Slices	Increase	91
	Hexose monophosphate shunt	Glucose-6-phosphate DH	Guinea pig	3 months—5 3/4 years	DNA	Slices	Increase	91
	Citric acid cycle	Isocitrate DH	Guinea pig	3 months—5 3/4 years	DNA	Slices	Increase	91
	Respiratory	Creatine phosphokinase	Guinea pig	3 months—5 3/4 years	DNA	Slices	Increase	91
	Hydrolytic, degradative	β-Glucuronidase	Man	21—40, 41—60, 61—80 years	Units		Decrease	92
		β-Acetylglucosaminidase	Man	21—40, 41—60, 61—80 years	Units		Decrease	92
		Myokinase	Guinea pig	3 months—5 3/4 years	DNA	Slices	Increase	91
Central nervous system								
Brain	Carbohydrate metabolism	Transacetylase	Rat	3, 11, 24 months		Homogenate	Decrease	93
	Hexose monophosphate shunt	Glucose-6-phosphate DH	Mouse	5, 25 months	Wet weight	Homogenate 100,000 g supernatant	Increase	94
	Protein metabolism	Glutaminase	Rat	3, 11, 24 months		Homogenate	Increase	93
		Glutamic-pyruvic transaminase	Rat	3, 11, 24 months		Homogenate	Increase	93
		Glutamic oxaloacetic transaminase	Rat	3,11,24 months		Homogenate	Increase	93

		Glutaminate dehydrogenase	Rat	2, 6, 13, 24 months	DNA, protein, organ	Homogenate 100,000 g supernatant	Increase, then decrease	95
		RNA polymerase	Rat	1, 5, 22 months			Decrease	96
		Protein methylase II	Rat	12, 24 months			No change	97
	Nuclear metabolism	Histone methylase	Rat	3, 12, 30 months	Units	Isolated nuclei	Decrease	98
	Detoxification	Superoxide dismutase	Rat	3, 13, 26 months	Protein	Homogenate	No change	99
Cerebral hemisphere	Carbohydrate metabolism	Lactate dehydrogenase	Rat	3, 10, 13, 24 months	Wet weight	Homogenate 12,000 g supernatant	Decrease	39
	Intermediary metabolism	Malate dehydrogenase	Rat	5, 24 months	Wet weight	Cytoplasmic mitochondrial fraction	Decrease	41
	Neurotransmission	Acetylcholinesterase	Rat	2, 6, 16 months			Decrease	100
Prosencephalon	Protein metabolism	Glutamic acid decarboxylase	Rat	2, 12, 26 months	Wet weight	Homogenate	No change	101
	Neurotransmission	Acetylcholinesterase	Rat	10, 12, 32, 36 months	DNA	Homogenate	No change	102
		$Na^{+}K^{+}$−ATPase	Rat	10, 12, 32, 36 months	DNA	Homogenate	No change	102
Cerebral cortex	Neurotransmission	Adenyl cyclase	Rat	3, 24 months			No change	103
		Adenyl cyclase	Rat	3, 6, 12, 24 months	Protein	Homogenate	No change	104
	Glial cell function	Carbonic anhydrase	Rat	6, 19 months	Protein, wet weight, DNA	Homogenate 700 g supernatant	Decrease	105
Cerebral medulla		Carbonic anhydrase	Rat	6, 19 months	Protein, wet weight, DNA	Homogenate 700 g supernantant	Decrease	105
Frontal cortex	Carbohydrate metabolism	Hexokinase	Human	20—100 years	Units	Unspecified	Increase	106
		Fructose-6-phosphate kinase	Human	20—100 years	Units	Unspecified	Decrease	106
	Hydrolytic degradative	β-Galactosidase	Human	24—89 years	Protein	Homogenate	No change	107
		β-Glucosidase	Human	24—89 years	Protein	Homogenate	No change	107
		β-Mannosidase	Human	24—89 years	Protein	Homogenate	No change	107
		Hexosaminidase	Human	24—89 years	Protein	Homogenate	No change	107

Table 1 (continued)

Organ or tissue	Function of enzyme	Enzyme	Species	Ages studied	Basis of specific activity measurements	Preparation of tissue	Effect of age	Ref.
		Acid phosphatase	Human	24—89 years	Protein	Homogenate	No change	107
	Neurotransmission	cAMP-protein kinase	Bovine	1, 8 years	Wet weight, protein	Homogenate and synaptosomal fraction	Decrease	108
		cAMP-protein kinase	Human	19—92 years	Units	Unspecified	Decrease	109
		Catechol-O-methyl transferase	Mouse	2, 6, 12, 18, 24 months	Wet weight	Homogenate	Decrease	110
Caudate	Hydrolytic degradative	β-Galactosidase	Man	24—89 years	Protein	Homogenate	No change	107
		β-Glucosidase	Man	24—89 years	Protein	Homogenate	No change	107
		β-Mannosidase	Man	24—89 years	Protein	Homogenate	No change	107
		Hexosaminidase	Man	24—89 years	Protein	Homogenate	No change	107
		Acid phosphatase	Man	24—89 years	Protein	Homogenate	No change	107
	Neurotransmission	Adenyl cyclase	Rat	3, 24 months			Increase	103
Hippocampus	Neurotransmission	Adenyl cyclase	Rat	3, 24 months			No change	103
		Choline acetyltransferase	Mouse	8, 24 months	Protein	Homogenate 40,000 g supernatant	Decrease	111
		Catechol-O-methyl transferase	Mouse	2, 6, 12, 18, 24, 30 months	Wet weight	Homogenate	Decrease	110
Hypothalamus	Neurotransmission	Catechol-O-methyl transferase	Mouse	2, 6, 12, 18, 24, 30 months	Wet weight	Homogenate	Decrease	110
Amygdala	Neurotransmission	Catechol-O-methyl transferase	Mouse	2, 6, 12, 18, 24, 30 months	Wet weight	Homogenate	Decrease	110
Inferior olive	Hydrolytic degradative	β-Galactosidase	Man	24—89 years	Protein	Homogenate	No change	107
		β-Glucosidase	Man	24—89 years	Protein	Homogenate	No change	107
		β-Mannosidase	Man	24—89 years	Protein	Homogenate	No change	107
		Hexosaminidase	Man	24—89 years	Protein	Homogenate	No change	107
		Acid phosphatase	Man	24—89 years	Protein	Homogenate	No change	107

Cerebellum	Protein metabolism	Glutamic acid decarboxylase	Rat	2, 12, 26 months	Wet weight	Homogenate	Increase	101
	Hydrolytic degradative	β-Galactosidase	Man	24—89 years	Protein	Homogenate	No change	107
		β-Glucosidase	Man	24—89 years	Protein	Homogenate	No change	107
		β-Mannosidase	Man	24—89 years	Protein	Homogenate	No change	107
		Hexosaminidase	Man	24—89 years	Protein	Homogenate	No change	107
		Acid phosphatase	Man	24—89 years	Protein	Homogenate	No change	107
	Neurotransmission	$Na^{+}K^{+}$-ATPase	Rat	10, 12, 32, 36 months	DNA	Homogenate	Decrease	102
		Acetylcholinesterase	Rat	10, 12, 32, 36 months	DNA	Homogenate	Decrease	102
		Acetylcholinesterase	Rat	2, 6, 16 months	Protein	Homogenate	No change	100
		Adenyl cyclase	Rat	3, 24 months			Increase	103
	Glial cell function	Carbonic anhydrase	Rat	6, 19 months	Wet weight; protein; DNA	Homogenate 700 g supernatant	Decrease	105
Hind brain	Neurotransmission	Monoamine oxidase	Human	25, 35, 45, 55, 65, 70 years	Protein	Unspecified	Increase	83
Brain stem	Protein metabolism	Glutamic acid decarboxylase	Rat	2, 12, 26 months	Wet weight	Homogenate	Increase	101
	Neurotransmission	$Na^{+}K^{+}$ATPase	Rat	10, 12, 32, 36 months	DNA	Homogenate	Increase	102
		Acetylcholinesterase	Rat	10, 12, 32, 36 months	DNA	Homogenate	Increase	102
CSF	Carbohydrate metabolism	Lactate dehydrogenase	Man	25, 35, 45, 55, 65, 75, 85 years	Units/mℓ		No change	112
		Malate dehydrogenase	Man	25, 35, 45, 55, 65, 75, 85 years	Units/mℓ		Increase	112
	Protein metabolism	Glutamic-oxaloacetic transaminase	Man	25, 35, 45, 55, 65, 75, 85 years	Units/mℓ		No change	112
	Hydrolytic degradative	β-Galactosidase	Man	24—89 years	Protein	Homogenate	No change	107
		β-Glucuronidase	Man	24—89 years	Protein	Homogenate	No change	107
		β-Mannosidase	Man	24—89 years	Protein	Homogenate	No change	107
		Hexosaminidase	Man	24—89 years	Protein	Homogenate	No change	107
		Acid phosphatase	Man	24—89 years	Protein	Homogenate	No change	107

Table 1 (continued)

Organ or tissue	Function of enzyme	Enzyme	Species	Ages studied	Basis of specific activity measurements	Preparation of tissue	Effect of age	Ref.
Eye lens	Carbohydrate metabolism	Phosphofructokinase	Bovine	4—13 years	Protein	Homogenate 18,000 g supernatant	No change	113
		Carbonic anhydrase	Bovine	2—9, 10 years		Homogenate	No change	114
Intestine	Carbohydrate metabolism	Fumarase	Mouse			Unspecified	No change	115
	Ion transport	Alkaline phosphatase	Mouse	11, 34 months	Nitrogen	Membrane fraction	Decrease	116
Kidney	Carbohydrate metabolism	Maltase	Rat	3, 24 months	Protein	Plasma membrane fraction	Decrease	117
	Glycolytic	Lactate dehydrogenase	Mouse	4, 18, 30 months	DNA; protein; wet weight	Homogenate	No change	13
	Hexose-monophosphate shunt	Glucose-6-phosphate DH	Mouse (female)	4, 18, 30 months	DNA; protein; wet weight	Homogenate	Decrease	13
		Glucose-6-phosphate DH	Mouse (male)	4, 18, 30 months	DNA; protein; wet weight	Homogenate	Increase	13
	Glycogenolysis	Glucose-6-phosphate DH	Mouse	5, 25 months	Wet weight	Homogenate 100,000 g supernatant	Increase	94
		Glucose-6-phosphatase	Mouse	4, 18, 30 months	DNA; protein, wet weight	Homogenate	Decrease	13
		Glucose-6-phosphatase	Rat	6, 24 months	Protein	Microsomal fraction	Increase	46
	Respiratory	Succinate dehydrogenase	Rat	13, 27 months	Wet weight	Homogenate	Decrease	43
		Succinoxidase	Rat	13, 27 months	Wet weight	Homogenate	Decrease	43
		Succinoxidase	Rat	13, 27 months	Protein	Mitochondrial fraction	No change	118
		Cytochrome oxidase	Rat	13, 27 months	Wet weight	Homogenate	Decrease	43
		Cytochrome oxidase	Rat	13, 27 months	DNA; protein; wet weight	Homogenate	No change	13

Lipid metabolism	NADH cytochrome *c* reductase	Rat	6, 24 months	Protein	Microsomal fraction	Decrease	46
	NADPH cytochrome *c* reductase	Rat	6, 24 months	Protein	Microsomal fraction	Decrease	46
	Succinate cytochrome *c* reductase	Rat	6, 24 months	Protein	Mitochondrial fraction	Decrease	46
	β-Hydroxy butyrate dehydrogenase	Rat	6, 24 months	Protein	Mitochondrial fraction	Decrease	46
Hydrolytic degradation	Acid phosphatase	Rat	6, 13, 24 months	Protein nitrogen	Homogenate	Decrease	119
	Acid phosphatase	Rat	6, 13, 25 months	Protein nitrogen	Homogenate	Increase	120
	Acid phosphatase	Mouse	4, 18, 30 months	DNA; protein; wet weight	Homogenate	No change	13
	Acid phosphatase	Mouse	3, 19 months	Wet weight	Homogenate	Decrease	121
	Acid DNase	Mouse	3, 19 months	Wet weight; cell number	Homogenate	Increase	121
	Acid DNase	Rat	3—25 months	Nitrogen	Homogenate	Increase	120
	Alkaline DNase	Mouse	3, 19 months	Wet weight; cell number	Homogenate	Decrease	121
	Alkaline DNase	Rat	3—25 months	Nitrogen	Homogenate	Increase	120
	Cathepsin	Rat	3, 12, 24 months	Wet weight	Homogenate	Increase	47
	β-Glucuromidase	Mouse	4, 18, 30 months	DNA; protein; wet weight	Homogenate	No change	13
Ion transport	Alkaline phosphatase	Mouse (male)	4, 18, 30 months	DNA; protein; wet weight	Homogenate	Increase	13
	Alkaline phosphatase	Mouse (female)	4, 18, 30 months	DNA; protein; wet weight	Homogenate	Decrease	13
	Alkaline phosphatase	Rat	Unspecified (up to 350 g)	Wet weight	Homogenate	Decrease	122
	Alkaline phosphatase	Rat	3, 24 months	Protein	Plasma membrane fraction	Decrease	117
		Rat	3, 24 months	Protein	Plasma membrane fraction	Decrease	117
	Na^+K^+-ATPase	Rat	3, 28 months	Protein	Homogenate	Decrease	123
	5′-nucleotidase	Mouse	4, 18, 30 months	DNA; protein; wet weight	Homogenate	Increase	13

Table 1 (continued)

Organ or tissue	Function of enzyme	Enzyme	Species	Ages studied	Basis of specific activity measurements	Preparation of tissue	Effect of age	Ref.
Liver	Carbohydrate metabolism	Hexokinase	Rat	3, 18 months	Protein	Homogenate 3,000 g supernatant	Decrease	124
	Glycolysis	Fructokinase	Rat	5, 21 months	Wet weight	Homogenate	Increase	125
		Phosphofructokinase	Rat	6, 10, 13 months	Wet weight	Homogenate	Increase	126
		Aldolase	Mouse	3, 31 months	Protein	Purified enzyme	Decrease	127
		Aldolase	Rat	3, 18 months	Protein	Homogenate 3,000 g supernatant	Decrease	124
		Aldolase	Rat	6, 10, 13 months	Wet weight	Homogenate	No change	126
		Aldolase	Rat	2, 24 months	Protein	Homogenate 40,000 g supernatant	No change	128
		Aldolase	Rabbit	2, 36 months	Protein	Homogenate 40,000 g supernatant	Decrease	129
		Fructose-1,6-diphophatase	Rat	3, 6, 9, 12, 15 months	Wet weight		Decrease	130
		Fructose-1,6 diphosphatase	Rat	3, 18 months	Protein	Homogenate 3000 g supernatant	Decrease	124
		Pyruvate kinase	Rat	6, 10, 13 months	Wet weight	Homogenate	Increase	126
		Lactate dehydrogenase	Rat	6, 21 months	Wet weight	Homogenate postnuclear supernatant	Increase	125
		Lactate dehydrogenase	Rat	2, 24 months	Wet weight	Homogenate 12,000 g supernatant	Decrease	39
		Lactate dehydrogenase	Mouse (male)	4, 18, 30 months	DNA; protein; wet weight	Homogenate	Increase	3
		Lactate dehydrogenase	Mouse (female)	4, 18, 30 months	DNA; protein; wet weight	Homogenate	No change	3

Hexose monophosphate shunt	Glucose-6-phosphate dehydrogenase	Rat	6, 10, 13 months	Wet weight	Homogenate	No change	126
	Glucose-6-phosphate dehydrogenase	Rat (Sprague-Dawley)	3, 24 months	Protein	Cytosol fraction	Decrease	131
	Glucose-6-phosphate dehydrogenase	Rat (Fischer 344)	3, 24 months	Protein	Cytosol fraction	Increase	131
	Glucose-6-phosphate debydrogenase	Mouse (male)	4, 18, 30 months	DNA; protein; wet weight	Homogenate	Increase	3
	Glucose-6-phosphate dehydrogenase	Mouse	5, 25 months	Wet weight	Homogenate 100,000 g supernatant	Increase	94
Citrate cycle	Malic enzyme	Rat	6, 10, 13 months	Wet weight	Homogenate	No change	126
	Malic dehydrogenase	Rat	6, 21 months	Wet weight	Homogenate	Increase	125
	Malate dehydrogenase	Mouse	3—6; 30—32 months	Protein	Homogenate; mitochondrial fraction	No change	5
	Isocitrate dehydrogenase	Rat	6, 10, 13 months	Wet weight	Cytosol	Decrease	126
Glycogenolysis	Glucose-6-phosphatase	Rat	3, 6, 9, 12, 15 months	Wet weight	Homogenate	Decrease	130
	Glucose-6-phosphatase	Rat	6, 24 months	Protein	Microsomal fraction	Decrease	46
	Glucose-6-phosphatase	Rat	3, 18 months	Protein	Homogenate 3000 g supernatant	Decrease	124
	Glucose-6-phosphatase	Mouse	9—27 months	Wet weight	Homogenate	No change	132
	Glucose-6-phosphatase	Mouse	4, 18, 30 months	DNA; protein; wet weight	Homogenate	Decrease	3
	Phosphoglucomutase	Mouse	4, 18, 30 months	DNA; protein; wet weight	Homogenate	Increase	3
	Glycogen phosphorylase	Mouse	4, 18, 30 months	DNA; protein; wet weight	Homogenate	No change	3
Lipogenesis	ATPcitrate lyase	Rat	6, 10, 13 months	Wet weight	Homogenate	Increase	126
	Aconitate hydratase	Rat	6, 10, 13 months	Wet weight	Cytosol	No change	126

Table 1 (continued)

Organ or tissue	Function of enzyme	Enzyme	Species	Ages studied	Basis of specific activity measurements	Preparation of tissue	Effect of age	Ref.
	Protein metabolism	D-Amino acid oxidase	Rat	6, 21 months	Wet weight	Homogenate	Increase	125
		L-Histidase	Rat	6, 21 months	Wet weight	Homogenate	Increase	125
		Tryptophan pyrrolase	Rat	6, 12, 24 months	Wet weight	Homogenate postnuclear supernatant	Decrease	133
		Tryptophan peroxidase	Rat	13, 26 months	Dry weight	Homogenate postnuclear supernatant	No change	134
		Tyrosine transaminase	Rat	13, 26 months	Dry weight	Homogenate postnuclear supernatant	No change	134
		Protein methylase I, III	Rat	2, 24 months	Protein	Homogenate	Decrease	135
		Protein methylase II	Rat	2, 24 months	Protein	Homogenate	No change	135
	Collagen biosynthesis	Prolyl hydroxylase	Rat	3, 8, 14 months	Protein	Homogenate postnuclear supernatant	Decrease	136
		Lysyl hydroxylase	Rat	3, 8, 14 months	Protein	Homogenate postnuclear supernatant	Decrease	136
		Collagen galactosyl transferase	Rat	3, 8, 14 months	Protein	Homogenate postnuclear supernatant	Increase	136
		Collagen glucosyl transferase	Rat	3, 8, 14 months	Protein	Homogenate postnuclear supernatant	Increase	136
	Respiratory	ATPase	Rat	16, 21 months	Wet weight	Homogenate	Increase	125
		Succinoxidase	Rat	12, 27 months	Wet weight	Homogenate	No change	43
		Succinate dehydrogenase	Rat	12, 27 months	Protein	Mitochondrial fraction	No change	118
		Succinate dehydrogenase	Rat	6, 21 months	Wet weight; dry weight	Homogenate	No change	125

	Succinate dehydrogenase	Mouse	4, 18, 30 months	DNA; protein; wet weight	Homogenate	Peak at 18 months	3
	Cytochrome oxidase	Mouse (female)	4, 18, 30 months	DNA; protein; wet weight	Homogenate	Peak at 18 months	3
	Cytochrome oxidase	Mouse (male)	4, 18, 30 months	DNA; protein; wet weight	Homogenate	Decrease	3
	Cytochrome oxidase	Mouse	3—6; 30—32 months	Protein	Homogenate; mitochondrial fraction	No change	5
	NAD diaphorase	Mouse	4, 18, 30 months	DNA; protein; wet weight	Homogenate	Decrease	3
Lipid metabolism	NADH cytochrome *c* reductase	Rat	6, 24 months	Protein	Microsomal fraction	Increase	46
	NADPH cytochrome *c* reductase	Rat	6, 24 months	Protein	Microsomal fraction	Decrease	46
	NADPH cytochrome *c* reductase	Rat	2, 12, 30 months	Protein	Microsomal fraction	Decrease	137
	Succinate cytochrome c reductase	Rat	6, 24 months	Protein	Mitochondrial fraction	Increase	46
	β-Hydroxybutyrate dehydrogenase	Rat	6, 24 months	Protein	Mitochondrial fraction	Decrease	46
Intermediary metabolism	Zoxazolamine hydroxylase	Rat	2, 12, 30 months	Wet weight	Microsomal fraction	Decrease	137
	Ornithine decarboxylase	Rat	3, 24 months	Protein	Homogenate 20,000 g supernatant	Increase	138
Nucleic acid control	tRNA methylase	Mouse	12, 18, 30 months	Protein	Homogenate 100,000 g supernatant	Decrease	139
	Glycine N-methyltransferase	Mouse	12, 18, 30 months	Protein	Homogenate 100,000 g supernatant	Increase	139
	Histone methylase	Rat	3, 12, 30 months	Wet weight	Nuclear fraction	Decrease	98
Hydrolytic degradative	Acid phosphatase	Rat	6, 21 months	Wet weight	Homogenate	No change	125
	Acid phosphatase	Rat	2—25 months	Nitrogen		Increase	120

Table 1 (continued)

Organ or tissue	Function of enzyme	Enzyme	Species	Ages studied	Basis of specific activity measurements	Preparation of tissue	Effect of age	Ref.
		Acid phosphatase	Rat	3, 12, 24, 30—35 months	Protein	Homogenate	Increased at 24 months, then decrease	6
		Acid phosphatase	Rat	3, 12, 24, 30—35 months	Protein	Isolated parenchymal cells	No change	6
		Acid phosphatase	Rat	3, 12, 24, 30—35 months	Protein	Isolated non-parenchymal cells	No change	6
		Acid phosphatase	Mouse	6, 24 months	Wet weight	Homogenate	No change	140
		Acid phosphatase	Mouse	6, 27 months	Wet weight	Unspecified	Increase	141
		Acid phosphatase	Mouse	4, 18, 30 months	DNA; protein; wet weight	Homogenate	Increase	3
		Acid phosphatase	Mouse	3—19 months	Wet weight	Homogenate	Decrease	142
		β-Glucuronidase	Mouse	4, 18, 30 months	Wet weight	Homogenate	Decrease	121
		β-Galactosidase	Mouse	4, 18, 30 months	DNA; protein; wet weight	Homogenate	Increase	3
		β-Galactosidase	Rat	3, 12, 24, 30—35 months	Protein	Homogenate	Increase at 12 and 24 months, then decrease	6
		β-Galactosidase	Rat	3,12, 24, 30—35 months	Protein	Isolated parenchymal cells	Decrease at 12 months	6
		β-Galactosidase	Rat	3, 12, 24, 30—35 months	Protein	Isolated non-parenchymal cells	Progressive decrease	6
		Arysulphatase B	Rat	6, 24 months	Wet weight		Increase	141

	Arysulphatase B	Rat	3, 12, 24, 30—35 months	Protein	Homogenate	Increase at 24 months, then decrease	6
	Arysulphatase B	Rat	3, 12, 24, 30—35 months	Protein	Isolated parenchymal cells	Increase at 24 months, then decrease	6
	Cathepsin D	Rat	3, 12, 24, 30—35 months	Protein	Isolated nonparenchymal cells	Increase at 12 months	6
	Cathepsin D	Rat	14, 35 months	Wet weight	Homogenate	Increase	143
	Cathepsin D	Rat	3, 12, 24, 30—35 months	Protein	Homogenate	Progressive increase	6
	Cathepsin D	Rat	3, 12, 24, 30—35 months	Protein	Isolated parenchymal cells	Increase at 24 and 35 months	6
	Acid DNase	Rat	3, 12, 24, 30—35 months	Protein	Isolated nonparenchymal cells	Decrease at 24 months	6
	Acid DNase	Rat	2, 25 months	Nitrogen	Homogenate	Increase	120
	Alkaline DNase	Mouse	3, 19 months	Wet weight	Homogenate	Increase	121
	Pyrophosphatase	Rat	6, 21 months	Wet weight	Homogenate	Decrease	125
	Aliesterase	Rat	6, 21 months	Wet weight	Homogenate	Increase	125
Ion transport	Alkaline phosphatase	Rat	6, 21 months	Wet weight	Homogenate	Decrease	125
	Alkaline phosphatase	Mouse	6, 27 months	Wet weight	Homogenate	No change	140
	Alkaline phosphatase	Mouse	6, 27 months	Wet weight	Homogenate	Increase	115
	Alkaline phosphatase	Mouse	4, 18, 30 months	DNA; protein; wet weight	Homogenate	Decrease	3
	Alkaline phosphatase	Mouse	4, 18, 12, 16, 20, 24 months	Wet weight	Homogenate 15,000 g supernatant	Decrease	36
	5′-Nucleotidase	Mouse (male)	4, 18, 30 months	DNA; protein; wet weight	Homogenate	Decrease	3

Table 1 (continued)

Organ or tissue	Function of enzyme	Enzyme	Species	Ages studied	Basis of specific activity measurements	Preparation of tissue	Effect of age	Ref.
		5′-Nucleotidase	Mouse (female)	4, 18, 30 months	DNA; protein; wet weight	Homogenate	No change	3
		Mg^{2+}-ATPase	Mouse	4, 18, 30 months	DNA; protein; wet weight	Homogenate	Increase	3
		Mg^{2+}-ATPase	Rat	2, 26 months		Plasma membrane fraction	Increase	31
		$Na^{+}K^{+}$ATPase	Rat	2, 26 months		Plasma membrane fraction	Increase	31
	Neurotransmission	Cholinesterase	Rat	27 months	Units		No change	87
		Monoamine oxidase	Rat	2, 18 months	Wet weight		Decrease	145
		Adenyl cyclase	Rat	2, 10 months	Protein	Homogenate	Decrease	48
		Guanyl cyclase	Rat	2, 10 months	Protein	Homogenate	Decrease	48
	Detoxification	Superoxide dismutase	Rat	3, 13, 26 months	Protein	Homogenate	No change	99
Lung	Carbohydrate metabolism	Lactate dehydrogenase	Mouse (male)	4, 18, 30 months	DNA; protein; wet weight;	Homogenate	Decrease	3
	Glycolysis	Lactate dehydrogenase	Mouse (female)	4, 18, 30 months	DNA; protein; wet weight	Homogenate	Peak at 18 months	3
	Hexose monophosphate shunt	Glucose-6-phosphate dehydrogenase	Mouse (female)	4, 18, 30 months	DNA; protein; wet weight	Homogenate	Peak at 18 months	3
		Glucose-6-phosphate dehydrogenase	Mouse (male)	4, 18, 30 months	DNA; protein; wet weight	Homogenate	No change	3
		Glucose-6-phosphate dehydrogenase	Mouse	5, 25 months	Wet weight	Homogenate 100,000 g supernatant	Increase	94
	Glycogenolysis	Glucose-6-phosphatase	Mouse	4, 18, 30 months	DNA; protein; wet weight	Homogenate	Decrease	3
		Phosphoglucomutase	Mouse	4, 18, 30 months	DNA; protein; wet weight	Homogenate	Increase	3
		Glycogen phosphorylase	Mouse	4, 18, 30 months	DNA; protein; wet weight	Homogenate	No change	3

	Respiratory	Succinate dehydrogenase	Mouse	4, 18, 30 months	DNA; protein; wet weight	Homogenate	Decrease	3
		Cytochrome oxidase	Mouse	4, 18, 30 months	DNA; protein; wet weight	Homogenate	Decrease	3
		NAD diaphorase	Mouse	4, 18, 30 months	DNA; protein; wet weight	Homogenate	Decrease	3
	Hydrolytic, degradative	Acid phosphatase	Mouse (male)	4, 18, 30 months	DNA; protein; wet weight	Homogenate	Decrease	3
		Acid phosphatase	Mouse (female)	4, 18, 30 months	DNA; protein; wet weight	Homogenate	No change	3
		Acid phosphatase	Mouse	2, 20 months	Protein	Homogenate	No change	146
		β-Glucuronidase	Mouse	4, 18, 30 months	DNA; protein; wet weight	Homogenate	Increase	3
		β-Glucuronidase	Mouse	2, 20 months	Protein	Homogenate	Increase	146
		Arylsulphatase	Mouse	2, 20 months	Protein	Homogenate	No change	146
		N-Acetyl-β-D-glucosaminidase	Mouse	2, 20 months	Protein	Homogenate	Increase	146
	Neurotransmission	Adenyl cyclase	Rat	2, 10 months	Protein	Homogenate	No change	48
		Guanyl cyclase	Rat	2, 10 months	Protein	Homogenate	No change	48
Muscle — skeletal	Carbohydrate metabolism	Lactate dehydrogenase	Rat	3, 30 months	Protein; wet weight	Homogenate	Decrease	147
	Glycolysis	Lactate dehydrogenase	Rat	2, 24 months	Wet weight	Homogenate 12,000 g supernatant	Decrease	39
		Aldolase	Human	24—84 years	Soluble protein; DNA	Homogenate 50,000 g supernatant	Decrease	148
		Creatine phosphokinase	Human	24—84 years	Soluble protein; DNA	Homogenate 50,000 g supernatant	Decrease	148
	Respiratory	ATPase	Rat	9, 16, 26 months	Wet weight	Homogenate 2,500 rpm supernatant	Decrease	149
	Ion transport	Mg^{2+}-ATPase	Rat	6, 29 months	Protein	Isolated actomyosin	Decrease	150
	Neurotransmission	Adenyl cyclase	Rat	2, 10 months	Protein	Homogenate	No change	48
		Guanyl cyclase	Rat	2, 10 months	Protein	Homogenate	No change	48

Table 1 (continued)

Organ or tissue	Function of enzyme	Enzyme	Species	Ages studied	Basis of specific activity measurements	Preparation of tissue	Effect of age	Ref.
Extensor digitorum longus	Carbohydrate metabolism	Triosephosphate dehydrogenase	Rat	3, 28—36 months	Wet weight	Homogenate	Decrease	20
	Glycolysis	Lactate dehydrogenase	Rat	3, 28—36 months	Wet weight	Homogenate	Decrease	20
		α-Glycerol-3-phosphate dehydrogenase	Rat	3, 28—36 months	Wet weight	Homogenate	Decrease	20
	Oxidative	Hexokinase	Rat	3, 28—36 months	Wet weight	Homogenate	Decrease	20
		Malate dehydrogenase	Rat	3, 28—36 months	Wet weight	Homogenate	No change	20
		Citrate synthase	Rat	3, 28—36 months	Wet weight	Homogenate	No change	20
Diaphragm	Glycolysis	Triose phosphate dehydrogenase	Rat	3, 28—36 months	Wet weight	Homogenate	Decrease	20
		Lactate dehydrogenase	Rat	3, 28—36 months	Wet weight	Homogenate	No change	20
		Citrate synthase	Rat	3, 28—36 months	Wet weight	Homogenate	Decrease	20
Soleus	Glycolytic	Triose phosphate dehydrogenase	Rat	3, 28—36 months	Wet weight	Homogenate	Decrease	20
		Lactate dehydrogenase	Rat	3, 28—36 months	Wet weight	Homogenate	Decrease	20
		α-Glycerol-3-phosphate dehydrogenase	Rat	3, 28—36 months	Wet weight	Homogenate	No change	20
	Oxidative	Hexokinase	Rat	3, 28—36 months	Wet weight	Homogenate	No change	20
		Malate dehydrogenase	Rat	3, 28—36 months	Wet weight	Homogenate	Decrease	20
		Citrate synthase	Rat	3, 28—36 months	Wet weight	Homogenate	Decrease	20
Pancreas	Carbohydrate metabolism	Amylase	Man	23—66 years	Units	Pancreatic secretion	Increase	151
		Amylase	Man	12—60, 60—96 years	Units	Duodenal juice	Decrease	152
	Protein metabolism	Trypsin	Man	23, 66 years	Units	Pancreatic secretion	No change	151
		Elastomucase	Rat	4, 8, 12, 16, 24, 28 months	Dry weight	Enzyme extract	No change	153
		Elastoproteinase	Rat	4, 8, 12, 16, 24, 28 months	Dry weight	Enzyme extract	Decrease	153

	Lipid metabolism	Lipase	Man	12—60, 60—96 years	Units	Duodenal juice	No change	152
		Lipase	Man	23, 66 years	Units	Pancreatic secretion	Decrease	151
Prostate gland	Carbohydrate metabolism	Lactate dehydrogenase	Mouse	9, 18, 24, 30 months	DNA; protein	Homogenate	Increase	154
		Glucose-6-phosphate dehydrogenase	Mouse	9, 18, 24, 30 months	DNA; protein	Homogenate	Increase	154
	Citrate cycle	Fumarase	Mouse	9, 18, 24, 30 months	DNA; protein	Homogenate	No change	154
		Isocitrate dehydrogenase	Mouse	9, 18, 24, 30 months	DNA; protein	Homogenate	Increase	154
	Respiratory	Succinate dehydrogenase	Mouse	9, 18, 24, 30 months	DNA; protein	Homogenate	Decrease	154
		Cytochrome oxidase	Mouse	9, 18, 24, 30 months	DNA; protein	Homogenate	Decrease	154
	Hydrolytic degradative	Acid phosphatase	Mouse	9, 18, 24, 30 months	DNA; protein	Homogenate	No change	154
		β-Acetyl glucosaminidase	Mouse	9, 18, 24, 30 months	DNA; protein	Homogenate	Decrease	154
	Ion transport	5′-Nucleotidase	Mouse	9, 18, 24, 30 months	DNA; protein	Homogenate	No change	154
Prostatic fluid	Carbohydrate metabolism	Lactate dehydrogenase	Man	40; 41—59; 60 years	Units/mℓ		Decrease	155
	Hydrolytic degradative	Acid phosphatase	Man	90 years	Wet weight		Decrease	156
Saliva	Carbohydrate metabolism	Ptyalin	Man	12—60, 60—96 years	Units		Decrease	152
Skin	Protein metabolism	Collagen galactosyl transferase	Man	20—80 years	Protein; wet weight	Homogenate 15,000 g supernatant	No change	157
		Collagen glucosyl transferase	Man	20—80 years	Protein; wet weight	Homogenate 15,000 g supernatant	No change	157
	Ion transport	Alkaline phosphatase	Rat	Unspecified (up to 230 days)	Wet weight	Homogenate	No change	21
Spleen	Carbohydrate metabolism	Glucose-6-phosphate dehydrogenase	Mouse	5, 25 months	Wet weight	Homogenate 100,000 g supernatant	Increase	94

Table 1 (continued)

Organ or tissue	Function of enzyme	Enzyme	Species	Ages studied	Basis of specific activity measurements	Preparation of tissue	Effect of age	Ref.
	Hydrolytic	Acid DNase	Mouse	3—19 months	Wet weight	Homogenate	Decrease	121
Stomach	Protein metabolism	Pepsin	Man	12—60, 60—96 years	Units	Gastric juice	Decrease	152
		Trypsin	Man	12—60, 60—96 years	Units	Gastric juice	Decrease	152
Testis	Protein metabolism	Protein methylase I, II, III	Rat	2, 12, 24 months	Protein	Homogenate	Decrease	135
	Testosterone biosynthesis	21-Hydroxylase	Mouse	3, 14 months	Protein	Homogenate	Increase	158
		17α-Hydroxylase	Mouse	3, 14 months	Protein	Homogenate 800 g supernatant	Increase	158
		20α-Hydroxysteroid oxidoreductase	Mouse	3, 14 months	Protein	Homogenate 800 g supernatant	Increase	158
		17-20 lyase	Mouse	3, 14 months	Protein	Homogenate 800 g supernatant	Increase	158
		17β-Hydroxysteroid oxidoreductase	Mouse	3, 14 months	Protein	Homogenate 800 g supernatant	Decrease	158
	Neurotransmission	Monoamine oxidase	Rat	1—12 months	Wet weight	Homogenate	Decrease	159
		Monoamine oxidase	Rat	1—12 months	Wet weight	Seminiferous tubules homogenate	Decrease	159
Thymus	Protein metabolism	Peptidase	Mouse	6, 10, 15 months	Units	Homogenate	Decrease	160
	Hydrolytic	Acid DNase	Mouse	3—19 months	Wet weight	Homogenate	Increase	121

REFERENCES

1. **Rowlatt, C., Chesterman, F. C., and Sheriff, M. U.,** Life span age changes and tumour incidence in an aging C57BL mouse colony, *Lab. Anim.*, 10, 419, 1976.
2. **Hollander, C. F.,** Current experience using the laboratory rat in aging studies, *Lab. Anim. Sci.*, 26, 320, 1976.
3. **Wilson, P. D.** Enzyme patterns in young and old mouse liver and lungs, *Gerontologia*, 18, 36, 1972.
4. **Wilson, P. D. and Franks, L. M.,** The effect of age on mitochondrial ultrastructure, *Gerontologia*, 21, 81, 1975.
5. **Wilson, P. D., Hill, B. T., and Franks, L. M.,** The effect of age on mitochondrial enzymes and respiration, *Gerontologia*, 21, 95, 1975.
6. **Knook, D. L. and Sleyster, E.,** Lysosomal enzyme activities in parenchymal and nonparenchymal liver cells isolated from young adult and old rats, *Mech. Ageing Dev.*, 5, 389, 1976.
7. **Florini, J.,** Differences in enzyme levels and physiological processes in mice of different ages, *Exp. Aging Res.*, 1, 137, 1975.
8. **Josephy, H.,** Acid phosphatase in the senile brain, *Arch. Neurol. Psychiatry*, 61, 164, 1949.
9. **Friede, R. L.,** Enzyme histochemical studies of senile plaques, *J. Neuropathol. Exp. Neurol.*, 24, 477, 1965.
10. **Morpurgo, M. and Severgnini, B.,** Regressive changes of aortic and cardiocirculatory aging, *J. Gerontol.*, 11, 107, 1963.
11. **Oka, M. and Angrist, A.,** Histoenzymatic studies of vascular changes in the aorta and coronary arteries of the aged rat, *J. Gerontol.*, 22, 23, 1967.
12. **Studor, H., Baumgartner, H. R., and Reber, K.,** Histochemical evidence of monoamine oxidase activity in rats of different ages, *Histochemie*, 4, 43, 1964.
13. **Wilson, P. D. and Franks, L. M.,** Enzyme patterns in young and old mouse kidneys, *Gerontologia*, 17, 16, 1971.
14. **Kaler, L. and Haensly, W.,** Kidney in the aging cat: neutral lipid and adenyl cylase histochemistry, *Am. J. Vet. Res.*, 38, 897, 1977.
15. **Kobayashi, H.,** Histochemical studies of enzymatic behavior in the hepatic cells of the senile rat liver, *Nagoya J. Med. Sci.*, 27, 167, 1965.
16. **Wilson, P. D.,** Differential enzyme distribution in lobules of livers from young and old mice and rats, *Gerontology*, 24, 348, 1978.
17. **Ghiringhelli, E. M. and Gerzeli, G.,** Histochemical activities of glandular cells in old rats, *J. Gerontol.*, 11, 1097, 1963.
18. **Suntzeff, V. and Angeletti, P.,** Histological and histochemical changes in intestine of mice with aging, *J. Gerontol.*, 16, 225, 1961.
19. **Bogart, B. I.,** The effect of aging on the histochemistry of the rat submandibular gland, *J. Gerontol.*, 22, 372, 1967.
20. **Bass, A., Gutmann, E., and Hanzlikova, V.,** Biochemical and histochemical changes in energy supply enzyme pattern of muscles of the rat during old age, *Gerontologia*, 21, 31, 1975.
21. **Valanju, S. and Rindani, T. H.,** Influence of age, sex, and gonadal hormone on skin metabolism. II. Alkaline phosphatase activity. *Indian J. Med. Res.*, 49, 470, 1961.
22. **Tonna, E. A.,** Posttraumatic variations in phosphatase and respiratory enzyme activities of the periosteum of aging rats, *J. Gerontol.*, 14, 159, 1959.
23. **Tonna, E. A. and Severson, A. R.,** Changes in localization and distribution of adenosine triphosphatase activity in skeletal tissue of the mouse concomitant with aging, *J. Gerontol.*, 26, 186, 1971.
24. **Brunk, V. and Ericsson, J.,** Electron microscopical studies on the rat brain neurons: localization of acid phosphatase and mode of formation of lipofuscin bodies, *J. Ultrastruct. Res.*, 38, 1, 1972.
25. **Holliday, R. and Tarrant, G. M.,** Altered enzymes in aging human fibroblasts, *Nature (London)*, 238, 26, 1972.
26. **Goldstein, S. and Moerman, E. J.,** Heat-labile enzymes in Werner's syndrome fibroblasts, *Nature (London)*, 255, 159, 1975.
27. **Yagil, G.,** Are altered G6PD molecules present in aged liver cells? *Exp. Gerontol.*, 11, 73, 1976.
28. **Gershon, H. and Gershon, D.,** Inactive enzyme molecules in ageing mice, *Proc. Natl. Acad. Sci. U.S.A.*, 70, 909, 1973.
29. **Grinna, L. S. and Barber, A.,** Age related changes in membrane lipid content and enzyme activities, *Biochim. Biophys. Acta*, 288, 347, 1972.
30. **Reiss, V. and Gershon, D.,** Comparison of cytoplasmic superoxide dismutase in liver, heart and brain of aging rats and mice, *Biochem. Biophys. Res. Commun.*, 73, 255, 1976.
31. **Hegner, D. and Platt, D.,** Effect of essential phospholipids on the properties of ATPases of isolated rat liver plasma membranes of young and old animals, *Mech. Ageing Dev.*, 4, 191, 1975.
32. **Grinna, L. S. and Barber, A.,** Kinetic analysis of the age-related differences in glucose-6-phosphatase activity, *Exp. Gerontol.*, 10, 319, 1975.

33. **Kahn, A., Guillouzo, A., Cottreau, D., Marie, J., Bourel, M., Boivin, P., and Dreyfus, J.,** Accuracy of protein synthesis and *in vitro* aging, *Gerontology,* 23, 174, 1977.
34. **Rubinson, H., Kahn, A., Boivin, P., Schapira, F., Gregori, C., and Dreyfus, J.,** Aging and accuracy of protein synthesis in man: search for inactive enzymatic cross-reacting material in granolocytes of aged people, *Gerontology,* 22, 438, 1976.
35. **Cooper, B. and Gregerman, R. I.,** Hormone sensitive fat cell adenylate cyclase in rat: influence of growth, cell size, and aging, *J. Clin. Invest.,* 57, 161, 1976.
36. **Samorajski, T. and Rolsten, C.,** Effect of age on alkaline phosphomonoesterase activity in the adrenals of male mice, *Anat. Rec.,* 163, 473, 1969.
37. **Shapiro, B. H. and Leathem, J. N.,** Aging and adrenal Δ^5-3β-hydroxysteroid dehydrogenase in female rats, *Proc. Soc. Exp. Biol. Med.,* 136, 19, 1971.
38. **Albrecht, E. D., Koos, R., and Wehreinberg, W.,** Aging and adrenal Δ^5-3-β-hydroxysteroid dehydrogenase in female mice, *J. Endocrinol.,* 73, 193, 1977.
39. **Singh, S. N. and Kanungo, M.,** Alterations in lactate dehydrogenase of the brain, heart, skeletal muscle, and liver of rats of various ages, *J. Biol. Chem.,* 243, 4526, 1968.
40. **Porter, H., Doty, P., and Bloor, C.,** Interaction of age and exercise on tissue lactic dehydrogenase activity in rats, *Lab. Invest,* 25, 572, 1971.
41. **Singh, S. N.,** Effect of age on the activity and citrate inhibition of malate dehydrogenase of the brain and heart of rats, *Experientia,* 15, 42, 1973.
42. **Lawrie, R.,** Biochemical differences between red and white muscle, *Nature (London),* 170, 122, 1952.
43. **Barrows, C. H., Yiengst, M. J., and Shock, N. W.,** Senescence and metabolism of various tissues of rats, *J. Gerontol.,* 13, 351, 1958.
44. **Gold, P., Gee, M., and Strehler, B.,** Effect of age on oxidation phosphorylation in the rat, *J. Gerontol.,* 23, 509, 1968.
45. **Honorati, M. and Ermini, M.,** Myofibrillar and mitochondrial ATPase activity of red, white diaphragmatic and cardiac muscle of young and old rats, *Experientia,* 30, 215, 1974.
46. **Grinna, L. S. and Barber, A.,** Age-related changes in membrane lipid content and enzyme activities, *Biochem. Biophys. Acta,* 288, 347, 1972.
47. **Barrows, C. H. and Roeder, L. M.,** Effect of age on protein synthesis in rats, *J. Gerontol.,* 16, 321, 1961.
48. **Williams, R. H. and Thompson, R. H.,** Effect of age upon guanyl cyclase, adenyl cyclase, and cyclic nucleotide phosphodiesterases in rats, *Proc. Soc. Exp. Biol. Med.,* 143, 382, 1973.
49. **Thompson, J., Su, C., Shih, J., Aures, D., Choi, L., Butcher, S., Loshota, W., Simon, M., and Silva, D.,** Effects of chronic nicotine administration and age on various neuro transmitters and associated enzymes in male Fischer 344 rats, *Toxicol. Appl. Pharmacol.,* 27, 41, 1974.
50. **Fuentes, J. A., Trepel, J., and Neff, N.,** Monoamine oxidase activity in the cardiovascular system of young and aged rats, *Exp. Gerontol.,* 12, 113, 1977.
51. **Chesky, J. A. and Rockstein, M.,** Reduced myocardial actomyosin adenosine triphosphatase activity in the aging male Fischer rat, *Cardiovasc. Res.,* 11, 242, 1977.
52. **Reiss, U. and Gershon, D.,** Comparison of cytoplasmic superoxide dismutase in liver, heart, and brain of aging rats and mice, *Biochem. Biophys. Res. Commun.,* 73, 255, 1976.
53. **Kirk, J. E.,** Enzyme activities of human arterial tissue, *Ann. N.Y. Acad. Sci.,* 72, 1006, 1959.
54. **Kirk, J. E.,** Enzyme chemistry of the vascular wall, in *Fundamentals of Vascular Grafting,* Weselowski, S. A. and Dennis, C., Eds., McGraw-Hill, New York, 1963, 32.
55. **Kirk, J. E.,** Enzyme activities and coenzyme concentration of human arterial tissue and their relation to age, *Gerontology,* 1, 288, 1957.
56. **Wang, I. and Kirk, J.,** The enolase activity of arterial tissues in individuals of various ages, *J. Gerontol.,* 14, 444, 1959.
57. **Kirk, J. E. and Ritz, E.,** The glyceraldehyde-3-phosphate and α-glycerophosphate dehydrogenase activities of arterial tissue in individuals of various ages, *J. Gerontol.,* 22, 427, 1967.
58. **Ritz, E. and Kirk, J. E.,** The phosphofructokinase and sorbitol dehydrogenase activities of arterial tissue in individuals of various ages, *J. Gerontol.,* 22, 433, 1967.
59. **Kirk, J. E.,** The phosphoglucomutase, phosphoglyceric acid mutase, and phosphomannose isomerase activities of arterial tissue of various ages, *J. Gerontol.,* 21, 420, 1966.
60. **Kirk, J. E.,** The 5-nucleotidase activity of human arterial tissue, *J. Gerontol.,* 14, 288, 1959.
61. **Kirk, J. E.,** The glycogen phosphorylase activity of arterial tissue in individuals of various ages, *J. Gerontol.,* 17, 154, 1962.
62. **Kirk, J. E.,** Isocitric dehydrogenase and TPN-malicenzyme activities of arterial tissue in individuals of various ages, *J. Gerontol.,* 15, 262, 1960.
63. **Kirk, J. E.,** The aconitase activity of arterial tissue in individuals of various ages, *J. Gerontol.,* 16, 25, 1961.
64. **Kirk, J. E.,** The glutamic dehydrogenase and glutathione reductase activities of arterial tissue in individuals of various ages, *J. Gerontol.,* 20, 357, 1965.

65. **Kirk, J. E.,** The leucine amino peptidase activity of arterial tissue in individuals of various ages, *J. Gerontol.*, 15, 136, 1960.
66. **Kirk, J. E.,** The glyoxolase I activity of arterial tissue in individuals of various ages, *J. Gerontol.*, 15, 139, 1960.
67. **Maier, N. and Haimovici, H.,** Metabolism of arterial tissue oxidative capacity of intact arterial tissue, *Proc. Soc. Exp. Biol. Med.*, 95, 425, 1957.
68. **Kirk, J. E.,** The diaphorase and cytochrome c reductase activities of arterial tissue in individuals of various ages, *J. Gerontol.*, 17, 276, 1962.
69. **Eisenberg, S., Stein, Y., and Stein, O.,** Phospholipases in arterial tissue. IV. The role of phosphatide acyl hydrolase, lysophosphatide acyl hydrolase, and sphingomyelin choline phosphohydrolase in the regulation of phospholipid composition in the normal human aorta with age, *J. Clin. Invest.*, 48, 2320, 1969.
70. **Kirk, J. E.,** The purine nucleoside phosphorylase activity of arterial tissue in individuals of various ages, *J. Gerontol.*, 16, 243, 1961.
71. **Platt, D.,** Interzellularstoffwechsel der Aortenwand in Abhangig — keit von Alter und Arteriosklerose, *Dtsch. Ges. Gerontol.*, 4, 171, 1970.
72. **Kirk, J. E.,** The adenyl pyrophophatase, inorganic pyrosphosphatase, and phosphomonoesterase activities of human arterial tissue in individuals of various ages, *J. Gerontol.*, 14, 181, 1959.
73. **Hermelin, B. and Pichard, J.,** Lysosomal N-acetyl-β-hexosaminidase and β-glucuronidase activities from arterial wall, *Gerontology*, 24, 405, 1978.
74. **Markkanen, T.,** Transketolase activity of red blood cells from infancy to old age, *Acta Haematol.* 42, 148, 1969.
75. **Kadlubowski, M. and Agutter, P.,** Changes in the activities of some membrane associated enzymes during *in vivo* aging of the normal human erythrocyte, *Brit. J. Haematol.*, 37, 111, 1977.
76. **Rider, J., Hodges, J., Swader, J., and Wiggins, A.,** Plasma and red cell cholinesterase in 800 healthy blood donors, *J. Lab. Clin. Med.*, 50, 376, 1957.
77. **Stern, K., Birmingham, M., Cullen, A., and Richer, R.,** Peptidase activity in leucocytes, erythrocytes, and plasma of young, adult, and senile subjects, *J. Clin. Invest.*, 30, 84, 1951.
78. **Meyer, J., Spier, E., and Neuwelt, F.,** Basal secretion of digestive enzymes in old age, *Arch. Interm. Med.*, 65, 171, 1940.
79. **Conconi, F., Manenti, F., and Benatti, G. D.,** Behavior of some enzyme activities in plasma in normal subjects in relation to age, *Acta Vitaminol.*, 17, 33, 1963.
80. **Reichard, H.,** Serumornithine transcarbarmylase activity in normal individuals, *Enzymol. Biol. Clin.*, 1, 47, 1961.
81. **Goldschmidt, L. and Whittier, J. R.,** Increase in N, N-dimethyl-p-phenylenediamine (DPP) oxidase positivity with aging in mental patients and controls, *J. Gerontol.*, 13, 132, 1958.
82. **Kayser and Legrand,** Sur l' oxydation de la para phenylene-diamine par le sérum du rat et son augmentation en fonction de l'age, *C. R. Acad. Sci. (Paris)*, 250, 1108, 1960.
83. **Robinson, D. S., Davis, J., Nies, A., Colburn, R., Bourne, H., Bunney, W., Shaw, D., and Coppen, A.,** Aging monoamine and monoamine-oxidase levels, *Lancet*, 1, 290, 1972.
84. **Sewell, S.,** Serum acid and alkaline phosphatase values in the adult male, *Am. J. Med. Sci.*, 240, 593, 1960.
85. **Clark, L. C., Beck, E. J., and Shock, N. W.,** Serum alkaline phosphatase in middle and old age, *J. Gerontol.*, 6, 7, 1951.
86. **Bertola, G. and Castellani, L.,** Cholinesterase activity of plasma in senility, *Arch. Pathol. Clin. Med.*, 13, 1577, 1957.
87. **Barrows, C. H., Shock, N. W., and Chow, B.,** Age differences in cholinesterase activity of serum and liver, *J. Gerontol.*, 13, 20, 1958.
88. **Freedman, L., Ohuchi, T., Goldstein, M., Axelrod, F., Fish, I., and Dancis, J.,** Changes in human serum dopamine β-hydroxylase activity with age, *Nature (London)*, 236, 310, 1972.
89. **Playfer, J. R., Powell, L., and Evans, D.,** Plasma paroxonase activity in old age, *Aging*, 6, 89, 1977.
90. **Resnitzky, P., Touma, M., and Danon, D.,** Neutrophilic turnover rate in human age groups evaluated by serum lysozyme activity, *Gerontology*, 24, 111, 1978.
91. **Silberberg, R., Stamp, W., Lesker, P., and Hasler, M.,** Aging changes in ultrastructure and enzymatic activity of articular cartilage of guinea pigs, *J. Gerontol.*, 25, 184, 1970.
92. **Platt, D.,** Die Bedeutung des katabolen Mucopolysaccharid-stoffwechsels in der Pathogeneses des degenerativen Rheumatisimus: in Ankylosierende Spondylitis, *Dtsch. Ges. Rheumatol.*, 1, 263, 1969.
93. **Oeriu, S.,** Research on the relation between vitamin coenzymes in relation to the age of the animal and under the influence of certain substances proper to the organism. *Biokhim.*, 28, 3, 1963.
94. **Wulf, J. and Cutler, R.,** Altered protein hypothesis of mammalian aging processes. I. Thermal stabilities of glucose-6-phosphate dehydrogenase in C57 BL/6J mouse tissue, *Exp. Gerontol.*, 10, 101, 1975.

95. **Kaur, G. and Kanungo, M.,** Alterations in glutamate dehydrogenase of the brain of rats of various ages, *Can. J. Biochem.*, 48, 203, 1970.
96. **Gibas, M. and Harman, D.,** Ribonucleic acid synthesis by nuclei isolated from rats of different ages, *J. Gerontol.*, 25, 105, 1970.
97. **Kim, S. and Paik, W.,** Age-dependent alterations of protein N- and O-methyltransferases in developing and aging brain, *Abstr. 10th Int. Congr. Gerontol.*, 2, 20, 1975.
98. **Lee, C. T. and Duerre, J. A.,** Changes in histone methylase activity of rat brain and liver with aging, *Nature (London)*, 251, 240, 1974.
99. **Kellogg, E. and Fridovich, I.,** Superoxide dismutase in the rat and mouse as a function of age and longevity, *J. Gerontol.*, 31, 405, 1976.
100. **Moudgil, V. and Kanungo, M.,** Induction of AChase by 17β-estradiol in the brain of rats of various ages, *Biochem. Biophys. Res. Commun.*, 52, 725, 1973.
101. **Epstein, M. and Barrows, C. H.,** The effects of age on the activity of glutamic acid decarboxylase in various regions of the brains of rats, *J. Gerontol.*, 24, 136, 1969.
102. **Hollander, J. and Barrows, C. H.,** Enzymatic studies in senescent rodent brains, *J. Gerontol.*, 23, 174, 1968.
103. **Walker, J. B. and Walker, J. P.,** Properties of adenylate cyclase from senescent rat brain, *Brain Res.*, 54, 391, 1973.
104. **Zimmerman, I. E. and Berg, A.,** Phosphodiesterase and adenyl cyclase activities in the cerebral cortex of the aging rat, *Mech. Ageing Dev.*, 4, 89, 1975.
105. **Koul, O. and Kanungo, M. S.,** Alterations in carbonic anhydrase of the brain of rats as a function of age, *Exp. Gerontol.*, 10, 273, 1975.
106. **Iwangoff, P., Armbruster, R., and Enz, A.,** The influence of aging on glycolytic enzymes in human and rat brain, *Experientia*, 33, 794, 1977.
107. **Brun, A. and Hultberg, B.,** Regional study of acid hydrolases and lysosomal membrane properties in the normal human brain at various ages, *Mech. Ageing Dev.*, 4, 201, 1975.
108. **Reichlmeier, K.,** Age-related changes of cyclic amp-dependent protein kinase in bovine brain, *J. Neurochem.*, 27, 1249, 1976.
109. **Reichlmeier, K., Schlecht, H. P., and Iwangoff, P.,** Enzyme activity changes in the aging human brain, *Experientia*, 33, 798, 1977.
110. **Eleftheriou, B. E.,** Regional brain catechol-o-methyl transferase age-related differences in the mouse, *Exp. Aging Res.*, 1, 99, 1975.
111. **Vijayan, N. K.,** Cholinergic enzymes in the cerebellum of the senescent mouse, *Exp. Gerontol.*, 12, 7, 1977.
112. **Hain, R. and Nutter, J.,** Cerebrospinal fluid enzymes as a function of age: its effect upon the significance of elevated values in various diseases of the nervous system, *Arch. Neurol. (Chicago)*, 2, 331, 1960.
113. **Bous, F., Hockwin, O., Ohrloff, C., and Bours, J.,** Investigations on phosphofructokinase (PFK) in bovine lenses in dependence on age, topographic distribution, and water soluble protein fractions, *Exp. Eye Res.*, 24, 383, 1977.
114. **Healy, R. and Reich, T.,** The effect of age on the carbonic anhydrase activity of bovine lenses, *J. Gerontol.*, 6, 100, 1951.
115. **Zorzoli, A.,** Enzymes and cellular metabolism, *Aging Life Processes*, Bakerman, Ed., Charles C Thomas, Springfield, 1969, 52.
116. **Sayeed, M. M. and Blumenthal, H. T.,** Age differences in the intestinal phosphomonoesterase activity of mice (33234), *Proc. Soc. Exp. Biol. Med.*, 129, 1, 1968.
117. **O'Bryan, D. and Lowenstein, L. M.,** Effect of aging on renal membrane-bound enzyme activities, *Biochem. Biophys, Acta*, 339, 1, 1974.
118. **Barrows, C. H., Falzone, J. H., and Shock, N. W.,** Age differences in the succinoxiclase activity of iromogenates and mitochondria from the livers and kidneys of rats, *J. Gerontol.*, 15, 130, 1960.
119. **Franklin, T. J.,** Activity of liver and kidney acid phosphatase at different stages in the life span of the rat, *Biochem. J.*, 79, 34, 1961.
120. **Franklin, T. J.,** The influence of age on the activity of some acid hydrolases in the rat liver and kidney, *Biochem. J.*, 82, 118, 1962.
121. **Kurnick, N. B. and Kernen, R. L.,** The effect of aging on the deoxyribose nuclease system, body and organ weight and cellular content, *J. Gerontol.*, 17, 245, 1962.
122. **Surtshin, A.,** The influence of age and renal ischemia at different levels on renal alkaline phosphatase in the rat, *J. Gerontol.*, 12, 161, 1957.
123. **Beauchene, R. E., Fanestil, D. D., and Barrows, C. H.,** The effect of age on active transport and sodium-potassium-activated ATPase activity in renal tissue of rats, *J. Gerontol.*, 20, 306, 1965.
124. **Bartoc, R., Bruhis, R., Klein, R., Moldoveanu, E., Oeriu, I., and Oeriu, S.,** Effect of age and −SH active groups on the activity of some enzymes involved in the carbohydrate metabolism, *Exp. Gerontol.*, 10, 161, 1975.

125. **Ross, M. H. and Ely, J. O.,** Aging and enzyme activity, *J. Franklin Inst.*, 285, 63, 1954.
126. **Webb, J. and Bailey, E.,** Changes in the activities of some enzymes associated with hepatic lipogenesis in the rat from weaning to old age and the effect of sucrose feeding, *Int. J. Biochem.*, 6, 813, 1975.
127. **Gershon, H. and Gershon, D.,** Inactive enzyme molecules in aging mice, *Proc. Natl. Acad. Sci.*, 70, 909, 1973.
128. **Anderson, P. J.,** The specific activity of aldolase in the livers of old and young rats, *Can. J. Biochem.*, 54, 194, 1976.
129. **Anderson, P. J.,** Aging effects on the liver aldolase of rabbits, *Biochem. J.*, 140, 341, 1974.
130. **Singhal, R. L.,** Effect of age on the induction of glucose-6-phosphatase and fructose-1,6-diphosphatase in rat liver, *J. Gerontol.*, 22, 77, 1967.
131. **Wang, R. and Mays, L.,** Opposite changes in rat liver glucose-6-phosphate dehydrogenase during aging in Sprague-Dawley and Fischer 344 male rats, *Exp. Gerontol.*, 12, 117, 1977.
132. **Zorzoli, A.,** The influence of age on mouse liver glucose-6-phosphatase activity, *J. Gerontol.*, 17, 359, 1962.
133. **Haining, J. L. and Correll, W. W.,** Turnover of tryptophan-induced tryptophan pyrrolase in rat liver as a function of age, *J. Gerontol.*, 23, 143, 1968.
134. **Gregerman, R. I.,** Adaptive enzyme responses in the senescent rat: trytophan peroxidase and tryosine transaminase, *Am. J. Physiol.*, 197, 63, 1959.
135. **Paik, W. K., Woo Lee, H., and Lawson, D.,** Age-dependency of various protein methylases, *Exp. Gerontol.*, 6, 271, 1971.
136. **Risteli, J. and Kivirikko, K. I.,** Intracellular enzymes of collagen biosynthesis in rat lines as a function of age and in hepatic injury induced by dimethylnitrosamine, *Biochem. J.*, 158, 361, 1976.
137. **Baird, M. B., Nicolos, R. J., Massie, H. R., and Samis, M. V.,** Microsomal mixed-function oxidase activity and senescence. I. Hexobarbital sleep time and induction of components of the hepatic microsomal enzyme system in rats of different ages, *Exp. Gerontol.*, 10, 89, 1975.
138. **Ferioli, M., Ceroti, G., and Comolli, R.,** Changes in rat liver ornithine decarboxylase activity during aging and effect of stimulation by dexamethasone, *Exp. Gerontol.*, 11, 153, 1976.
139. **Mays, L. L., Borek, E., and Finch, C. E.,** Glycine N-methyltransferase is a regulatory enzyme which increases in aging animals, *Nature (London)*, 243, 411, 1973.
140. **Zorzoli, A.,** The influence of age on mouse liver acid and alkaline phosphatase, *J. Gerontol.*, 6, 171, 1951.
141. **Elens, A. and Wattiaux, R.,** Age-correlated changes in lysosomal enzyme activities: an index of aging? *Exp. Gerontol.*, 4, 131, 1969.
142. **Zorzoli, A.,** The influence of age on phosphatase activity in the liver of the mouse, *J. Gerontol.*, 10, 156, 1955.
143. **Barrows, C. H., Roeder, L. M., and Falzone, J. A.,** Effect of age on the activities of enzymes and the concentrations of nucleic acids, *J. Gerontol.*, 17, 144, 1962.
144. **Read, S. F. and McKinley, W. P.,** A comparison of the esterases in liver and kidney homogenates, *J. Assoc. Off. Agric. Chem.*, 46, 863, 1963.
145. **Gandhi, B. S. and Kanungo, M.,** Effect of cortisone on monoamine oxidase of the liver of young and old rats, *Ind. J. Biochem. Biophys.*, 11, 102, 1974.
146. **Traurig, H. H.,** Lysosomal acid hydrolase activities in the lungs of fetal, neonatal, adult, and senile mice, *Gerontology*, 22, 419, 1976.
147. **Schmukler, M. and Barrows, C. H., Jr.,** Age differences in lactic and malic dehydrogenase in the rat, *J. Gerontol.*, 21, 109, 1966.
148. **Steinhagen-Thiessen, E. and Hilz, H.,** The age-dependent decrease in creative kinase and aldolase activities in human striated muscle is not caused by an accumulation of faulty proteins, *Mech. Ageing Dev.*, 5, 447, 1976.
149. **Rockstein, M. and Brandt, K. F.,** Changes in the phosphorus metabolism of the gastrocnemius muscle in aging white rats, *Proc. Soc. Exp. Biol. Med.*, 107, 377, 1961.
150. **Kaldor, G. and Min, B.,** Enzymatic studies on the skeletal myocin A and actomocsin of aging rats, *Fed. Proc.*, 34, 191, 1975.
151. **Necheles, H., Plotke, F., and Meyer, J.,** Studies on old age. V. Active pancreatic secretion in the aged. *Am. J. Dig. Dis.*, 9, 157, 1942.
152. **Meyer, J., Golden, J., Steiner, N., and Necheles, H.,** The ptyalin content of human saliva in old age, *Am. J. Physiol.*, 119, 600, 1937.
153. **Loewen, W. A. and Baldwin, M.,** Elastolytic enzymes and elastin in the aging rat. I. Pancreatic elastolytic enzymes, *Gerontologia*, 17, 170, 1971.
154. **Mainwaring, W. I. P.,** The aging process in the mouse ventral prostate gland: a preliminary biochemical survey, *Gerontologia*, 13, 177, 1967.
155. **Grayhack, J. T. and Kropp, K.,** Changes with aging in prostatic fluid; citric acid, acid phosphatase; and lactic dehydrogenase concentration in man, *J. Urol.*, 93, 258, 1965.

156. **Kirk, J. E.,** The acid phosphatase concentration of the prostatic fluid in young, middle-aged, and old individuals, *J. Gerontol.*, 3, 98, 1948.
157. **Anttinen, H., Oikarinen, A., and Kivirikko, K. I.,** Age-related changes in human skin collagen galactosyltransferase and collagen glucosyltransferase activities, *Clin. Chim. Acta*, 76, 95, 1977.
158. **Slonim, A. and Bedrak, E.,** Activity of enzymes associated with the biosynthesis of testosterone by gonads of the old mouse, *Exp. Gerontol.*, 12, 35, 1977.
159. **Urry, R., Dougherty, K., and Ellis, L.,** Alterations with age in rat seminiferous tubule monoamine oxidase activity when compared with whole testicular tissue, *Proc. Soc. Exp. Biol. Med.*, 148, 805, 1975.
160. **Birmingham, M. K. and Grad, B.,** Peptidase activity in the thymus of a normal and a leukemic strain of mice during growth and aging, *Cancer Res.*, 14, 352, 1954.
161. **Knook, D. L.,** personal communication.

CROSS-LINKING OF MACROMOLECULES

J. H. Waite and M. L. Tanzer

INTRODUCTION

Definitions

Proteins, polysaccharides, and polynucleotides are common biological macromolecules if one accepts a macromolecule as having a molecular weight greater than 10,000[1]. A macromolecular cross-link is a chemical entity that mediates the covalent association of at least two macromolecules. The formation of cross-links in biological systems is spontaneous or enzyme-catalyzed, but cross-links can also be induced by radiation or the presence of bifunctional agents. Here, we shall describe well-characterized cross-links that occur in proteins, polysaccharides, and polynucleotides of animals; those that covalently unite fully synthesized macromolecules. Excluded are linkages between proteins and carbohydrates, e.g., the protein moiety serves as an initiation point for the assembly of polysaccharides.

Function

By its nature, a cross-link confers stability to macromolecules, but it also confines them by diminishing their relative relative dynamic mobility, and hence, potential entropy. This is the double-edged blade of cross-linking. It is reasonable to speculate that cross-links have been evolved and widely exploited by organisms to confer upon the macromolecules of supporting and protecting structures those properties that are best suited to coping with the stresses of function, habitat, and life history.[2] More or less than optimal cross-linking in a cross-linked network of macromolecules could produce undesirable or inferior structural properties that might ultimately contribute to the death of the organism. The *de novo* induction of cross-links in functionally uncross-linked macromolecules is likely to have an even more drastic effect on the organism. A knowledge about the abundance and types of cross-links in macromolecular structures can thus provide important insights into the relationship of structure to function in animals, and the effects of age on these parameters.

Identification

The present *modus operandi* for determining the presence of cross-links in biological materials is arbitrary and presumptive. One chooses a solvent or series of solvents in which macromolecules are known to be soluble and by which they are denatured, but not degraded. Examples of such solvents are 8 *M* urea, 6 *M* guanidine hydrochloride, weak acid or alkali, concentrated salt solutions, phenol, detergents, etc. Materials resisting solubilization in these are assumed to be stabilized by covalent cross-links. Solubility of macromolecules in these solvents, however, does not necessarily imply the absence of cross-links. This is particularly true of interstrand cross-links in DNA or protein-DNA cross-links which may affect the solubility of the macromolecules only slightly. For details concerning the isolation of cross-links from particular macromolecules, it is necessary to consult specific papers in the cited literature.

In contrast to the solubility considerations, the chemical identification of a new structure (such as a cross-link) is rigorous and comprehensive. To be truly convincing, the characterization of a macromolecular cross-link should include the following: (1) preparation by two different routes of hydrolysis, (2) purification to homogeneity, (3) demonstrated identity with a synthetic compound using physical and chemical criteria such as mass spectra, NMR, IR and UV absorbance, chromatography, etc., (4) biosynthesis from known precursors, and (5) isolation of the cross-linked region after extensive enzymatic digestion. Unfortunately, the last criterion can not yet be met in cross-linked macromolecules completely resistant to known degradative enzymes.

Background

The history of the study of macromolecular cross-links in animals has until very recent years been largely an exercise in hopeless frustration. In 1950, Brown[3] reviewed protein stabilizing forces and mentioned only two covalent cross-links — the disulfide bond and the quinone cross-link. Initial progress in the chemistry of disulfides was largely the product of keratin research[4,5] and has since contributed immensely to the biochemistry of proteins in general. The quinone cross-link, on the other hand, remains putative and has never been isolated or characterized. In the 1960s, great strides were made by the identification of cross-links in the insoluble proteins, elastin and resilin.[6,7] Further advances were made possible by the application of sodium borohydride reduction and isotope labeling techniques to the labile cross-links in collagen and elastin.[8,9] Total enzymatic digestion of macromolecules has enabled the isolation of labile cross-links in proteins and polynucleotides.[10,11] At present, about 20 naturally occurring cross-links have been identified in biological macromolecules. Several more can be induced in vivo by radiation or bifunctional chemicals. In the following tables and text, we shall describe the properties, chemical basis, abundance, precursors, and stability of biological cross-links that have been characterized in the literature. Although we have limited the scope of this review to cross-links in macromolecules of animal origin, bacterial and viral cross-links are also mentioned wherever relevant.

TYPES OF CROSS-LINKS

Protein-Protein Cross-Links

Collagen and Elastin Cross-links

The connective tissue proteins, collagen and elastin, are synthesized as monomeric molecules which polymerize in the extracellular regions. The polymeric forms become cross-linked once the enzyme lysyl oxidase[12] has catalyzed the conversion of specific ε-NH_2 groups into aldehydes. In elastin the majority of the ε-NH_2 groups become aldehydes,[13] while in collagen only two or three aldehydes per molecule are formed, predominantly from lysines and hydroxylysines near the NH_2- and COOH-termini.[14] Structures cross-linking these molecules are specified in Table 1 (numbers 1, 2, 6, 7, and 10 through 19).

Lysyl oxidase is essential for cross-linking of elastin and collagen; irreversible inhibition of the enzyme by lathrogens such as β-aminopropionitrile causes connective tissue fragility and rupture.[15] Lysyl oxidase deficiency can also be produced by a copper-free diet; the enzyme requires Cu^{++} for activity. Lysyl oxidase binds avidly to collagen and elastin, and may be added to these proteins as they emerge from the cell. Progressive catalysis by lysyl oxidase may occur in the substrate polymers since these polymers can initially be solubilized under mild conditions, and the soluble forms contain lesser amounts of cross-links and aldehydes.

Once aldehydes are formed in collagen and elastin, cross-linking appears to occur spontaneously, involving the aldehydes and unconverted ε-NH_2 groups of lysines or hydroxylysines (in collagen) as well as the imidazole of histidine (in collagen).[16] Two general classes of compounds are formed, those which are reducible with borohydride (BH_4) and related compounds, and those which cannot be reduced. Some of these latter substances are viewed as "permanent" or "final" cross-links, especially in collagen. However, reducibility is not necessarily a criterion of instability since the desmoisines of elastin (Table 1, numbers 1 and 16) which are quite stable, can be reduced with BH_4.[17]

Table 1
CROSS-LINKS IN PROTEINS

	Postulated structure	Molecular[a] weight	Trivial name	Systematic name[b]	Structural evidence
1. 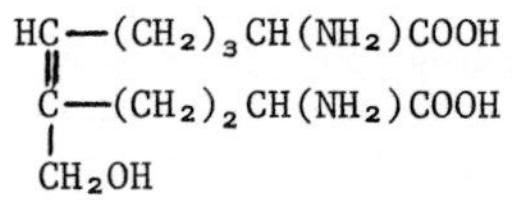	HC—(CH₂)₃CH(NH₂)COOH ‖ C—(CH₂)₂CH(NH₂)COOH │ CH₂OH	274.32	Aldol condensation product	2,10-Diamino-5-(hydroxymethyl)-5-undecenedioic acid	Mass spectra, derivatives (ethylester and periodate),
2. 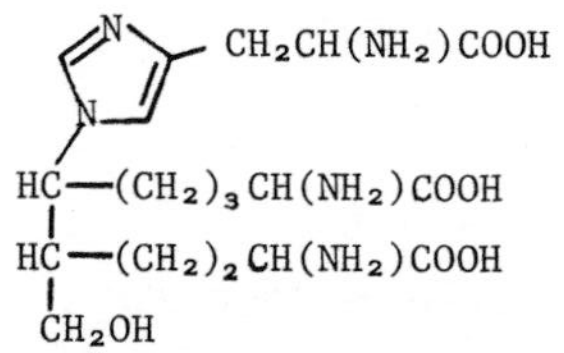	(imidazole ring, N) CH₂CH(NH₂)COOH; N—HC—(CH₂)₃CH(NH₂)COOH │ HC—(CH₂)₂CH(NH₂)COOH │ CH₂OH	429.49	Aldol histidine	2,10-Diamino-6-(N^3-histidinyl)-5-(hydroxymethyl)-undecanedioic acid	Mass spectra, derivatives (permethyl acetyl ester, trifluoroacetyl methyl ester), ^{1}H-NMR, UV, cross-linked
3. 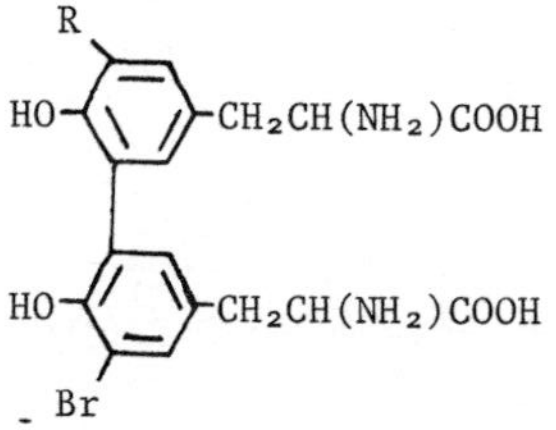	R; HO—(ring)—CH₂CH(NH₂)COOH │ HO—(ring)—CH₂CH(NH₂)COOH; Br	439.6 (R = H) 518.2 (R = Br)	Bromodityrosine	3,3′-5-Bromo-bityrosine 3,3′; 5,5′-Dibromo-bityrosine	Mass spectra, derivatives (acetyl methyl ester), UV spectrum, fluorescence, synthesis, chromatography[49]
4. 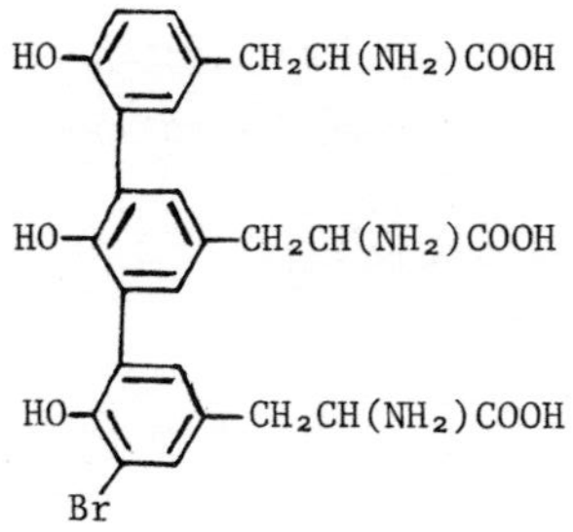	HO—(ring)—CH₂CH(NH₂)COOH │ HO—(ring)—CH₂CH(NH₂)COOH │ HO—(ring)—CH₂CH(NH₂)COOH; Br	629.5	Bromotrityrosine	3,3′; 5′,3″; 5-bromo-tertyrosine	Mass spectra, derivatives (acetyl methyl ester), UV spectrum, fluorescence, chromatography[49]

Table 1 (continued)
CROSS-LINKS IN PROTEINS

	Postulated structure	Molecular[a] weight	Trivial name	Systematic name[b]	Structural evidence
5.	$S-CH_2CH(NH_2)COOH$ / $S-CH_2CH(NH_2)COOH$ (S–S bonded)	240.29	Cystine	2,2′-Diamino-3,3′-dithio-bis (propionic acid)	Derivatives, IR spectrum; synthesis, crystallization,
6.	Pyridinium ring (N⁺) bearing $(CH_2)_3CH(\overset{+}{N}H_3)COO^-$, $(CH_2)_2CH(\overset{+}{N}H_3)COO^-$, $(\overset{+}{N}H_3)CH(COO^-)(CH_2)_2$–, and on N: $(CH_2)_4CH(NH_2)COO^-$	879.43	Desmosine	4-(4-Amino-4-carboxybutyl)-1-(5-amino-5-carboxypentyl)-3, 5-bis (3-amino-3-carboxy propyl) pyridinium	Elemental analysis, UV absorption, ^{1}H-NMR, synthetic analogues, biosynthesis, cross-linked peptides, chromatography, fluorescence[6,163-168]
7.	$HN<$ ($CH_2CHOH(CH_2)_2CH(NH_2)COOH$)$_2$	307.35	Dihydroxylysinonorleucine	N^6-(5-Amino-5-carboxy-2-hydroxypentyl)-5-hydroxylysine	Mass spectra, derivatives (isobutoxycarbonyl permethylester; trifluoroacetyl methyl ester), synthesis, chromatography, cross-linked peptide[171-172,174]

	Abundance[c]	Proposed precursors	Stability	Misc.
1.	Elastin: mature bovine (4—5), chick embryo aorta (5—7),[153] collagen: chick skin[154,155] rat skin (4 residues per 10^5 mol wt	α-Amino-adipic acid δ-semialdehyde, twice; spontaneous reaction	Reduced aldehyde; stable in 2 N NaOH	BH_4-reduced aldehyde; intramolecular cross-link in β_{12} collagen[154,155]
2.	Collagen: bovine skin, tendon, bone, basement membrane, ovine basement membrane	Aldol condensation product and histidine,[156] spontaneous reaction	Reduced aldehyde stable to 3 M HC1	No reaction with Pauly reagent; BH_4-reduced aldehyde[156]

3. Exocuticle, crab[49]	Tyrosine (×2); bromine; peroxidase-catalyzed	6 N HCl, 110°C	λ^{pH2}_{max} = 286 nm (R = H)[49] λ^{pH11}_{max} = 319 nm λ^{pH2}_{max} = 288 nm (R = Br) λ^{pH11}_{max} = 319 nm
4. Exocuticle, crab[49]	Tyrosine; dityrosine, bromine; peroxidase-catalyzed	6 N HCl, 110°C	λ^{pH2}_{max} = 288 nm[49] λ^{pH11}_{max} = 319 nm
5. Collagen: *Ascaris* cuticle (27),[58] Type III,[59] basement membrane,[60] procollagen,[61] collagen-acetylcholinesterase(161); keratin: mohair wool (96), human hair (163), rabbit (137), seal fur (149), red kangaroo (123), koala (117), platypus (136), echidna (157),[57] Erythrocyte membrane: protein[162]	Cysteine (×2); spontaneous reaction	Alkali-labile; reduced to -SH by thioglycollic acid; oxidized to cysteic acid by performic acid	Highest sulfur-containing protein in keratin fiber matrix[57]
6. Elastin: aortae of rabbit (4.2),[169] pig (1.3), swan (1.3), turtle (1,2), frog (1.0), lung-fish (0.5), coelocanth (1.1), sturgeon (0.9), gar (1.0), cod (0.3), hammerhead (1.7),[170] human (2.1),[55] bovine lung, ligamentum nuchae mature (3), calf (2.25), fetus (1.5);[167] absent in invertebrates and cyclostomes[170]	Lysine and α-amino adipic acid-δ-semialdehyde (×3); spontaneous reaction[167,168]	6 N HCl, 100°C; BH_4-reducible; cleaved by permanganate and alkali ferricyanide	λ^{pH2}_{max} = 235; 269 nm (ε = 4900 M^{-1} cm^{-1}) λ^{pH11}_{max} = 237; 270 nm[6,163] λ_{max} (emission) = 350/420 λ_{max} (excitation) = 280/305
7. Collagen: bovine skin, tendon, scalpula dentin, basement membrane, cartilage; chick tendon, bone, cartilage; human bone, dentin, skin; guinea pig skin; cod fish, skin, scales, swim bladder; sea urchin body wall; sea cucumber body wall; sponge; dogfish elastoidin; earthworm cuticle[16]	Hydroxylysine and δ-hydroxy-α-amino adipic acid δ-semialdehyde; spontaneous reaction[171]	Reduced Schiff base is acid stable; cleaved by periodate; unreduced compound stable to heat 2 min, 70°C; dilute acids, α-amino-β-thiols	BH_4-reduced; may occur as O-glycosylated form[173]

Table 1 (continued)
CROSS-LINKS IN PROTEINS

	Postulated structure	Molecular[a] weight	Trivial name	Systematic name[b]	Structural evidence
8.	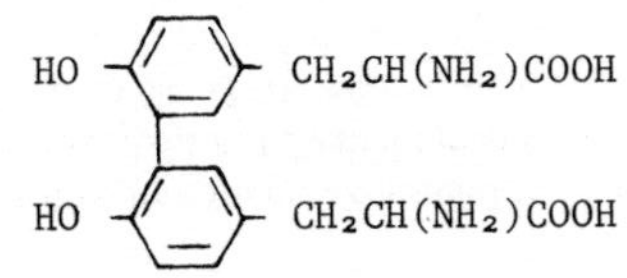 HO–(benzene ring)–$CH_2CH(NH_2)COOH$ / HO–(benzene ring)–$CH_2CH(NH_2)COOH$	360.4	Dityrosine	3,3′-Bityrosine	Mass spectra, derivative (acetyl methyl ester), UV and IR absorption; synthesis, fluorescence, chromatography[7,33,79,175]
9.	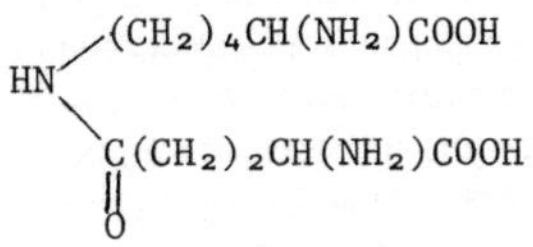 HN<$(CH_2)_4CH(NH_2)COOH$ / $C(=O)(CH_2)_2CH(NH_2)COOH$	275.31	ε(γ-Glutamyl)-lysine	N^6-(4-Amino-4 carboxy-1-oxobutyl) lysine	Synthesis, cross-linked peptide, chromatography, biosynthesis[10,23,180-182]
10.	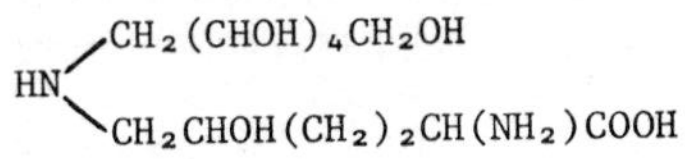 HN<$CH_2(CHOH)_4CH_2OH$ / $CH_2CHOH(CH_2)_2CH(NH_2)COOH$	326.35	N^ϵ-Hexosylhydroxylysine	N^6-(2,3,4,5,6-pentahydroxyhexyl)5-hydroxylysine	Mass spectra, derivatives (acetyl, permethyl; isobutyloxy carbonyl, permethyl), synthesis, chromatography[113]
11.	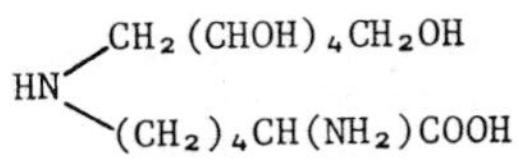 HN<$CH_2(CHOH)_4CH_2OH$ / $(CH_2)_4CH(NH_2)COOH$	310.35	N^ϵ-Hexosylysine	N^6-(2,3,4,5,6-pentahydroxyhexyl) lysine	Mass spectra, derivative (trifluoroacetyl methyl ester), synthesis, chromatography[114]
12.	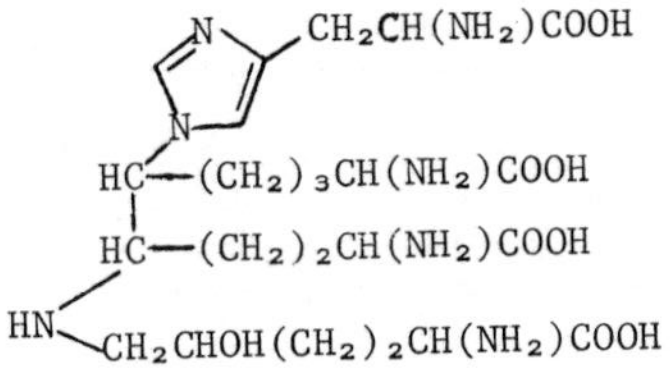 (imidazole ring)–$CH_2CH(NH_2)COOH$; N–HC–$(CH_2)_3CH(NH_2)COOH$; HC–$(CH_2)_2CH(NH_2)COOH$; HN–$CH_2CHOH(CH_2)_2CH(NH_2)COOH$	573.65	Histidino-hydroxymero desmosine	2,10-Diamino-6-(N^3-histidinyl)-5-[[(2-hydroxy-5-amino-5-carboxy pentyl) amino]methyl] undecanedioic acid	Mass spectra, derivatives (acetyl, permethyl; trifluoroacetyl methyl ester; pentafluoropropionyl methyl ester) ^1H- and ^{13}C-NMR, chromatography[156,193,194]

	Structure		Name	Chemical name	Identification
13.	$CH_2CHOH(CH_2)_2CH(NH_2)COOH$ | $C—(CH_2)_2CH(NH_2)COOH$ ‖ CH | N-imidazole ring — $CH_2CH(NH_2)COOH$	427.5	Hydroxyaldol-histidine	2,10-Diamino-5-[(N^3-histidinyl)methylene]-7-hydroxy-undecanedioic acid	Mass spectra, derivative (trifluoroacetyl methyl ester), ^{1}H-NMR, cross-linked peptide, chromatography[195]
14.	$HC—(CH_2)_3CH(NH_2)COOH$ ‖ $CH_2—C—(CH_2)_2CH(NH_2)COOH$ | $HN—CH_2CHOH(CH_2)_2CH(NH_2)COOH$	418.5	Hydroxymerodesmosine	2,10-Diamino-5-[(2-hydroxy-5-amino-5- pentyl) amino]methyl-6-undecanedioic acid	Mass spectra, derivative (trifluoroacetyl methyl ester), chromatography[196]

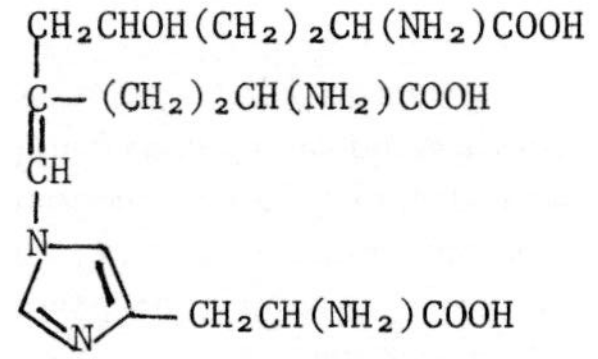

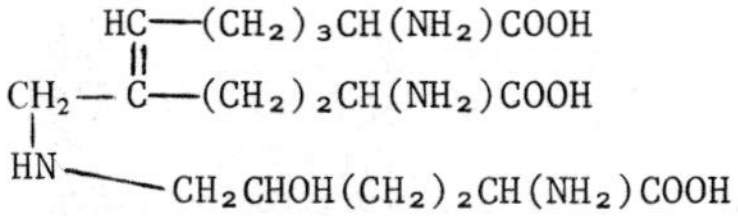

	Abundance[c]	Proposed precursors	Stability	Misc.
8.	Resilin (7.7);[7] wool keratin (1),[48] elastin acidic protein (6);[176,177] tussah silk (10);[48] adhesive protein-byssus (25.5);[45,46] egg cases: dragon fly,[38] trematode,[47] fruit fly,[178] sea urchin (6); [41, 42] bovine skin collagen (1)[53] crab carapace,[79] *Ascaris* cuticulin (3 mol/mol protein),[179] cataractous lens protein (human)[43, 44]	Tyrosine (×2); peroxidase[7,41,42] tyrosinase-catalyzed[38]	6 N HC1, 100°C; NaOH; nonreducible with BH_4	λ^{pH2}_{max} = 283.5 nm (ε = 5400 M^{-1} cm^{-1}) 293 nm (ε = 5340) λ^{pH11}_{max} = 316; λ^{borate}_{max} = 252; 292[7,175] Fluorescence: emission λ_{max} = 410 nm, excitation λ^{pH2}_{max} = 290 nm; λ^{pH11}_{max} = 320 nm

Table 1 (continued)
CROSS-LINKS IN PROTEINS

	Abundance[c]	Proposed precursors	Stability	Misc.
9.	Fibrin: bovine, human, monkey (3—5.2 mol/mol protein);[31,181,182] fibrinogen: lobster (3 mol/mol protein)[183] seminal fluid clot (43.5)[25] hair medulla protein (13),[184] cornified skin protein (1 mol/mol protein),[185] spines, echidna, porcupine (2—10),[186] wool keratin (15 μmol/g),[187] cell proteins:[189] fibroblasts,[30] *Paramecium aurelia Physarum polycephalum*,[188] spectrin,[26,190] myosin;[191] fibronectin;[127] egg capsule (gastropod);[192] bovine colostrum[29]	Lysine and glutamine: transglutamidase-catalyzed[22] (fibroligase)	Acid- alkali-labile; nonreducible with BH_4	Prepared by enzymatic digestion of proteins; detectable as fraction of lysines unreactive to acrylonitrile,[181] often formed as artefact in denatured proteins[28]
10.	Collagen: insoluble calf skin and nasal cartilage[113]	Hexose and hydroxylysine; spontaneous reaction[113]	Reduced compound stable; destroyed by periodate	BH_4-reduced Schiff base; identity of hexose epimers not yet known; possibly a cross-link between proteoglycans and collagen[113]
11.	Collagen: bovine skin[114]	Hexose and lysine; spontaneous reaction[114]	Reduced compound stable to 6 N HCl, 110°C; destroyed by periodate	BH_4-reduced Schiff base; hexoses may be mannose and glucose; possibly a cross-link between proteoglycans and collagen[114]
12.	Collagen: bovine skin, tendon, cartilage, cornea; rabbit selera, cornea; rat skin, tendon; chick skin, tendon; mouse fibroblasts; human bone, skin; guinea pig skin; fish skin, scales; dogfish elastoidin[16]	Hydroxylysine, histidine, aldol condensation product; spontaneous reactions[16]	Reduced compound stable to 6 N HCl, 107°C; unstable to NH_4OH and periodate; Schiff base is acid-labile	BH_4-reduced Schiff base; not abundant in bone

13. Collagen: bovine skin (mature), calf skin[195]	Histidine, α-amino adipic acid-δ-semialdehyde, α-amino-δ-hydroxyadipic acid-δ-semialdehyde; spontaneous reactions[195]	Stable to 6 N HCl, 108°C	not BH_4-reducible
14. Collagen: calf skin, basement membrane; sheep basement membrane[196]	Hydroxylysine, aldol condensation product; spontaneous reactions[196]	Reduced compound stable to 6 M HCl, 107°C; unstable to NH_4OH and periodate; Schiff base is acid-labile	BH_4-reduced Schiff base

	Postulated structure	Molecular[a] weight	Trivial name	Systematic name[b]	Structural evidence
15.	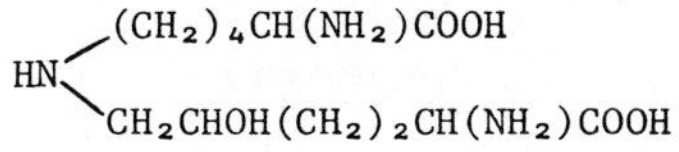 HN<(CH₂)₄CH(NH₂)COOH / CH₂CHOH(CH₂)₂CH(NH₂)COOH	291.35	Hydroxylysinonorleucine	N^6-(5-Amino-5-carboxypentyl)-5-hydroxylysine	Mass spectra, derivatives (trifluoroacetyl, methyl ester; acetyl, permethyl ester), synthesis, chromatography, cross-linked peptide[174,197,198]
16.	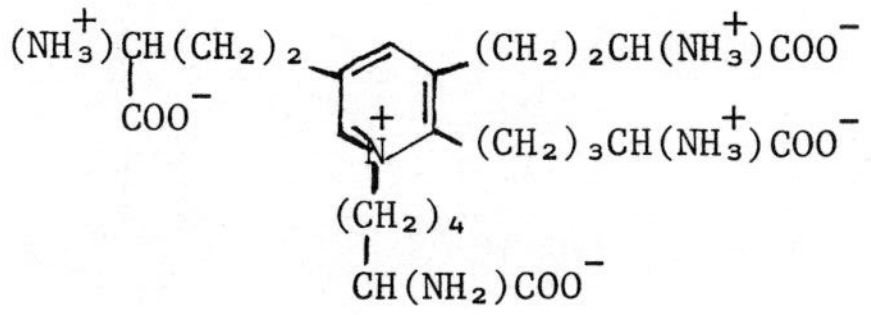 $(\overset{+}{N}H_3)CH(COO^-)(CH_2)_2$– pyridinium ring with $(CH_2)_2CH(\overset{+}{N}H_3)COO^-$, $(CH_2)_3CH(\overset{+}{N}H_3)COO^-$, and N-$(CH_2)_4CH(NH_2)COO^-$	879.43	Isodesmosine	2-(4-Amino-4-carboxybutyl)-1-(5- amino-5-carboxypentyl)-3,5-bis(3-amino-3-carboxypropyl) pyridinium	Elemental analysis, UV absorption, synthetic analogues, biosynthesis, ^1H-NMR; cross-linked peptides[10, 163-168]
17.	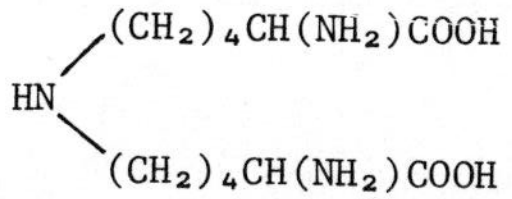 HN<(CH₂)₄CH(NH₂)COOH / (CH₂)₄CH(NH₂)COOH	275.35	Lysinonorleucine	N^6-(5-Amino-5-carboxypentyl) lysine	Mass spectra, derivatives (acetyl, permethyl); chromatography, ^1H-NMR; chromatography[199-203]
18.	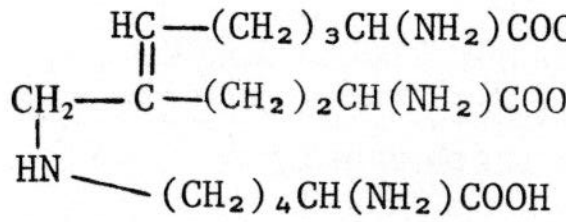 HC—(CH₂)₃CH(NH₂)COOH ‖ CH₂—C—(CH₂)₂CH(NH₂)COOH; CH₂—HN—(CH₂)₄CH(NH₂)COOH	402.5	Merodesmosine	2,10-Diamino-5-[(5-amino-5-carboxypentyl) amino methyl] 6-undecenedioic acid	Mass spectra; derivatives (trifluoroacetyl, methyl ester; tributyl, ethyl ester), IR absorbance, ^1H-NMR, chromatography[204]

Table 1 (continued)
CROSS-LINKS IN PROTEINS

	Postulated structure	Molecular[a] weight	Trivial name	Systematic name[b]	Structural evidence
19.	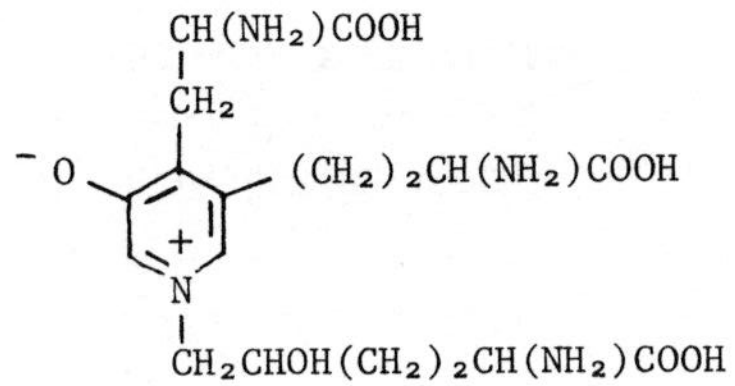 $CH(NH_2)COOH$ – CH_2 – pyridinium ring (^-O, $(CH_2)_2CH(NH_2)COOH$, N^+–$CH_2CHOH(CH_2)_2CH(NH_2)COOH$)	429	Pyridinoline	4-(2-Amino-2-carboxyethyl)-3-(3-amino-3-carboxypropyl)-5-hydroxy-1-(2-hydroxy-5-amino-5-carboxypentyl) pyridinium	Mass spectra; derivative (trifluoroacetyl methyl ester); ^{1}H-NMR, ^{13}C-NMR, ^{13}C-NMR, IR; UV absorbance, chromatography, synthetic analogoes, cross-linked peptide[205-207]
20.	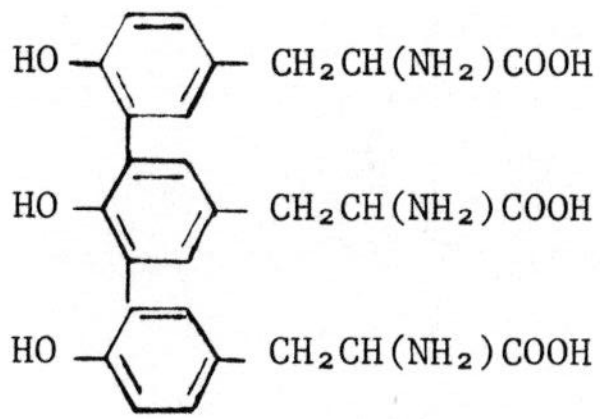 HO–(ring)–$CH_2CH(NH_2)COOH$ / HO–(ring)–$CH_2CH(NH_2)COOH$ / HO–(ring)–$CH_2CH(NH_2)COOH$	540.6	Trityrosine	3,3′;5′,3″-tertyrosine	Mass spectra; derivatives (acetyl, methyl ester), UV absorbance; chromatography, synthesis, fluorescence, titration[7,33,79,175]

	Abundance[c]	Proposed precursors	Stability	Misc.
15.	Collagen: bovine tendon, scapula, skin, cartilage, cornea, dentin; chick bone, tendons; human bone, cartilage, skin; rat tendon, skin; codfish scales, swimbladder; dogfish elastoidin; earthworm cuticle, sea urchin body wall; sponge[16]	Hydroxylysine and α-amino-adipic acid-δ-semialdehyde, or lysine and α-amino-δ-hydroxyadipic acid-δ-semialdehyde; spontaneous reactions[198]	Reduced compound stable to 6 M HCl, 110°C; cleaved by periodate	BH_4-reduced Schiff base; may occur as O-glycosylated form[173]

16. Elastin: aorta rabbit (2.8), pig (1.9), swan (1.8), turtle (1.5), frog (1.0), lungfish (0.7), coelacanth (1.1), sturgeon (0.9), gar (1.0), cod (0.3), hammerhead (1.9) 170; human aorta (1.1), pleura (1.0)[55]; bovine lung (3); ligamentum michae (3), fetal (1.5), calf (2.25;[167] absent in invertebrates and cyclostomes[170]	Lysine and α-amino adipic acid δ-semialdehyde (×3); [167,168] spontaneous reactions	6 N HC1, 100°C; BH_4-reducible	λ^{pH2}_{max} = 280 nm (ε = 7850 M^{-1} cm^{-1}) λ^{pH11}_{max} = 282 nm[10,163]
17. Collagen: bovine tendon, scapula, skin, nasal cartilage, basement membrane; human skin; mouse fibroblasts; rabbit selera, cornea; rat tendon skin; sponge; fish scales and swim bladder; dogfish elastoidin,[16] elastin: bovine lung (mature) (1), embryonic (1.7); rabbit aorta (1.2); human aorta (1.3)[55]	Lysine and α-amino-adipic acid-δ-semialdehyde; spontaneous reactions	Reduced compound stable to 6 N HC1, 110°C; unreduced, acid-labile	BH_4-reduced Schiff base in collagen; in elastin, reduced form occurs naturally; reduced/unreduced = 3[200]
18. Elastin: bovine ligamentum nuchae (0.25), visceral pleura; duck aorta; naturally reduced in bovine ligamentum nuchae: mature (0.1), calf (0.8)[204]	Lysine and aldol condensation compound; spontaneous reactions[204]	Reduced compound is acid-, alkali-stable; unreduced is acid-labile	BH_4-reduced Schiff base; reduced/unreduced (in elastin) = 1; [204] unreduced not found in collagen
19. Collagen: rat tendon (0.02); costal cartilage (0.15); bovine achilles tendon (0.16); human (20 years) costal cartilage (0.2); tendon (0.2); varies widely with animal and age[19]	Hydroxylysine and α-amino-δ-hydroxyadipic acid-δ-semialdehyde (×2); spontaneous reactions[207]	Stable to 6 N HCl, 110°C; unstable in water under air 110°C, 24 hr[207]	Nonreducible with BH_4; fluorescent $\lambda_{max}{}^{(exc)}{}_{(em)}$ = ${}^{295\ nm}{}_{395\ nm}$; λ^{pH2} = 295 nm (ε = 8300 M^{-1} cm^{-1}), λ^{pH11}_{max} = 325 nm
20. Resilin (3.9); [7] adhesive protein-byssus; (13.9)[46] crab exocuticle;[79] sea urchin egg case[42]	Tyrosine (×3); peroxidase-tyrosinase-catalyzed[7,41,42]	Stable to 6 N HC1, 110°C	λ^{pH2}_{max} = 286 nm (ε = 8000; 9000 M^{-1} cm^{-1}) λ^{pH10}_{max} = 322; 315 nm; λ^{borate}_{max} = 292 nm; fluorescent[7,175]

[a] Assumed to be anhydrous.
[b] According to nomenclature proposed by IUPAC-IUB commision.[152]
[c] Numbers without units in parentheses correspond to residues per 1000.

Most of the original lysines in elastin become cross-linked while the majority of the lysines and hydroxylysines in collagen are not involved in cross-linking reactions. With age, the collagen polymer becomes progressively insoluble and the population of reducible cross-links diminishes.[18] Although a reciprocal increase in stable cross-links has been postulated during aging, this postulate has not been directly proven. In the best documented case, pyridinoline (Table 1, number 19) content of collagen in rat costal cartilage and achilles tendon increases with age while it diminishes in the same human collagens after mid-life (about 40 years).[19] Adult bovine tendons do not appear to change their content of cross-linked peptides with age, suggesting that the maximum density of cross-linking develops by adulthood.[20] Elastin cross-linking seems to develop more rapidly than collagen cross-linking since elastin is insoluble at most ages except for a small soluble proportion in embryonic tissues.

Information has been garnered concerning the locations of cross-links in elastin and collagen; the primary structures of cross-linked peptides from both proteins have been reported. In the case of elastin, the desmosines and isodesmosines bridge across two polypeptide chains;[21] the other elastin cross-links have not been located. In the case of collagen, the reduced Schiff-base cross-links have been localized in several different peptides. Most of the peptides originate from bridges between the collagen helix and the NH_2- or COOH-terminal regions.[14] The composite picture supports the "quarter stagger" packing mode of collagen monomers in the collagen polymer; eventually it may be possible to construct a detailed map of molecular packing in the highly organized collagen polymer. Since elastin seems to be organized in a more random fashion, it is not likely that a similar type of map will be obtained.

In summary, we may conclude that the chemistry of collagen and elastin maturation has taken a significant leap forward in the past decade. We may optimistically expect that future studies will elucidate the details of both lysyl oxidase catalysis and cross-link location and the means by which cross-link structure develops and changes with age.

Proteins with ε-(γ-Glutamyl) Lysine Cross-Links

ε-(γ-Glutamyl) lysine cross-links (Table 1, number 9) have been detected throughout the phylogenetic scale and in many different types of proteins. The compound was first isolated from enzymatically digested bovine fibrin clots.[10] Its formation in blood is catalyzed by the thrombin-activated blood coagulation factor XIII, also called fibroligase, transglutamidase, and endo-γ-glutamine: ε-lysine transferase.[22,23] It is a calcium-requiring enzyme which transfers the ε-NH_2 groups of particular lysine residues of one fibrin molecule to specific glutaminyl residues of another, thus forming an isopeptide-bonded polymeric network. Fibroligases are also present in other tissues and fluids where ε-(γ-glutamyl) lysine cross-links are formed, such as in skin,[24] seminal fluid,[25] and membrane proteins.[26, 27] Asquith et al.,[28] however, have cautioned that the cross-link is known to arise spontaneously in some heat-denatured proteins. ε-(γ-Glutamyl) lysine is a highly labile cross-link. It is not reduced with borohydride, but destroyed by treatment with acid and alkali. It can be directly detected after extensive proteolysis of cross-linked protein, or indirectly by amino acid analysis before and after cyanoethylation of free lysines. We note that a preliminary report of β-aspartyl-ε-lysine in insoluble bovine colostrum has appeared.[29]

No conclusive evidence regarding the formation of this cross-link and aging has been reported. However, variations from normal cross-linking frequencies have been demonstrated in transformed lung fibroblasts.[30] Defects in cross-link formation have also been implicated in hyaline membrane disease, thrombosis, atherosclerosis,[31] and bronchial sputum.[32]

Proteins with Dityrosine Cross-Links

Dityrosine is a versatile protein cross-link which occurs throughout the animal kingdom (Table 1, numbers 3, 4, 8, and 20). It was first isolated by Andersen[7,33] from the protein resilin, a component of the wing hinge of locusts. The compound is quite stable, fluorescent, and has strong UV absorbance; these properties have contributed to its ease of detection. Dityrosine cross-linked proteins, however, tend to be extremely insoluble and resistant to proteolytic digestion. This has hampered attempts to demonstrate the location of intermolecular cross-links.[7]

The formation of di- or trityrosine cross-links in vivo is unclear in most instances. In vitro, they can be formed by the action of peroxidase (E.C. 1.11.1.7) on tyrosine[34] or tyrosine-containing proteins,[35-37] tyrosinase (E.C. 1.14.18.1) on insect egg-case proteins.[38] and UV irradiation of tyrosine[39] and tyrosine-containing peptides.[40] Only in the egg fertilization membrane of the sea urchin *Strongylocentrotus purpuratus* has the formation of di- and trityrosine cross-links been clearly associated with the release of ovoperoxidase activity.[41,42] Formation of dityrosine in human cataractous lens protein may be related to UV irradiation.[43-44] Cross-links in *Mytilus* byssus,[45,46] trematode egg shell,[47] tussah silk,[48] and crab carapace[49] could be related to the presence of phenoloxidase in these materials,[50-52] but this connection is at best tenuous.

The effect of aging or maturation on the formation of dityrosine needs to be studied. Waykole and Heidemann[53] detected dityrosine only in old bovine skin. Fluorescence attributed to dityrosine was found to increase in human elastin with increasing age.[54,55]

Proteins with Cystine Cross-Links

Cystine cross-links (Table 1, number 5) are ubiquitous and important as both intra- and intermolecular protein bonds. In extracellular fibrous proteins, they occur in hair, skin, feathers, and horn, contributing to stabilization of the β-pleated sheet structures.[56,57] Extensive cystine cross-linking is also present in the cuticle collagen of *Ascaris*,[8] in type III collagen,[59] basement membranes,[60] and all procollagens.[61] The presence of these cross-links in globular proteins is too extensive to enumerate; the reader is referred to several reviews.[62,63]

Cystine cross-links are formed spontaneously in proteins by the oxidation of nearby cysteine residues. They can be easily cleaved by reduction or oxidation.[62,63] Little is known about cystine cross-links and aging. Anderson and Spector[64] have recently noted that insoluble cataractous lens protein contains a higher than normal amount of disulfides.

Protein Cross-Linked by Synthetic Bifunctional Agents

Several bifunctional reagents are available for the covalent cross-linking of proteins.[65-68] At this time, it is difficult to assess what or how much such cross-linkers might contribute to the function of proteins in vivo.

Proteins with Uncharacterized Cross-Links

The term "quinone-tanned" protein was probably introduced by Pryor[69] who observed that o-diphenols are released from the left colleterial gland of the cockroach, and oxidized to quinones by phenoloxidase. The quinones subsequently bring about the rapid sclerotization and darkening of cockroach egg-case proteins.[70] Quinone-tanned proteins have since been proposed to exist in many other protein structures including silks,[51] insect cuticles,[71,72] structural proteins of molluscs and annelids,[73] helminth egg cases,[50] and others[74] too numerous to mention here. It is important to recognize that even though the o-diphenols have been identified in most allegedly tanned systems, no quinone cross-link has been identified to date.

The reason for this probably lies in the complexity of possible reactions between quinones and proteins.[75] Andersen recently published evidence for the existence of two possible cross-linking pathways in insect cuticles.[76] The first, termed β-sclerotization involves protein addition to the side chain of the cross-linker N-acetyldopamine; the second involves addition to the aromatic ring. The ratio of the two cross-linking functions varies among different insects, and even within different cuticular regions of the same insect. No definitive protein cross-links have yet been proposed.

In molluscs, cross-linked extracellular proteins include the periostracum, byssus, operculum, and hinge ligament. Hunt[77] has described 2,4-quinoline-dicarboxylic acid in hydrolysates of insoluble gastropod operculum. Although the biochemical origin of this compound is unknown, Hunt suggests that it may be a difunctional cross-link forming isopeptide-like bonds with the primary NH_2 groups of proteins. The presence of dityrosine in molluscan byssus was mentioned earlier. The cross-link 3,3′-methylenebis-tyrosine was reported in the hinge ligament of bivalve molluscs,[78] but has since been recognized as an artefact of hydrolysis.[79] An unidentified, intensely fluorescent compound in partially solubilized peptide fragments of the hinge protein is now presumed to be the cross-linking species.[80] Periostracum, the insoluble shell protein of bivalve molluscs, is composed of cross-linked 3,4-dihydroxyphenylalanine-containing (DOPA) proteins.[81-83] DOPA has been shown to disappear rapidly with the age and insolubility of the protein.[84] The reactions consuming DOPA, however, are unknown.

An important unidentified cross-link in mammals occurs in the brown insoluble proteins of senile cataractous lenses. At one time these proteins were considered quinone-tanned.[85,86] Recent evidence, however, indicates the presence of both cystine and dityrosine bonds.[44,64] A third type of cross-link has been suggested by the release of a fluorescent chromophore, identified as β-carboline, in alkaline hydrolysates of the insoluble protein.[87] A fluorescent tryptic peptide has been prepared from the insoluble lens protein, and should soon enable identification of this cross-link.[64]

Protein-Polynucleotide Cross-Links

Until a few years ago, little was known about covalent interactions between DNA or RNA and proteins. In 1978, Rothberg et al.[88] and Ambros and Baltimore[89] identified a protein bound through a tyrosine hydroxyl in a phosphodiester linkage to the 5′ uridine terminus of polio viral RNA. There have been other reports of protein linked to the 5′ termini of RNA and DNA.[90-94] Nomoto et al.,[95] however, suggest the function of the protein to be an initiation site of replication or transcription. In this light, the O^4-(5-uridylyl)-tyrosine linkage is not a true cross-link.

Proteins can be cross-linked to DNA/RNA in vivo by UV or gamma irradiation[96-100] and bifunctional alkylating agents.[101,102] Although no cross-links have yet been chemically identified, Möller et al.[11] have isolated an oligonucleotide-peptide fragment from UV-irradiated 30 S ribosomes after extensive enzymatic digestion. Model experiments suggest a possible free-radical coupling of cysteine and pyrimidine.[103,104] Such studies should provide much insight about the spatial arrangement of proteins in DNA and RNA.

The biological significance of lesions produced by the chemical- and radiation-induced cross-linkage of proteins and DNA is the subject of much speculation and research, and is critical to several theories of cell aging and mutagenesis.[99,105,106]

Protein-Polysaccharide Cross-Links

Covalent protein-carbohydrate interactions mediated by the linkage of the nonreducing end of the sugar to serine, threonine, asparagine, and hydroxylysine residues of proteins abound in biochemistry and are thoroughly reviewed in the literature.[107-110] Such glycoprotein linkages, however, are not true cross-links since the two macromolecules are not postsynthetically cross-linked; rather, the protein serves as an initiation site for the polymerization of sugars.

Brandt et al.[111] have shown that *p*-quinone can cross-link dextrans and proteins. Similar reactions are presumed to occur between chitin and protein in quinone-tanned arthropod cuticles, but there has been no direct evidence for this.[112]

N^6-hexosyl-hydroxylysine and N^6-hexosyl-lysine have been suggested as cross-links between collagen and proteoglycans.[113, 114] If this is confirmed by the isolation of enzymatically digested cross-linked oligosaccharide-peptide fragments, then these compounds would be the first known examples of protein-polysaccharide cross-links occurring in animal tissues.

Polynucleotide-Polynucleotide Cross-Links

The two strands of the double helix of DNA are normally linked by the extensive hydrogen bonding of the complementary purine-pyrimidine base pairs. However, covalent cross-links between the two strands of DNA (Table 2, numbers 1 through 4) can be induced by a variety of agents including UV irradiation,[115,116] nitrous acid,[117] mitomycin *c*[118,119] furocoumarins,[120-124] bifunctional alkylating agents,[125-127] and platinum coordination compounds.[128,129] The experimental induction of cross-links in DNA and the organism's subsequent ability to repair such lesions form the basis of the research behind many of the current theories about aging and mutagenesis.[130,131]

The formation of interstrand cross-links is experimentally determined by measuring the renaturation,[115] viscosity,[120,132] sedimentation equilibrium,[115,116] or light scattering properties[133] of denatured DNA. Interstrand cross-links can often be visualized by electron microscopy.[134]

The simplest method of forming cross-links in DNA is by UV irradiation at 254 nm. In vitro experiments indicate that DNA must be partially denatured for interstrand cross-linking to occur. This condition could be satisfied in vivo during replication or transcription. The major photodimer isolated from UV-irradiated DNA is the cis, syn isomer of the cyclobutyl dimer of thymine[135-138](Table 2, number 1). This is thought to be primarily an intrastrand cross-link formed by the free-radical coupling of adjacent thymines.[131] Cyclobutyl dimers of thymine-uracil and uracil-uracil also occur.[133,139,140] Uracil in DNA is derived by deamination from cytosine.[140] The trans, syn isomer of the thymine dimer (Table 2, number 1) has been isolated from irradiated, denatured DNA, and hence may represent an interstrand cross-link.[141] A second type of photodimer is the thymine adduct, 5-hydroxy-6,4′-(5-methyl-pyrimidin-2′-one) dihydrothymine[142] (Table 2, number 3). This is also presumed to be an intrastrand cross-link, although its involvement in interstrand cross-links is not categorically discounted. This type of adduct can also occur between thymine and cytosine (Table 2, number 4) and two cytosines.[143] The third type of photodimer from UV-irradiated DNA, 5-thyminyl-5,6-dihydrothymine[144,145] (Table 2, number 2), occurs only in spore DNA and frozen DNA. The location of this cross-link is uncertain; its formation is favored by low humidity.

Other types of interstrand cross-links have not yet been chemically characterized. The photoactivated cross-link formed by furocoumarins with native DNA presumably involves a cyclobutane-type coupling with the 4,5-double bond of two pyrimidines.[121,122] Lawley and Brookes[125,127] and Zwieb et al.[146] have proposed that bifunctional mustards and nitrosamines cross-link DNA via the 7N of guanines; however, chemical evidence for this is not compelling. Research on the cross-linking action of mitomycin *c*[118,119] and platinum[128,129] is just beginning. RNA is also prone to the formation of UV- and chemically induced cross-links.[146] The biological significance of the chemical modification of DNA and RNA has been discussed in recent reviews.[130,147]

Polynucleotide-Polysaccharide Cross-Links

There are no known examples of this type of cross-link.

Table 2
CROSS-LINKS IN POLYNUCLEOTIDES

	Postulated structure	Molecular[a] weight	Trivial name	Systematic name[b]	Structural evidence
1.	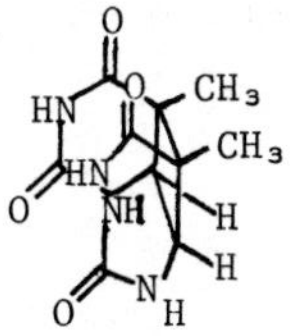 cis,syn; 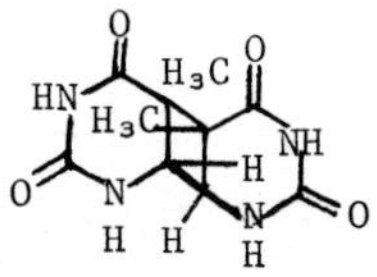 trans,syn	252	Cyclobutylthymine dimers	Cis-cyclobuta [1, 2-d; 4, 3-d']dithymine; trans-cyclobuta [1,2-d; 4.3-d']dithymine	Mass spectrum, derivative, UV and IR absorbance, ^{1}H-NMR, crystallography, synthesis, chromatography[139-141,207,208]
2.	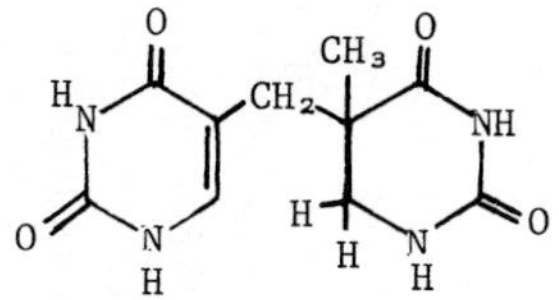	252	Spore photo-product	5,5' [5'-Pyrimidine-2',4'-dione)methyl]-5,6-dihydrothymine	Mass spectrum, IR and UV absorbance, ^{1}H-NMR, chromatography, synthesis[144,145]
3.	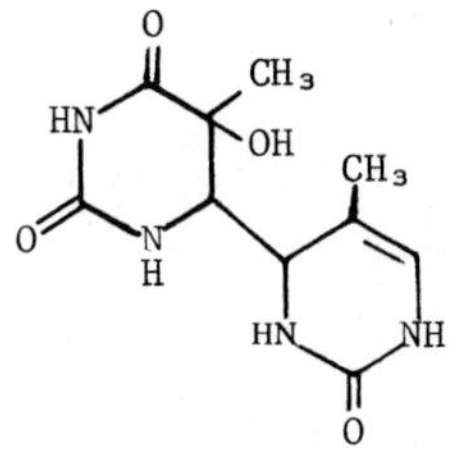	252	Thymine adduct	5-Hydroxy-6,4'-(5'-methyl pyrimidine-2'-one)-5,6-dihydrothymine	Mass spectra, UV and IR absorbance, ^{1}H-NMR, crystallography, synthesis, chromatography[142,211]

4.	220	Thymine adduct	6,4′-(Pyrimidine-2′-one) thymine	Mass spectra, derivative, UV and IR absorbance, ^{1}H-NMR synthesis, chromatography[143,212]

	Abundance	Proposed precursors	Stability	Misc.
1.	DNA: *Escherichi coli; Saccharomyces cervesiae; Tetrahymena pyriformis; Paramecium aurelia;* salmon sperm; calf thymus; Chinese hamster cells; human skin cells (xeroderma pigmentosum)[139,140, 208-210]	Thymine (×2); coupling of free radicals induced by λ 254 nm irridation	Stable to $HC10_4$, 100°C; labile to bromine (alkali); photo reversible to UV light 200—289 nm; BH_4-reducible; trans-syn isomer not reversed by yeast photolyase; Stable 6 N HC1, 85°C, 15 min[141]	Cis, syn is major (90%) DNA photoproduct; primarily intramolecular cross-link; λ_{230} ε = 2100 M^{-1} cm^{-1};[138,140] trans, syn isomer favored in partially denatured DNA;[141] ratio trans, syn/cis, syn < 0.02 in native DNA
2.	DNA: bacterial spores; bacteria (low-temperature); frozen calf thymus[144,145]	Thymine (×2); coupling of free radicals induced by UV (254 nm) irradiation	Stable to CF_3COOH, 170°C, 90 min; not photo reversible; labile to formic acid[144,145]	Major photoproduct in spore and frozen DNA; $\lambda^{pH2}{}_{max}$ = 265 nm (ε = 8200 M^{-1} cm^{-1}) $\lambda^{pH11}{}_{max}$ = 290 nm (ε = 7500 M^{-1} cm^{-1})[144,145] formation favored by low humidity; probably intrastrand cross-link
3.	DNA: calf thymus; bacteria[142]	Thymine (× 2); coupling of free radicals induced by UV irradiation (254 nm); initially forms oxetidine intermediate[142]	Heat, acid unstable; photo reversible at 310—340 nm; reversible with yeast DNA photolyase; degrades to dehydration product in acid[210]	Largely intrastrand cross-links; $\lambda^{pH2}{}_{max}$ = 316 nm (ε = 4920 M^{-1} cm^{-1}), $\lambda^{pH12}{}_{max}$ = 306 nm (ε = 5680 M^{-1} cm^{-1}); formation enhanced in frozen or dry DNA; reduced in denatured DNA[142]
4.	DNA: bacteria, calf thymus	Thymine and cytidine (deaminated), from azetidine intermediate; induced by irradiation at 254 nm; reversed at 313 nm	Acid stable	$\lambda^{pH2}{}_{max}$ = 316 nm (ε = 5380 M^{-1} cm^{-1}), $\lambda^{pH12}{}_{max}$ = 304 nm (ε = 7000 M^{-1} cm^{-1},[212]

[a] Assumed to be anhydrous.
[b] According to nomenclature proposed by IUPAC-IUB commission.[213]

Polysaccharide-Polysaccharide Cross-Links

A classic synthetic example of this type of cross-linkage is formed upon treatment of dextrans with epichlorhydrin.[148] The only known examples of cross-linked polysaccharides in nature occur in the cell envelopes of gram-negative bacteria. In these, peptide linkages mediate the cross-linkage of a polymeric network of polysaccharides.[149-151]

REFERENCES

1. **Miall, L. M. and Sharp, D. W. A., Eds.,** *A New Dictionary of Chemistry,* 4th ed., John Wiley & Sons, New York, 1968, 355.
2. **Wainwright, S. A., Biggs, W. D., Curry. J. D., and Gosline, J. M.,** *Mechanical Design in Organisms,* John Wiley & Sons, New York, 1976, 423.
3. **Brown, C. H.,** A review of the methods available for the determination of the forces stabilizing structural proteins in animals, *Q. J. Microsc. Sci.,* 91, 331, 1950.
4. **Folin, O. and Looney, J. M.,** Colorimetric methods for the separate determination of tyrosine, tryptophane, and cystine in proteins, *J. Biol. Chem.,* 51, 421, 1922.
5. **Goddard, D. R. and Michaelis, L.,** A study on keratin, *J. Biol. Chem.,* 106, 605, 1934.
6. **Partridge, S. M., Elsden, D. F., and Thomas, J.,** Constitution of cross-linkages in elastin, *Nature,* 197, 1297, 1963.
7. **Andersen, S. O.,** Covalent cross-links in a structural protein, resilin, *Acta Physiol. Scand.,* 66, (Suppl. 763), 1, 1966.
8. **Starcher, B. C., Partridge, S. M., and Elsden, D. F.,** Isolation and partial characterization of a new amino acid from reduced elastin, *Biochemistry,* 6, 2425, 1967.
9. **Blumenfeld, O. O. and Gallop, P. M.,** Amino aldehydes in collagen: the nature of a probable cross-link, *Proc. Natl. Acad. Sci. U.S.A.,* 56, 1260, 1966.
10. **Matačic, S. S. and Loewy, A. G.,** The identification if isopeptide cross-link in insoluble fibrin, *Biochem. Biophys. Res. Commun.,* 30, 356, 1968.
11. **Möller, K., Zwieb, C., and Brimacombe, R.,** Identification of the oligonucleotide and oligopeptide involved in an RNA protein cross-link induced by UV irradiation of *Escherichia coli* 30 S ribosomal subunits, *J. Mol. Biol.,* 126, 489, 1978.
12. **Siegel, R. C.,** Lysyl oxidase, in *International Review of Connective Tissue Research,* Hall, D. A. and Jackson, D. S., Eds., Academic Press, New York, in press.
13. **Franzblau, C., Faris, B., Lent, R. W., Salcedo, L. L., Smith, B., Jaffe, R., and Crombie, G.,** Chemistry and biosynthesis of cross-links in elastin, in *Chemistry and Molecular Biology of the Intercellular Matrix,* Vol. 1, Balazs, E. A., Ed., Academic Press, New York, 1970, 617.
14. **Stimler, N. P. and Tanzer, M. L.,** Location of intermolecular cross-linking sites in collagen, *Adv. Exp. Med. Biol.,* 86B, 675, 1976.
15. **Tanzer, M. L.,** Experimental lathyrism, in *International Review of Connective Tissue Research,* Vol. 3, Hall, D. A., Ed., Academic Press, New York, 1965, 91.
16. **Tanzer, M. L.,** Cross-linking, in *Biochemistry of Collagen,* Ramachandran, G. N. and Reddi, A. H., Eds., Plenlum Press, New York, 1976, chap. 4.
17. **Gallop, P. M. and Paz, M. A.,** Posttranslational modifications with special attention to collagen and elastin, *Physiol. Rev.,* 55, 418, 1975.
18. **Fujii, K. and Tanzer, M. L.,** Age-related changes in the reducible cross-links of human tendon collagen, *FEBS Lett.,* 43, 300, 1972.
19. **Moriguchi, T. and Fujimoto, D.,** Age-related changes in the content of the collagen cross-link, pyridinoline, *J. Biochem.,* 84, 933, 1978.
20. **Davison, P. F.,** Bovine tendons: aging and collagen cross-linking, *J. Biol. Chem.,* 253, 5635, 1978.
21. **Franzblau, C., Foster, J. A., and Faris, B.,** Role of cross-linking in fiber formation, *Adv. Exp. Med. Biol.,* 79, 313, 1977.
22. **Lorand, L. and Stenberg, P.,** Endo-γ-glutamine: ε-lysine transferase, in *Handbook of Biochemistry and Molecular Biology,* Vol. 2, 3rd ed., Fasman, G. D., Ed., CRC Press, Boca Raton, Fla., 1976, 669.
23. **Lorand, L., Downey, J., Gotoh, T., Jacobsen, A., and Tokura, S.,** The transpeptidase system which cross-links fibrin by γ-glutamyl ε-lysine bonds, *Biochem. Biophys. Res. Commun.,* 31, 222, 1968.

24. **Rice, R. H. and Green, H.**, The cornified envelope of terminally differentiated human epidermal keratinocytes consists of cross-linked protein, *Cell*, 11, 417, 1977.
25. **Williams-Ashman, H. G., Notides, A. C., Pabalan, S. S., and Lorand, L.**, Transamidase reactions involved in enzymatic coagulation of semen: isolation of γ-glutamyl ε-lysine dipeptide from clotted secretion protein of guinea pig seminal veside, *Proc. Natl. Acad. Sci. U.S.A.*, 69, 2322, 1972.
26. **Siefring, G. E., Apostol, A. B., Velasco, P. T., and Lorand, L.**, Enzymatic basis for the Ca^{++}-induced cross-linking of membrane proteins in intact human erythrocytes, *Biochemistry*, 17, 2598, 1978.
27. **Keski-Oja, J., Mosher, D., and Vaheri, A.**, Cross-linking of fibronectin catalyzed by blood coagulation factor XIII, *Cell*, 9, 29, 1976.
28. **Asquith, R. S., Otterburn, M. S., and Sinclair, W. J.**, Isopeptide cross-links — their occurrence and importance in protein structures, *Angew. Chem. Int. Ed. Eng.*, 13, 514, 1974.
29. **Klostermeyer, H., Rabbel, K., and Reimedes, E. H.**, Vorkommen der isopeptide bindugen N^{ϵ}(β-aspartyl)lysine and N^{ϵ}(γ-glutamyl) lysine in rindercolostrum, *Hoppe Seyler's Z. Physiol. Chem.*, 357, 1197, 1976.
30. **Birckbichler, P. J., Carter, H. A., Orr, G. R., Conway, E., and Patterson, M. R.**, ε-(γ-glutamyl) lysine isopeptide bonds in normal and virus-transformed human fibroblasts, *Biochem. Biophys. Res. Commun.*, 84, 232, 1978.
31. **Folk, J. E. and Finlayson, J. S.**, ε-(γ-glutamyl) lysine, *Adv. Protein Chem.*, 31, 1, 1977.
32. **Barton, A. D. and Lourenco, R. V.**, γ-glutamyl transpeptidase and possible cross-linking in bronchial secretions, *Fed. Proc.*, 30 (Abstr.,) 1146, 1971.
33. **Andersen, S. O.**, Cross-links in resilin identified as dityrosine and trityrosine, *Biochim. Biophys. Acta*, 93, 213, 1967.
34. **Gross, A. J. and Sizer, I. W.**, The oxidation of tyramine, tyrosine, and related compounds by peroxidase, *J. Biol. Chem.*, 234, 1611, 1959.
35. **LaBella, F. S., Waykole, P., and Queen, P.**, Formation of insoluble gels and dityrosine by the action of peroxidase insoluble collagens, *Biochem. Biophys. Res. Commun.*, 30, 333, 1968.
36. **Müllerova, A., Michlik, I., and Blazěj, A.**, Formation of dityrosine in collagen and elastin, *Das Leder*, 25, 85, 1974.
37. **Aeschbach, R., Amado, R., aand Neukom, H.**, Formation of dityrosine cross-links in proteins by oxidation of tyrosine residues, *Biochim. Biophys. Acta*, 439, 292, 1976.
38. **Kawasaki, H., Sato, H., and Suzuki, M.**, Structural proteins in the egg envelopes of the dragonflies, *Sympetrum infuscatum* and *S. frequens, Insect Biochem.*, 4, 99, 1974.
39. **Shimizu, O.**, Excited states of aqueous tyrosine at room temperature, *Photochem. Photobiol.*, 18, 125, 1973.
40. **Lehrer, S. S. and Fasman, G. D.**, Ultraviolet irradiation effects in poly-L-tyrosine and model compounds: identification of bityrosine as a photoproduct, *Biochemistry*, 6, 757, 1967.
41. **Foerder, C. A. and Shapiro, B. M.**, Release of ovoperoxidase from sea urchin eggs hardens fertilization membrane with tyrosine cross-links, *Proc. Natl. Acad. Sci. U.S.A.*, 74, 4214, 1977.
42. **Hall, H. G.**, Hardening of the sea urchin envelope by peroxidase-catalysed phenolic coupling of tyrosines, *Cell*, 15, 343, 1978.
43. **Garcia-Castineiras, S., Dillon, J., and Spector, A.**, Detection of bityrosine in cataractous human lens protein, *Science*, 199, 897, 1978.
44. **Garcia-Castineiras, S., Dillon, J., and Spector, A.**, Nontryptophan fluorescence associated with human lens proteins apparent complexity, isolation of bityrosine and anthranilic acid, *Exp. Eye Res.*, 26, 407, 1978.
45. **Chandrakasan, G., Geetha, B., Krishnan, G., and Joseph, K. T.**, Studies of invertebrate collagens. I. Nature of the collagenous protein in byssus threads of *Mytilus edulis, Ind. J. Biochem. Biophys.*, 14, 132, 1977.
46. **De Vore, P. P. and Gruebel, R. J.**, Dityrosine in adhesive formed by the sea mussel, *Mytilus edulis, Biochem. Biophys. Res. Commun.*, 993, 1978.
47. **Ramalingam, K.**, The chemical nature of the egg shell of helminths. I. Absence of quinone-tanning in the egg shell of the liver fluke, *Fasciola hepatica, Int. J. Parasitol.*, 3, 67, 1973.
48. **Raven, D. J., Garland, C., and Little, M.**, The occurrence of dityrosine in tussah silk fibroin and keratin, *Biocbim. Biophys. Acta*, 251, 96, 1971.
49. **Welinder, B. S., Roepstorff, P., and Andersen, S. O.**, The crustacean cuticle. VI. Isolation and identification of cross-links from *Cancer pagurus* cuticle, *Comp. Biochem. Physiol.*, 53B, 529, 1976.
50. **Smyth, J. D.**, A technique for the demonstration of polyphenoloxidase and its application to egg shell formation in helminths and byssus formation in *Mytilus, Q. J. Microsc. Sci.*, 95, 139, 1954.
51. **Brunet, P. C. J. and Coles, B. C.**, Tanned silks, *Proc. R. Soc. London*, 187, 133, 1974.
52. **Stevenson, J. R. and Adomako, T. Y.**, Diphenol-oxidase in the crayfish cuticle: localization and changes in activity during the moulting cycle, *J. Insect Physiol.*, 13, 1803, 1967.
53. **Waykole, P. and Heidemann, E.**, Dityrosine in collagen, *Connect. Tissue Res.*, 4, 219, 1976.
54. **LaBella, F. S.**, Enzymic vs. nonenzymic factors in the deterioration of connective tissue, *Adv. Exp. Med. Biol.*, 43, 377, 1974.

55. **John, R. and Thomas, J.**, Chemical compositions of elastins isolated from aortas and pulmonary tissues of humans of various ages, *Biochem. J.*, 127, 261, 1972.
56. **Crewther, W. G., Fraser, R. D. B., Lennox, F. G.**, and Lindley H., The chemistry of keratins, *Adv. Protein Chem.*, 20, 191, 1965.
57. **Bradbury, J. H.**, The structure and chemistry of keratin fibers, *Adv. Protein Chem.*, 27, 111, 1973.
58. **McBride, O. W. and Harrington, W. F.**, *Ascaris* cuticle collagen: on the disulfide cross-bridges and molecular properties of the subunits, *Biochemistry*, 6, 1484, 1967.
59. **Fessler, J. H., Greenberg, D. G., and Fessler, L. I.**, Processing of procollagen, in *Biology and Chemistry of Basement Membranes*, Kefalides, N. A., Ed., Academic Press, New York, 1978, 373.
60. **Alper, R. and Kefalides, N. A.**, The use of hydroxylamine cleavage as a probe of the supramolecular organization of bovine anterior lens capsule basement membrane, in *Biology and Chemistry of Basement Membranes*, Kefalides, N. A., Ed., Academic Press, New York, 1978, 239.
61. **Fessler, L. I., Morris, N. P., and Fessler, J. H.**, Procollagen: biological scission of amino and carboxy extension peptides, *Proc. Natl. Acad. Sci. U.S.A.*, 72, 4905, 1975.
62. **Fluharty, A. L.**, in *The Chemistry of the Thiol Group*, Patai, S., Ed., John Wiley & Sons, New York, 1974, 589.
63. **Cecil, R. and McPhee, J. R.**, The sulfur chemistry of proteins, *Adv. Protein Chem.*, 14, 256, 1959.
64. **Anderson, E. I. and Spector, A.**, The state of sulfhydryl groups in normal and cataractous human lens proteins. I. Nuclear region, *Exp. Eye Res.*, 26, 407, 1978.
65. **Fasold, H., Klappenberger, J., Meyer, C., and Remold, H.**, Bifunctional reagents for the cross-linking of proteins, *Angew. Chem. Int. Eng. Ed.*, 10, 795, 1971.
66. **Lutter, L. C., Ortanderl, F., and Fasold, H.**, Use of a new series of cleavable protein cross-linkers on the *E. coli* ribosome, *FEBS Lett.*, 48, 288, 1974.
67. **Uy, R. and Wold, F.**, Introduction of artificial cross-links into proteins, *Adv. Exper. Med. Biol.*, 86A, 169, 1977.
68. **Wold, F.**, Bifunctional reagents, in *Methods in Enzymology*, Vol. 25, Hirs, C. H. W. and Timasheff, S. N., Eds. Academic Press, New York, 1972, 623.
69. **Pryor, M. G. M.**, On the hardening of the ootheca of *Blatta orientalis*, *Proc. R. Soc. London Ser. B:* 128, 378, 1940.
70. **Pau, R. N., Brunet, P. C. J., and Williams, M. J.**, The isolation and characterization of proteins from the left colleterial gland of the cockroach, *Periplaneta americana* (L.), *Proc. R. Soc. London Ser. B:* 177, 565, 1971.
71. **Hackman, R. H. and Goldberg, M.**, Molecular cross-links in cuticles, *Insect Biochem.*, 7, 175 1977.
72. **Andersen, S. O.**, Cuticular enzymes and sclerotization in insects, in *The Insect Integument*, Hepburn, H. R., Ed., Elsevier, Amsterdam, 1976, 121.
73. **Brown, C. H.**, Quinone-tanning in the animal kingdon, *Nature*, 165, 275, 1950.
74. **Brown, C. H.**, *Structural Materials in Animals*, John Wiley & Sons, New York, 1975, 448.
75. **Morrison, M., Steele, W., and Danner, D.**, The reaction of benzoquinone with amines and proteins, *Arch. Biochem. Biophys.*, 134, 512, 1969.
76. **Andersen, S. O.**, Evidence for two mechanisms of sclerotization in insect cuticle, *Nature*, 251, 507, 1976.
77. **Hunt, S.**, Operculin, a molluscan scleroprotein: 2,4-Quinoline-dicarboxylic acid, a possible cross-link, *Comp. Biochem. Physiol.*, 62B, 55, 1979.
78. **Andersen, S. O.**, Isolation of a new type of cross-links from the hinge ligament protein of molluscs, *Nature*, 216, 1029, 1967.
79. **Welinder, B. S., Roepstorff, P., and Andersen, S. O.**, The crustacean cuticle. IV. Isolation and identification of cross-links from *Cancer pagurus* cuticles, *Comp. Biochem. Physiol.*, 53B, 529, 1976.
80. **Thornhill, D. P.**, Abduction: locus and spectral characteristics of a brown fluorescent protein chromophore, *Biochemistry*, 10, 2644, 1975.
81. **Waite, J. H.**, Evidence for the mode of sclerotization in a molluscan periostracum, *Comp. Biochem. Physiol.*, 58B, 157, 1977.
82. **Waite, J. H. and Andersen, S. O.**, Dihydroxyphenylalanine in an insoluble shell protein of *Mytilus edulis*, *Biochim. Biophys. Acta*, 541, 107, 1978.
83. **Waite, J. H., Saleuddin, A. S. M., and Andersen, S. O.**, Periostracin, a soluble precursor of sclerotized periostracum in *Mytilus edulis*, L., *J. Comp. Physiol.*, 130, 301, 1979.
84. **Waite, J. H. and Andersen, S. O.**, 3,4-dihydroxyphenylalanine (DOPA) and sclerotization of periostracum in *Mytilus edulis* L., *Biol. Bull.*, 158, 164, 1980.
85. **Pirie, A.**, Reaction of tyrosine oxidation products with proteins of the lens, *Biochem. J.*, 109, 701, 1968.
86. **Srivastava, S. K. and Beutler, E.**, Cataract produced by tyrosinase systems in rabbit lens *in vitro*, *Biochem. J.*, 112, 421, 1969.
87. **Dillon, J., Spector, A., and Nakanishi, K.**, Identification of β-carbolines isolated from fluorescent human lens protein, *Nature*, 259, 422, 1976.

88. **Rothberg, P. G., Harris, T. J. R., Nomoto, A., and Wimmer, G.,** O^4(5′-uridylyl) tyrosine is the bond between tbe genome linked protein and the linked protein and the RNA of poliovirus, *Proc. Natl. Acad. Sci. U.S.A.*, 75, 4868, 1978.
89. **Ambros, V. and Baltimore, D.,** Protein is linked to the 5′ end of polio virus RNA by a phosphodiester linkage to tyrosine, *J. Biol. Chem.*, 253, 5263, 1978.
90. **Stanley, J., Rottier, P., Davies, J. W., Zabel, P., and van Kammen, A.,** A protein linked to the 5′ termini of both RNA components of the cowpea virus genome, *Nucl. Acid. Res.*, 5, 4505, 1978.
91. **Sonenberg, N., Morgen, M. A., Merrick, W. C., and Shatkin, A. J.,** A polypeptide in eukaryotic initiation factors that cross-links specifically to the 5′-terminal cap in mRNA, *Proc. Natl. Acad. Sci. U.S.A.*, 75, 4843, 1978.
92. **Harding, N. E., Ito, J., and David, G. S.,** Identification of the protein firmly bound to the ends of bacteriophage ∅ 29 DNA, *Virology*, 84, 279, 1978.
93. **Galas, M., Mellado, R. P., Viñuela, E., and Sogo, J. M.,** Characterization of a protein covalently linked to the 5′-termini of the DNA of *Bacillus subtilis* phage ∅ 29, *J. Mol. Biol.*, 119, 209, 1978.
94. **Sangar, D. V., Rowland, D. J., Harris, T. J. R., and Brown, F.,** Protein covalently linked to hoof-and-mouth disease virus RNA, *Nature*, 268, 648, 1978.
95. **Nomoto, A., Detjen, B., Pozzatti, R., and Wimmer, E.,** The location of the polio genome protein in viral RNAs and its implication for RNA synthesis, *Nature*, 268, 208, 1977.
96. **Shoemaker, H. J. P., Budzik, G. P., Giege, R. C., and Schimmel, P. R.,** Three photo cross-linked complexes of yeast phenylalanine-specific transfer RNA with its cognate amino acyl transfer RNA synthetases, *J. Biol. Chem.*, 250, 4440, 1975.
97. **Gordon, M. P.,** Role of protein in the inactivation of viruses by ultraviolet light, in *Aging, Carcinogenesis and Radiation Biology*, Smith, K. C., Ed., Plenum Press, New York, 1976, 105.
98. **Smith, K. C.,** The radiation induced addition of proteins and other molecules to nucleic acids, in *Photochemistry and Photobiology of Nucleic Acids*, Vol. II, Wang, W. Y., Ed., Academic Press, New York, 1976, 187.
99. **Kornhauser, A.,** UV-induced DNA-protein cross-links *in vitro* and *in vivo*, *Photochem. Photobiol.*, 23, 457, 1976.
100. **Hawkins, R. B.,** Quantitative determination of cross-linkage of bacteriophage DNA and protein by ionizing radiation, *Int. J. Radiat. Biol.*, 33, 425, 1978.
101. **Thomas, C. B., Kohn, K. W., and Bonner, W. M.,** Characterization of DNA-protein cross-links formed by treatment of L1210 cells and nuclei with bis-(2-chloroethyl) methylamine, *Biochemistry*, 17, 3954, 1978.
102. **Thomas, J. O.,** Chemically induced DNA-protein cross-links, in *Aging Carcinogenesis and Radiation Biology*, Smith, K. C., Ed., Plenum Press, New York, 1976, 193.
103. **Berman, H., Zacharias, D., Carrell, H., and Varghese, A. J.,** α-S-cysteinyl thymine: a model for protein-nucleic acid cross-linking, *Biochemistry*, 15, 463, 1976.
104. **Ito, S., Saito, I., Nakata, A., and Matsuura, T.,** Photochemical synthesis of model compounds for nucleic acid-protein adducts, *Nucl. Acid. Res.*, 5, s321, 1978.
105. **Cutler, R. G.,** Cross-linkage hypothesis of aging: DNA adducts in chromatin as a primary aging process, in *Aging, Carcinogenesis and Radiation Biology*, Smith, K. C., Ed., Plenum Press, New York, 1976, 443.
106. **Paterson, M. C.,** Use of purified lesion-recognizing enzymes to monitor DNA repair *in vivo*, *Adv. Radiat. Biol.*, 7, 1, 1978.
107. **Zinn, A. B., Plantner, J. J., and Carlson, D. M.,** Nature of linkages between protein core and oligosaccharides, in *The Glycoconjugates*, Vol. 1, Horowitz, M. I. and Pigman, W., Ed., Academic Press, New York, 1977, 69.
108. **Spiro, R. G.,** Glycoproteins, *Adv. Protein Chem.*, 27, 350, 1973.
109. **Kornfeld, R. and Kornfeld, S.,** Comparative aspects of glycoprotein structure, *Annu. Rev. Biochem.*, 45, 217, 1976.
110. **Hunt, S.,** *Polysaccharide-Protein Complexes in Invertebrates*, Academic Press, London, 1970, 329.
111. **Brandt, J., Anderson, L. O., and Porath, J.,** Covalent attachment of proteins to polysaccharide carriers by means of benzoquinone, *Biochim. Biophys. Acta*, 386, 196, 1975.
112. **Jeuniaux, C.,** Chitinous structures, *Compr. Biochem.*, 26C, 595, 1971.
113. **Tanzer, M. L., Fairweather, R., and Gallop, P. M.,** Collagen cross-links: isolation of reduced N^{ϵ}-hexosylhydroxylysine from boro-hydride-reduced insoluble calf skin collagen, *Arch. Biochem. Biophys.*, 151, 137, 1972.
114. **Robins, S. P. and Bailey, A. J.,** Age-related changes in collagen: the identification of reducible lysine-carbohydrate condensation products, *Biochem. Biophys. Res. Commun.*, 48, 76, 1972.
115. **Glišin, V. R. and Doty, P.,** The cross-linking of DNA by UV radiation, *Biochim. Biophys. Acta*, 142, 314, 1967.
116. **Marmur, J. and Grossman, L.,** UV light-induced linking of deoxyribonucleic acid strands and its reversal by photo-reactivating enzyme, *Proc. Natl. Acad. Sci. U.S.A.*, 47, 778, 1961.

117. **Geiduschek, G. P.,** Reversible DNA, *Proc. Natl. Acad. Sci. U.S.A.,* 47, 950, 1961.
118. **Iyer, V. N. and Szybalski, W.,** A molecular mechanism of mitomycin action: linking of complementary DNA strands, *Proc. Natl. Acad. Sci. U.S.A.,* 50, 355, 1963.
119. **Ogawa, K., Nomura, A., Fujiwara, T., and Tomita, K.,** Structural studies of mitomycin *c* and cross-linking mechanism to double-stranded DNA, *Nucl. Acid. Res.,* 3, s79, 1977.
120. **Cole, R. S.,** Psoralen monoadducts and interstrand cross-links in DNA, *Biochim. Biophys. Acta,* 254, 30, 1971.
121. **Dall'Acqua, F., Marciani, S., Gavetta, L., and Rodighiero, G.,** Formation of interstrand cross-linkages in the photo reactions between furo-coumarins and DNA, *Z. Naturforsch.,* 326, 561, 1971.
122. **Dall'Acqua, F., Marciani, S., Vedaldi, D., and Rodighiero, G.,** Studies on the photo reactions between DNA and some methyl psoralens, *Biochim. Biophys. Acta,* 353, 267, 1974.
123. **Ley, R. D., Grube, D. D., and Fry, R. J. M.,** Photosensitizing effects of 8-methoxypsoralen on the skin of hairless mice. I. Formation of interstrand cross-links in epidermal DNA, *Photochem. Photobiol.,* 25, 265, 1977.
124. **Yoakum, G. H. and Cole, R. S.,** Cross-linking and relaxation of supercoiled DNA by psoralen and light, *Biochim. Biophys. Acta,* 521, 529, 1978.
125. **Brookes, P. and Lawley, P. D.,** The reaction of mono- and difunctional alkylating agents with nucleic acids, *Biochem. J.,* 80, 496, 1961.
126. **Ewig, R. A. and Kohn, K. W.,** DNA-protein and DNA-interstrand cross-linking by halo ethyl nitroso ureas in L-1210 cells, *Cancer Res.,* 38, 3197, 1978.
127. **Lawley, P. D. and Brookes, P.,** Interstrand cross-linking of DNA by difunctional alkylating agents, *J. Mol. Biol.,* 25, 143, 1967.
128. **Kelman, A. D. and Buchbinder, M.,** Platinum — DNA cross-linking: platinum antitumor drug interactions with native lambda bacteriophage DNA using a restriction endonuclease, *Biochimie,* 60, 893, 1978.
129. **Zwelling, L. A., Anderson, T., and Kohn, K. W.,** DNA-protein and DNA-interstrand cross-linking by cis- and trans-platinum (II) diammine dichloride in L-1210 mouse leukemia cells and relation to cytotoxiety, *Cancer Res.,* 39, 365, 1979.
130. **Jagger, J.,** Ultraviolet inactivation of biological systems, in *Photochemistry and Photobiology of Nucleic Acids,* Vol. 2, Wang, W. Y., Ed., Academic Press, New York, 1976, 147.
131. **Setlow, J. K.,** The effects of ultraviolet radiation and photo-reactivation, in *Comprehensive Biochemistry,* Vol. 27, Florkin, M. and Stotz, G. H., Eds., Elsevier, Amsterdam, 1967, 157.
132. **Triebel, H., Reinert, K. E., Bär, H., and Lang, H.,** Structural changes of ultraviolet irradiated-DNA derived from hydrodynamic measurements, *Biochim. Biophys. Acta,* 561, 59, 1979.
133. **Patrick, M. H. and Rahn, R. O.,** Photochemistry of DNA and polynucleotides: photoproducts, in *Photochemistry and Photobiology of Nucleic Acids,* Vol. 2, Wang, W. Y., Ed., Academic Press, New York, 1976, 35.
134. Bohr, V., Wadskov, S., Sønderbaard, J., and Lerche, A., DNA interstrand cross-links in normal human skin visualised by electron microscopy, *Acta Derm. Venereol.,* 58, 379, 1978.
135. **Beukers, R. and Behrend, W.,** Isolation and identification of the irradiation product of thymine, *Biochim. Biophys. Acta,* 41, 550, 1960.
136. **Blackburn, G. M. and Davies, R. J. H.,** Photochemistry of nucleic acids. III. The structure of the DNA-derived thymine photodimer, *J. Am. Chem. Soc.,* 89, 5941, 1967.
137. **Blackburn, G. M. and Davies, R. J. H.,** Structure of the DNA-derived thymine dimer, *Biochem. Biophys. Res. Commun.,* 22, 704, 1966.
138. **Varghese, A. J. and Wang, S. Y.,** Cis-syn thymine homodimer from ultraviolet-irradiated calf thymus DNA, *Nature,* 213, 909, 1967.
139. **Dellweg, H. and Wacker, A.,** Strahlenchemische Veränderung von Thymin and Cytosin in der DNA durch UV-Licht, *Z. Naturforsch.,* 176, 827, 1962.
140. **Setlow, R. B. and Carrier, W. L.,** Pyrimidine dimers in ultraviolet-irradiated DNAs, *J. Mol. Biol.,* 17, 237, 1966.
141. **Ben-Hur, E. and Ben-Ishai, R.,** Trans-syn thymine dimers in ultraviolet-irradiated denatured DNA: identification and photoreactivity, *Biochim. Biophys. Acta,* 166, 9, 1968.
142. **Varghese, A. J. and Wang, S. Y.,** Thymine-thymine adduct as a photoproduct of thymine, *Science,* 160, 186, 1968.
143. **Varghese, A. J.,** Photochemical reactions of cytosine nucleosides in frozen aqueous solution and in DNA, *Biochemistry,* 10, 2194, 1971.
144. **Donnellan, J. E. and Setlow, R. B.,** Thymine photoproducts but not thymine dimers found in ultraviolet-irradiated spores, *Science,* 149, 308, 1965.
145. **Varghese, A. J.,** 5-Thyminyl-5,6-dihydrothymine from DNA irradiated with ultraviolet light, *Biochem. Biophys. REs. Commun.,* 38, 484, 1970.
146. **Zwieb, C., Ross, A., Rinke, J., Meinke, M., and Brimacombe, R.,** Evidence for RNA-RNA cross-link formation in *E. coli* ribosomes, *Nucl. Acid Res.,* 5, 2705, 1978.

147. **Roberts, J. J.**, The repair of DNA modified by cytotoxic mutagenic and carcinogenic chemicals, *Adv. Radiat. Biol.*, 7, 212, 1978.
148. **Porath, J.**, Cross-linked dextrans as molecular sieves, *Adv. Protein Chem.*, 17, 209, 1962.
149. **Ghuysen, J. M., Strominger, J. L., and Tipper, D. J.**, Bacterial cell walls, *Compr. Biochem.*, 26A, 53, 1967.
150. **Braun, V. and Hantke, K.**, Biochemistry of bacterial cell envelopes, *Annu. Rev. Biochem.*, 43, 89, 1974.
151. **Dezelee, P. and Shockman, G. D.**, Studies on the formation of peptide cross-links in the cell wall of peptidoglycan of *Streptococcus faecalis*, *J. Biol. Chem.*, 250, 6806, 1975.
152. IUPAC commission on the nomenclature of organic chemistry and IUPAC-IUB commission on biochemical nomenclature, nomenclature of α-amino acids *Biochemistry*, 14, 449, 1974.
153. **Lent, R. W., Smith, B., Salcedo, L. L., Faris, B., and Franzblau, C.**, Studies on the reduction of elastin. II. Evidence for the presence of α-amino adipic acid-δ-semi aldehyde and its aldol condensation product, *Biochemistry*, 8, 2837, 1969.
154. **Kang, A. H., Faris, B., and Franzblau, C.**, Intramolecular cross-link of chick skin collagen, *Biochem. Biophys. Res. Commun.*, 36, 345, 1969.
155. **Rojkind, M., Gutierrez, A. M., Zeichner, M., and Lent, R. W.**, The nature of the intramolecular cross-link in collagen, *Biochem. Biophys. Res. Commun.*, 36, 350, 1969.
156. **Tanzer, M. L., Housley, T., Berube, L., Fairweather, R., Franzblau, C., and Gallop, P. M.**, Structure of two histidine-containing cross-links from collagen, *J. Biol. Chem.*, 248, 393, 1973.
157. **Loring, H. S. and duVigneaud, V.**, The isolation and characterization of meso-cystine, *J. Biol. Chem.*, 102, 287, 1933.
158. **Wright, N.**, The infrared adsorption spectrum of the stereoisomers of cystine, *J. Biol. Chem.*, 120, 641, 1937.
159. **Roberts, G. C. V. and Jardetzky, O.**, Nuclear magnetic resonance spectroscopy of amino acids, peptides, and proteins, *Adv. Protein Chem.*, 24, 447, 1970.
160. **Ryle, A. P., Sanger, F., Smith, L. F., and Kitai, R.**, The disulphide bonds of insulin, *Biochem. J.*, 60, 541, 1955.
161. **Rosenberry, T. L. and Richardson, J. M.**, Structure of 18S and 14S acetyl-cholinesterase: identification of collagen-like subunits that are linked by disulfide bonds to catalytic subunits, *Biochemistry*, 16, 3550, 1977.
162. **Liu, S. C., Fairbanks, G., and Palck, J.**, Spontaneous reversible protein cross-linking in the human erythrocyte membrane, *Biochemistry*, 16, 4066, 1977.
163. **Thomas, J., Elsden, D. F., and Partridge, S. M.**, Degradation products from elastin, *Nature*, 200, 651, 1963.
164. **Partridge, S. M., Elsden, D. F., Thomas, J., Dorfman, A., Telser, A., and Ho, P. L.**, Biosynthesis of the desmosine and isodesmosine cross-bridges in elastin, *Biochem. J.*, 93, 30, 1964.
165. **Bedford, G. R. and Katritzky, A. R.**, Proton magnetic resonance spectra of degradative products from elastin, *Nature*, 200, 652, 1963.
166. **Anwar, R. A.**, Desmosine peptides: amino acid sequence and role of these sequences in cross-link formation, *Adv. Exp. Med. Biol.*, 71, 329, 1977.
167. **Francis, G., John, R., and Thomas, J.**, Biosynthetic pathway of desmosines in elastins, *Biochem. J.*, 136, 45, 1973.
168. **Partridge, S. M.**, Biosynthesis and nature of elastin structures, *Fed. Proc.*, 3, 1023, 1966.
169. **Foster, J. A., Mecham, R., Imberman, M., Faris, B., and Franzblau, C.**, A high molecular weight species of soluble elastin-proelastin, *Adv. Exp. Med. Biol.*, 79, 351, 1977.
170. **Sage, G. H. and Gray, W. R.**, Evolution of elastin structure, *Adv. Exp. Med. Biol.*, 79, 291, 1977.
171. **Mechanic, G. and Tanzer, M. L.**, Biochemistry of collagen cross-linking: isolation of a new cross-link hydroxylysine hydroxynonleucine and its reduced precursor dehydroxylysinonorleucine from bovine tendon, *Biochem. Biophys. Res. Commun.*, 41, 1597, 1970.
172. **Mechanic, G., Gallop, P. M., and Tanzer, M. L.**, The nature of cross-linking in collagens from mineralized tissues, *Biochem. Biophys. Res. Commun.*, 45, 644, 1971.
173. **Eyre, D. R. and Glimcher, M. J.**, Analysis of a cross-linked peptide: evidence that hydroxylysyl glycoside participates in the cross-link, *Biochem. Biophys. Res. Commun.*, 52, 663, 1973.
174. **Henkel, W., Rauterberg, J., and Stirtz, T.**, Isolation of a cross-linked cyanogen bromide peptide from insoluble rabbit collagen, *Eur. J. Biochem.*, 69, 223, 1976.
175. **Andersen, S. O.**, Resilin, in *Comprehensive Biochemistry*, Vol. 26C, Florkin, M. and Stotz, G. H., Eds., Elsevier-North-Holland, Amsterdam, 1971, 633.
176. **Downie, J. W., LaBella, F. S., and Whitaker, S.**, The relationship between elastin and acidic protein in mammalian uterus, *Connect. Tissue Res.*, 2, 37, 1973.
177. **Keeley, F. W. and LaBella, F. S.**, Isolation of dityrosine from an alkali-soluble tissue protein, *Biochim. Biophys. Acta*, 263, 52, 1972.

178. **Petri, W. H., Wyman, A. R., and Kafatos, F. C.**, Specific protein synthesis in cellular differentiation. III. The eggshell proteins of *Drosophila melanogaster* and their program of synthesis, *Dev. Biol.*, 49, 185, 1976.
179. **Fujimoto, D.**, Occurrence of dityrosine in cuticulin, a structural protein from *Ascaris* cuticle, *Comp. Biochem. Physiol.*, 51B, 205, 1975.
180. **Doolittle, R. F.**, Structural aspects of the fibrinogen to fibrin conversion, *Adv. Protein Chem.*, 27, 2, 1973.
181. **Pisano, J. J., Finlaysen, J. S., and Peyton, M. P.**, Chemical and enzymic detection of protein cross-links: measurement of ε-(γ-glutamyl)-lysine in fibrin polymerised by factor XIII, *Biochemistry*, 8, 871, 1969.
182. **Pisano, J. J., Bronzert, J. J., Peyton, M. P., and Finlayson, J. S.**, ε-(γ-glutamyl)-lysine crosslinks: determination in fibrin from normal and factor XIII-deficient individuals, *Ann. N.Y. Acad. Sci.*, 202, 98, 1972.
183. **Fuller, G. M. and Doolittle, R. F.**, Studies of invertebrate fibrinogen. II. Transformation of lobster fibrinogen into fibrin, *Biochemistry*, 10, 1311, 1971.
184. **Harding, H. W. J. and Rogers, G. E.**, Isolation of peptides containing citrulline and the cross-link ε(γ-glutamyl) lysine from hair medulla protein, *Biochem. Biophys. Acta*, 427, 315, 1976.
185. **Abernathy, J. L., Hill, R. L., and Goldsmith, L. A.**, ε(γ-glutamyl) lysine cross-links in human stratum corneum, *J. Biol. Chem.*, 252, 1837, 1977.
186. **Harding, H. W. J. and Rogers, G. E.**, The occurrence of the ε-(γ-glutamyl) lysine cross-link in the medulla of hair and quill, *Biochem. Biophys. Acta*, 257, 37, 1972.
187. **Asquith, R. S., Otterburn, M. S. Buchanan, J. H., Cole, M., Fletcher, J. C., and Gardner, K. L.**, The identification of ε-N(γ-glutamyl)-L-lysine cross-links in native wool keratins, *Biochim. Biophys. Acta*, 221, 342, 1970.
188. **Loewy, A. G., Matačic, S. S., and Showe, M.**, The isopeptide bond — its distribution and possible functions, *Fed. Proc.*, 30 (Abstr. 1299), 1275, 1971.
189. **Birckbichler, P. J., Dowben, R. M., Matačic, S., and Loewy, A. G.**, Isopeptide bonds in membrane proteins from eukaryotic cells, *Biochim. Biophys. Acta*, 291, 149, 197.
190. **Lorand, L., Weissmann, L. B., Epel, D. L., and Brunner-Lorand, J.**, Role of intrinsic trans-glutaminases in the Ca^{++}-mediated cross-linking of erythrocyte proteins, *Proc. Natl. Acad. Sci. U.S.A.*, 73, 4479, 1976.
191. **Cohen, I., Young-Bandala, L., Blankenberg, T. A., Siefring, G. E., and Brunner-Lorand, J.**, Fibroligase-catalyzed cross-linking of myosin from platelet and skeletal muscle, *Arch. Biochem. Biophys.*, 192, 100, 1979.
192. **Price, N. R. and Hunt, S.**, Studies on the cross-linking regions of whelk egg capsule proteins, *Biochem. Soc. Trans.*, 1, 158, 1973.
193. **Franzblau, C., Kang, A. H., and Faris, B.**, *In vitro* formation of intermolecular cross-links in chick skin collagen, *Biochem. Biophys. Res. Commun.*, 40, 437, 1970.
194. **Hunt, E. and Morris, H. R.**, Collagen cross-links: a mass spectrometric and ^{1}H- and ^{13}C-nuclear resonance study, *Biochem. J.*, 135, 833, 1973.
195. **Housley, T. J., Tanzer, M. L., and Henson, E., and Gallop, P. M.**, Collagen cross-linking: isolation of hydroxy aldol histidine, a naturally occurring cross-link, *Biochem. Biophys. Res. Commun.*, 67, 824, 1975.
196. **Tanzer, M. L., Fairweather, R., and Gallop, P. M.**, Isolation of the cross-link, hydroxymerodesmosine, from borohydride-reduced collagen, *Biochim. Biophys. Acta*, 310, 130, 1973.
197. **Tanzer, M. L., Mechanic, G., and Gallop, P. M.**, Isolation of hydroxylysinonorleucine and its lactone from reconstituted collagen fibrils, *Biochim. Biophys. Acta*, 207, 548, 1970.
198. **Bailey, A. J. and Peach, C. M.**, Isolation and structural identification of a labile intermolecular cross-link in collagen, *Biochem. Biophys. Res. Commun.*, 33, 812, 1968.
199. **Franzblau, C., Sinex, F. M., Faris, B., and Lampidus, R.**, Identification of a new cross-linking amino acid in elastin, *Biochem. Biophys. Res. Commun.*, 21, 575, 1965.
200. **Franzblau, C., Faris, B., and Papaioannou, R.**, Lysinonorleucine: a new amino acid from hydrolysates of elastin, *Biochemistry*, 8, 2833, 1969.
201. **Franzblau, C., Sinex, F. M., and Faris, B.**, Isolation of an unknown component from hydrolysates of elastin, *Nature*, 205, 802, 1965.
202. **Tanzer, M. L. and Mechanic, G.**, Isolation of lysinonorleucine from collagen, *Biochem. Biophys. Res. Commun.*, 39, 183, 1970.
203. **Kang, A. H., Faris, B., and Franzblau, C.**, The *in vitro* formation of intermolecular cross-links in chick skin collagen, *Biochem. Biophys. Res. Commun.*, 39, 175, 1970.
204. **Paz, M. A., Henson, E., Blumenfeld, O. O., Seifter, S., and Gallop, P. M.**, Dehydromerodesmosine and merodesmosine in elastin, *Biochem. Biophys. Res. Commun.*, 44, 1518, 1971.
205. **Fujimoto, D., Akiba, K., and Nakamura, N.**, Isolation and characterization of a fluorescent material in bovine achilles tendon collagen, *Biochem. Biophys. Res. Commun.*, 76, 1124, 1977.

206. **Fujimoto, D. and Moriguchi, T.**, Pyridinoline, a non-reducible cross-link of collagen, *J. Biochem.*, 83, 863, 1978.
207. **Fujimoto, D., Moriguchi, T., Ishida, T., and Hayashi, H.**, The structure of pyridinoline, a collagen cross-link, *Biochem. Biophys. Res. Commun.*, 84, 52, 1978.
208. **Weinblum, D.**, Characterization of photodimers from DNA, *Biochem. Biophys. Res. Commun.*, 27, 384, 1967.
209. **Wacker, A., Dellweg, H., and Weinblum, D.**, Strahlenchemische Veranderung der Bakteriendesoxynbonucleinsaure, *Naturwissenschaften*, 47, 477, 1960.
210. **Johnson, B. E.**, Formation of thymine containing dimers in skin exposed to ultraviolet radiation, *Bull. Cancer*, 65, 283, 1978.
211. **Brunk, C. F.**, Distribution of dimers in ultraviolet irradiated DNA, *Nature (London) New Biol.*, 241, 74, 1973.
212. **Varghese, A. J. and Wang, S. Y.**, Ultraviolet irradiation of DNA *in vitro* and *in vivo* produces a third thymine-derived product, *Science*, 156, 955, 1967.
213. **Karle, I. L., Wang, S. Y., and Varghese, A. J.**, Crystal and molecular structure of a thymine-thymine adduct, *Science*, 164, 183, 1969.
214. **Wang, S. Y. and Varghese, A. J.**, Cytosine-thymine addition product from DNA irradiated with ultraviolet light, *Biochem. Biophys. Res. Commun.*, 29, 543, 1967.
215. **Cohn, W. E., Leonard, N. J., and Wang, S. Y.**, Abbreviations for pyrimidine photoproducts, *Photochem. Photobiol.*, 19, 89, 1974.

LIPOFUSCIN

H. Donato and R. S. Sohal

RELATIONSHIP OF LIPOFUSCIN ACCUMULATION TO AGING

Accumulation of lipofuscin or age pigment is the most prominent age-associated change observed in a variety of cell types from phylogenetically divergent organisms. In particular, the long-lived postmitotic cells, such as neurons and cardiac myocytes, progressively and almost universally exhibit deposition of lipofuscin in relation to aging. For example, lipofuscin deposits were observed in nerve cells of all 47 different species examined by Dayan.[1] Structures resembling lipofuscin were also observed in tissues of several invertebrates.[2-5] In a study on autopsied human hearts of different ages, Strehler et al. noted that the pigment was absent in the young, whereas it was invariably present in the old.[6] Pigment increased with age without correlation to any specific myopathic conditions. The authors suggested that lipofuscin accumulation may represent a basic feature of cellular aging. The rate of lipofuscin accumulation in the hearts of dogs has been found to be approximately 5.5 times faster than in humans, which roughly corresponds to the differences in the life spans of dog and man.[7] The existence of a specific relationship between the rate of aging and lipofuscin accumulation was demonstrated by Sohal and Donato in the housefly *Musca domestica*.[8,9] The life span of the housefly is inversely proportional to metabolic rate.[10-12] Median and maximum life spans were experimentally prolonged approximately twofold by varying flight activity. The rate of lipofuscin accumulation was faster in the short-lived flies undergoing accelerated rates of aging, as compared to the slow-aging, long-lived flies.[8] The maximal lipofuscin content reached, however, was similar in both groups, albeit at different ages.

PROPERTIES OF LIPOFUSCIN

Numerous studies have been made of the structure, composition, and origin of lipofuscin.

Morphology

At the light microscopic level, lipofuscin granules appear rounded or oblong in shape and are 1 to 5 μm in diameter, increasing in size with age. In heart cells, they are located in the perinuclear region, but are randomly distributed in the perikarya of nerve cells. In unstained sections, lipofuscin is brownish in color. In electron micrographs (Figure 1), lipofuscin granules appear bounded by a limiting membrane surrounding a pleomorphic mass of membranous lamallae, osmiophilic granules, and vacuoles.[13] There is considerable variation in the ultrastructural appearance of lipofuscin even within the nerve cell. Hasan and Glees have recognized six different structural categories of lipofuscin granules.[14]

Cytochemical Characterization

Information on the chemical composition of lipofuscin has mainly been derived from histochemical analysis, and has been reviewed extensively.[15-17] Lipofuscin has been histochemically characterized as follows: basophilic due to the presence of acidic groups with pk_a of about 3 to 4; periodic acid-Schiff positive probably due to the presence of unsaturated lipids or carbon chains with adjacent hydroxyl groups; resistant to alcoholic dehydration and extraction; stained by lipid stains, such as Sudan

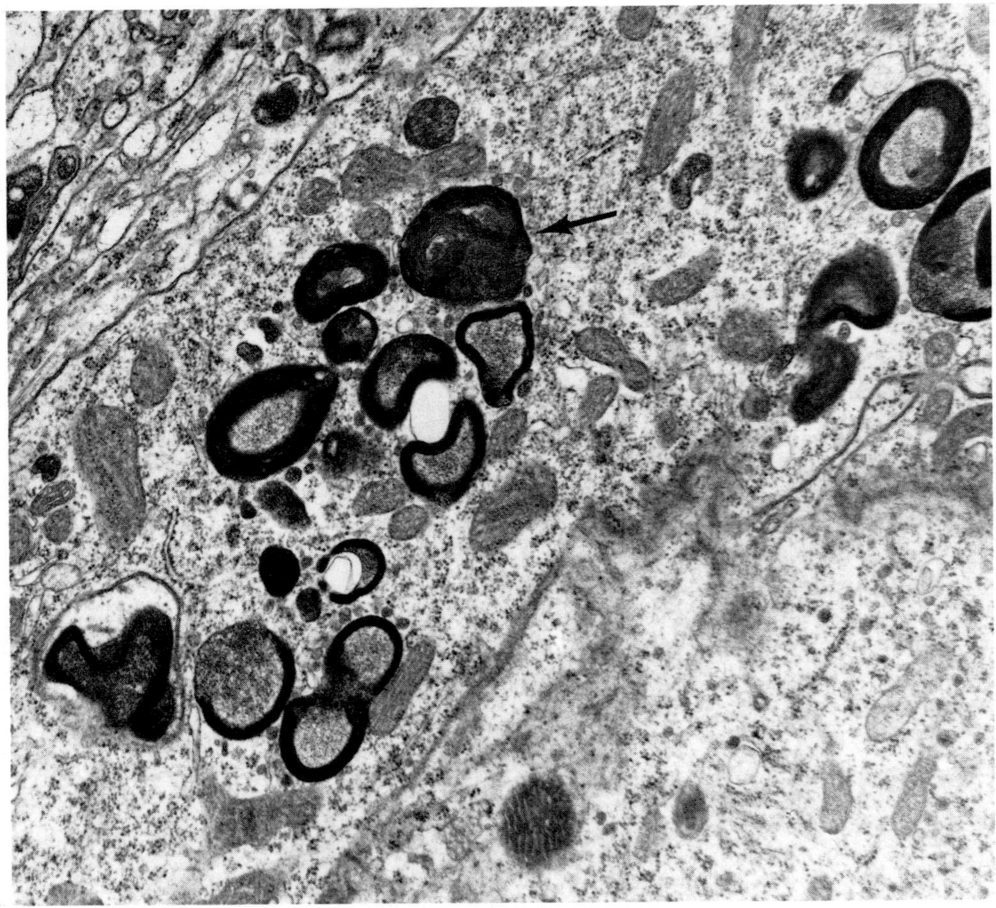

FIGURE 1. An electron micrograph of a section of the brain of the housefly *Musca domestica* showing lipofuscin (arrow) granules. Bar = 0.05 μm.

black B and performic acid-Schiff test, and by reagents specific for proteins; emission of yellow-green to orange fluorescence when excited with near ultraviolet light; reduction by silver salts; and presence of several hydrolytic enzymes.[15-18] The staining reactions of cardiac lipofuscin are described in Table 1.

Isolation and Composition

Several procedures employing density gradient and/or differential centrifugation for isolating lipofuscin granules from tissues have been reported.[19,20] The purity of the preparations is customarily judged by light or electron microscopic examination, or by measurements of lipid-soluble fluorescent material.[19] Chemical analyses of isolated lipofuscin granules have indicated the presence of three major components: 19 to 51% lipids, 30 to 50% proteins, and 9 to 30% acid hydrolysis-resistant residues.[19-21] Extracts of purified lipofuscin in chloroform:methanol mixtures contain a variety of lipids.[16] The fluorescent substances in these mixtures have been related to conjugated Schiff-bases derived from lipid peroxidation of the membranous material.[22] The bulk of the residue remaining after extraction with a chloroform:methanol mixture can be solubilized by acid hydrolysis, and primarily yields a mixture of amino acids. As of yet, the composition of the remaining residue (resistant to acid hydrolysis) is unknown.[19] Li-

Table 1
HISTOCHEMICAL CHARACTERISTICS OF CARDIAC LIPOFUSCIN[16]

Test	Method	Staining intensity
Protein	Hg-bromophenol blue	+ + +
	Ninhydrin-Schiff	+
	CTR	+ +
	DNFR	+
Lipids	Sudan black	+ +
	Fettrot O	+ +
	Sudan III, IV	+ +
Lipids (after extraction with chloroform:methanol)	Sudan III, IV	+ +
Phospholipids	Luxol	+ +
	Baker method	+ +
Plasmalogen	$HgCl_2$-Schiff	+ +
Unsaturated lipids	UV-Schiff	+
	Performic acid-Schiff	+
Acid groups (acid-fast)	Lang-Ziel-Nielsen	+ + +
Acid groups	Toluidine blue (pH 4.0)	+
Acid mucopolysaccharides	Toluidine blue metachromasia	—
Acidic groups (iron-binding)	Hale	+
Basic groups	Solochromecyanin	—
Vicinal poly-OH groups	PAS	+ +
Vicinal poly-OH groups (after diastase)	PAS	+ +
Vicinal poly-OH groups (after hyaluronidase)	PAS	+ +
Reducing groups	Ag reduction	+

pofuscin granules also contain a variety of lysosomal enzymes. Hence, they are considered to be a component of the intracellular lysosomal system.[23]

ORIGIN OF LIPOFUSCIN

A great deal of attention has been devoted to the possible mode of origin of lipofuscin granules. At the morphological level, an overwhelming body of evidence suggests that lipofuscin arises by a process of autophagocytosis involving lysosomes.[13,16,23-26] Presumably, focal areas of the cytoplasm are initially isolated within limiting membranes which arise from preexisting cisternae of endoplasmic reticulum (albeit other sources of limiting membranes have also been suggested) resulting in the formation of autophagic vacuoles.[27] These vacuoles fuse with primary or secondary lysosomes whereupon hydrolytic enzymes induce the degradation and digestion of the enclosed organelles.[23] The undigested residues are generally indistinguishable from lipofuscin.[23,24,28,29]

A chemical hypothesis concerning the origin of lipofuscin (which has been developed in the past decade) postulates that lipofuscin is an end product of lipid peroxidation.[22] The sequence of reactions outlined in Figure 2 presumably originates from univalent reduction of oxygen in cells, and the consequent generation of free radicals.

The role of free radicals as a source of incessant cellular damage during aging was

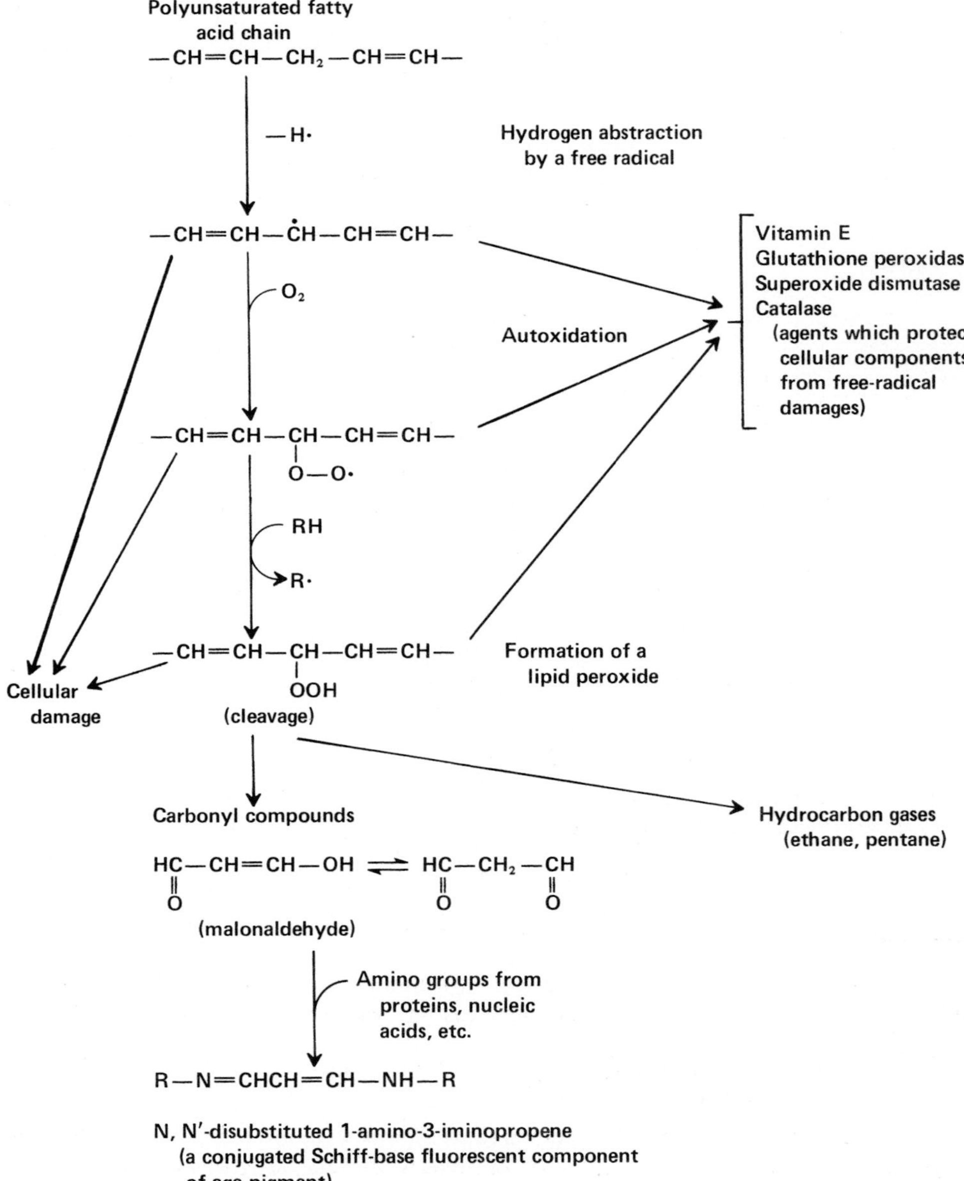

FIGURE 2. A model for the formation of fluorescent components of lipofuscin.

originally postulated by Harman.[30] Free radicals are thought to react with unsaturated lipids in the cells, forming fatty acid-free radicals which combine with oxygen to form a highly reactive fatty acid peroxy-free radicals.[31] The peroxidized lipid-free radicals tend to abstract a hydrogen from another fatty acid molecule, converting the latter into yet another free radical. In its turn, the second oxidized fatty acid molecule can react with oxygen in a chain reaction which, if uninterrupted, can cause disruption of lipoidal structures, e.g., membranes of cell organelles. The production of free radicals during lipid peroxidation can also possibly lead to damaging reactions due to indiscriminate attacks on cellular substances such as proteins and nucleic acids. The peroxidized lipids (especially malonaldehyde, a major product of unsaturated fatty acid peroxidation) can cross-link proteins by reacting with the primary amino groups of the proteins. This reaction results in the formation of the fluorescent Schiff-base products with the structure: RN=CH−CH=CH−NHR′.[22] Similar fluorescent products can also be produced by the reaction of malonaldehyde with amino groups of nucleic acids and with phospholipids. Schiff-base compounds have a fluorescent excitation maximum of 360 to 390 nm, and an emission maximum of about 450 to 470 nm which is similar to that exhibited by the major fluorescent substance in chloroform:methanol extracts of lipofuscin from mammalian and insect tissues.[3,20,32]

Experimental evidence supporting the concept that free radical-induced lipid peroxidation is a source of molecular damage which leads to the formation of fluorescent chromophores in the cells is primarily based on in vitro studies.[22] It has been shown that amino acids (or their esters) and n-hexylamine can react with malonaldehyde to yield conjugated Schiff-bases.[33] Similarly, lipid peroxidation intermediates and malonaldehyde in the in vitro preparation caused inactivation of ribonuclease A activity by intra- and intermolecular cross-lining of the enzyme molecules.[34] The fluorescence produced as a result of the cross-linking was attributed to the conjugated imine structure formed in the proteins between two amino groups and malonaldehyde with a marked similarity to the fluorescence spectrum of the age pigment. However, the mechanism by which peroxidation damage to cell organelles would lead to the formation of autophagic vacuoles and their fusion with the lysosomes is unknown. It is conceivable that the damaged organelles may be selectively invaded by the lysosomes. The secondary lysosomes thus formed would undergo progressive protein digestion and autoxidation of lipids with the condensation of the resulting oxidized compounds into solid polymers of increasing insolubility.[3]

It has been suggested that the amount of fluorescent material present in lipofuscin is a measure of the extent to which peroxidation reactions have occurred in cells or tissues.[22] Fletcher et al. have developed a method for quantifying the relative amount of age pigment present in tissues based on the relative fluorescent intensity of chloroform:methanol extracts.[35] Using this technique, it has been shown that chloroform:methanol extracts of the nematode *Caenorhabditis elegans, Drosophila melanogaster, Neurospora crassa,* the housefly *Musca domestica,* and rat testis undergo an increase in fluorescence intensity (at wavelengths characteristic of age pigment fluorescence) as a function of the age of the organisms.[32,36-41]

Some attempts have been made to isolate and identify the fluorescing components of the chloroform:methanol extracts of rat tissues. Using silicic acid column and thin-layer chromatography, Trombly and Tappel and Trombly et al. found three major fractions of extracts of rat testes which manifested the characteristic fluorescence spectra of age pigment.[42,43] Shimasaki et al. have shown by a thin-layer chromatographic method, that chloroform:methanol extracts of old rat tissues contain a fluorescent substance not present in extracts from young rats.[44] The chemical nature of these compounds has not, however, been determined.

Whether lipofuscin granules themselves are toxic to cells or merely harmless byproducts of metabolism is not known. However, as mentioned above, the lipid peroxidative reactions which lead to the formation of age pigments are known to cause considerable disruption of cellular function. Age-associated changes in enzymes, proteins, nucleotides, DNA, and cell membranes may be attributed (to a varying extent) to reactions initiated by lipid peroxides.[45] Other free radicals which play a role in lipid peroxidation (e.g., the superoxide anion and O_2^-) are thought to be responsible for cellular damage, and may also be responsible for the toxic effects of high concentrations of oxygen.[46]

A correlation between rate of oxygen consumption and concentration of fluorescent age pigment has been demonstrated in houseflies.[8]

ACKNOWLEDGMENT

The authors are supported by Robert A. Welch Foundation grant 719 to H. Donato, and National Institutes of Health grant AG-00171 to R. S. Sohal. The assistance of Ms. Terese Hirth in completing this manuscript is gratefully acknowledged.

REFERENCES

1. **Dayan, A. D.,** Comparative neuropathology of aging: studies on the brain of 47 species of vertebrates, *Brain,* 94, 31, 1971.
2. **Abolins-Krogis, A.,** Fluorescence and histochemical studies of the calcification-initiating lipofuscin-type pigment granules in the shell-repair membrane of the snail, *Helix pomatia* l, *Z. Zellforsch.,* 142, 205, 1973.
3. **Miquel, J., Oro, J., Bensch, K., and Johnson, J.,** Lipofuscin: fine-structural and biochemical studies, in *Free Radicals in Biology,* Pryor, W. A., Ed., Academic Press, New York, 1975.
4. **Sohal, R.,** Fine structural alterations with age in the fat body of the adult male housefly, *Musca domestica, Z. Zellforsch.,* 140, 169, 1973.
5. **Sohal, R. and Sharma, S.,** Age-related changes in the fine structure and number of neurons in the brain of the housefly, *Musca domestica, Exp. Gerontol.,* 7, 243, 1972.
6. **Strehler, B., Mark, D., Mildwan, A., and Gee, M.,** Rate and magnitude of age pigment accumulation in the human myocardium, *J. Gerontol.,* 14, 430, 1959.
7. **Munnel, J. and Getty, R.,** Rate of accumulation of cardiac lipofuscin in the aging canine, *J. Gerontol.,* 23, 154, 1968.
8. **Sohal, R. and Donato, H.,** Effects of experimentally altered life spans on the accumulation of fluorescent age pigment in the housefly, *Musca domestica, Exp. Gerontol.,* 13, 335, 1978.
9. **Sohal, R. and Donato, H.,** Effect of experimental prolongation of life span of lipofuscin content and lysosomal enzyme activity in the brain of the housefly, *Musca domestica, J. Gerontol.,* 34, 489, 1979.
10. **Ragland, S. and Sohal, R.,** Mating behavior, physical activity and aging in the housefly, *Musca domestica, Exp. Gerontol.,* 8, 135, 1973.
11. **Ragland, S. and Sohal, R.,** Ambient temperature, physical activity and aging in the housefly, *Musca domestica, Exp. Gerontol.,* 10, 279, 1975.
12. **Sohal, R. S.,** Metabolic rate and life span, *Interdiscip. Top. Gerontol.,* 9, 25, 1976.
13. **Samorajski, T., Ordy, J., and Keefe, J.,** The fine structure of lipofuscin age pigment in the nervous system of aged mice, *J. Cell Biol.,* 26, 779, 1965.
14. **Hasan, M. and Glees, P.,** Electron microscopical appearance of neuronal lipofuscin using different preparative techniques including freeze-etching, *Exp. Gerontol.,* 7, 345, 1972.
15. **Pearse, A.,** *Histochemistry,* Vol. 2, 3rd ed., Williams & Wilkins, Baltimore, 1972.
16. **Strehler, B.,** On the histochemistry and ultrastructure of age pigment, in *Advanced Gerontological Research,* Strehler, B., Ed., Academic Press, New York, 1964.
17. **Wolman, M.,** Biological peroxidation of lipids and membranes, *Isr. J. Med. Sci.,* 11, 1, 1975.
18. **Barka, T. and Anderson, P.,** *Histochemistry,* Harper & Row, New York, 1965.
19. **Bjorkerud, S.,** Isolated lipofuscin granules — a survey of new field, in *Advanced Gerontological Research,* Strehler, B., Ed., Academic Press, New York, 1964.
20. **Siakotos, A. and Koppang, N.,** Procedures for the isolation of lipopigments from brain, heart, and liver and their properties: a review, *Mech. Ageing Dev.,* 2, 177, 1973.
21. **Hendley, D., Mildvan, A., Reporter, M., and Strehler, B.,** The properties of isolated human cardiac age pigment. II. Chemical and enzymatic properties, *J. Gerontol.,* 18, 250, 1963.
22. **Tappel, A.,** Lipid peroxidation and fluorescent molecular damage to membranes, in *Pathobiology of Cell Membranes,* Trumps, B. and Arstila, A., Eds., Academic Press, New York, 1975.
23. **DeDuve, C. and Wattiaux, R.,** Functions of lysosomes, *Annu. Rev. Physiol.,* 28, 435, 1966.
24. **Brandes, D.,** Lysosomes and aging pigment, in *Topics in the Biology of Aging,* Krohn, P., Ed., Interscience, New York, 1966.

25. **Essner, E. and Novikoff, A.,** Human hepatocellular pigments and lysosomes, *J. Ultrastruct. Res.,* 3, 374, 1960.
26. **Koenig, H.,** The autofluorescence of lysosomes: its value for the identification of lysosomal constituents, *J. Histochem. Cytochem.,* 11, 556, 1963.
27. **Arstila, A. and Trump, B.,** Autophagocytosis: origin of membrane and hydrolytic enzymes, *Virchows Arch. B:,* 2, 85, 1969.
28. **Frank, A. L. and Christensen, A.,** Localization of acid phosphatase in lipofuscin granules and possible autophagic vacuoles in interstitial cells of the guinea pig testis, *J. Cell Biol.,* 36, 1, 1968.
29. **Quatacker, J.,** Formation of autophagic vacuoles during human corpus luteum involution, *Z. Zellforsch.,* 122, 479, 1971.
30. **Harman, T.,** Aging: a theory based on free radical and radiation chemistry, *J. Gerontol.,* 11, 298, 1956.
31. **Dormandy, T.,** Biological rancidification, *Lancet,* 2, 684, 1969.
32. **Donato, H. and Sohal, R.,** Age-related changes in lipofuscin-associated fluorescent substances on the adult male housefly, *Musca domestica, Exp. Gerontol.,* 13, 335, 1978.
33. **Chio, K. S. and Tappel, A. L.,** Synthesis and characterization of the fluorescent products derived from malonaldehyde and amino acids, *Biochemistry,* 8, 2821, 1969.
34. **Chio, K. S. and Tappel, A.,** Inactivation of ribonuclease and other enzymes by peroxidizing lipids and by malonaldehyde, *Biochemistry,* 8, 2827, 1969.
35. **Fletcher, B. L., Dillard, C., and Tappel, A.,** Measurement of fluorescent lipid peroxidation products in biological systems and tissues, *Anal. Biochem.,* 52, 1, 1973.
36. **Klass, M.,** Aging in the nematode *Caenorhabditis elegans:* major biological and environmental factors influencing life span, *Mech. Ageing Dev.,* 6, 413, 1977.
37. **Miquel, J., Tappel, A., Dillard, C., Herman, M., and Bensch, K.,** Fluorescent products and lysosomal components in aging *Drosophila melanogaster, J. Gerontol.,* 29, 622, 1974.
38. **Sheldahl, J. and Tappel, A.,** Fluorescent products from aging *Drosophila melanogaster:* an indicator of free radical lipid peroxidation damage, *Exp. Gerontol.,* 9, 33, 1974.
39. **Rana, R. and Munkres, K.,** Lipid peroxidation and decay of respiratory enzymes in an inositol auxotroph, *Mech. Ageing Dev.,* 7, 241, 1978.
40. **Donato, H., Hoselton, M., and Sohal, R.,** Lipofuscin accumulation: effects of individual variation and selective mortality on population averages, *Exp. Gerontol.,* 14, 141, 1979.
41. **Miquel, J., Lundgren, P., and Johnson, J.,** Spectrophotometric and electron microscopic study of lipofuscin accumulation in the testes of aging mice, *J. Gerontol.,* 33, 5, 1978.
42. **Trombly, R. and Tappel, A.,** Fractionation and analysis of fluorescent products of lipid peroxidation, *Lipids,* 10, 441, 1975.
43. **Trombly, R., Tappel, A., Coniglio, J., Grogan, W., and Rhamy, R.,** Fluorescent products and polyunsaturated fatty acids of human testes, *Lipids,* 10, 591, 1975.
44. **Shimasaki, H., Nozawa, T., Privett, O., and Anderson, W.,** Detection of age-related fluorescent substances in rat tissues, *Arch. Biochem. Biophys.,* 183, 443, 1977.
45. **Bland, J.,** Biochemical consequences of lipid peroxidation, *J. Chem. Educ.,* 55, 151, 1978.
46. **Gregory, E. and Fridovich, I.,** Induction of superoxide dismutase by molecular oxygen, *J. Bacteriol.,* 114, 54, 1973.

Control Processes

AGING EFFECTS ON HORMONE CONCENTRATIONS AND ACTIONS

Gail D. Riegle and Anna E. Miller

INTRODUCTION

As one of the two major regulators of body function, the endocrines are recognized to influence all aspects of body function. The effects of age alterations in endocrine function have always fascinated gerontologists. Aging changes in endocrine function have often been considered to be closely associated with the effect of age on diverse physiological systems. In fact, many early investigators postulated that age deterioration of gonadal function was the cause of biological aging.

In recent years we have witnessed major advances in our understanding of the biochemistry, physiology, and pharmacology of all endocrine systems. Significant age-related alterations in resting hormone function and decreases in the ability of endocrine control systems to respond appropriately to stress or stimulation have been identified in most endocrine control systems. Clinicians and scientists have been adept at combining clinical skills with biochemical tests to identify and treat many age-related alterations in endocrine function, often with spectacular results.

REPRODUCTIVE CONTROL SYSTEMS

Aging changes in reproduction and reproductive endocrine control systems have been extensively studied and are more well-documented than aging effects on most other endocrine systems. Although the loss of reproductive function with increased age is of concern for many animal breeders, age effects on reproduction have not been of major concern in our society since most men and women have procreated their desired offspring before they reach the age when fertility has been significantly reduced. On the other hand, the effect of age on reproductive hormones and human sexuality is of major concern in human societies. No other effect of aging on endocrine function is as dramatic as that which occurs with menopause in women. However, it must be remembered that aging effects on reproduction are continuous, and important changes in reproductive control systems occur throughout the biological life span of all mammals.

Similar time-course relationships between aging effects on reproductive hormone systems and age-related deterioration of functions of other physiological systems have been demonstrated in many species. This relationship suggests that a better understanding of aging changes in reproductive hormonal control systems will allow the development of clinical procedures that may affect not only aging changes in reproductive hormones, but also the quality if not the quantity of life for the aged. A wealth of new information and understanding regarding the anatomical and physiological parameters that are associated with reproductive control mechanisms has been obtained in recent years. Major advances have been made in understanding the relationships between the hypothalamus and pituitary, and the mechanisms by which these tissues interact with the gonads to control both gametogenesis and steroidogenesis. It has become clear that there are significant differences in the effect of age on parameters of the reproductive control system among various species. In the following paragraphs, representative data related to the effect of biological aging on reproductive control systems will be summarized.

Male

Increasing age is accompanied by decreased sexual activity.[100] Several psychological

Table 1
SERUM TESTOSTERONE CONCENTRATIONS IN MALES

Species	Age	Serum testosterone (nmol)[a]	Ref.
Human	<50 years	17.7	183
	>65 years	9.6	
	<40 years	17.1	8
	>71 years	8.0	
	21—50 years	22.0	15
	>50 years	17.0	
Rat	3—6 months	9.1	67
	>24 months	4.5	
	4 months	14.8	
	13 months	6.9	127
	22 months	4.6	
Mouse	6 months	15.9	48
	28 months	15.1	
	6 months	32.0	54
	28 months	26.2	

[a] Calculated from published values on the basis of a molecular weight of 275 daltons; thus, a concentration of 10 nmol corresponds to 2.75 ng/mℓ.

factors including marital state, health of spouse, and previous levels of sexual activity have been shown to be correlated with sexual function in men.[115,136] Although aged males have decreased sexual function, individual males have been shown to be fertile at advanced age.[18,161] Since many of the effects of increased age on reproduction are consistent with effects which would be expected with decreased testosterone secretion, it has long been assumed that aging is associated with decreasing testicular endocrine function. Aged human Leydig cells show variable amounts of anatomical changes with age.[18] The effect of age on serum testosterone concentrations is not uniform between and within mammalian species (Table 1). Several studies have shown no effects of age on blood testosterone concentrations in men and mice.[48,54,101] On the other hand, other experiments have shown substantially decreased serum testosterone in aged men and rats.[3,20,37] One study in aged men also found increased testosterone binding protein compared to young men, which resulted in an even greater reduction in free testosterone than in total blood testosterone.[37]

The reduction in testosterone secretion in the aged male rat could reflect either an age-related loss of the ability of testicular interstitial cells to respond to luteinizing hormone (LH) secretion or a reduction in gonadotropin secretion in the aged male. The aged male rat has reduced testicular Δ^5-3β-hydroxysteroid dehydrogenase activity which can be restored with HCG stimulation;[108] 7 days of subcutaneous HCG injection (5 IU HCG/100 g bw) induced similar increases in serum testosterone and testicular responsiveness to acute HCG stimulation in young and aged male rats.[127] These findings suggest that the aged male rat is capable of sustaining higher testosterone secretion, and the decrease in testosterone secretion is due to reductions with age in LH stimulation of the testes.

In summary, age-related decreases in sexual function occur in males of all tested mammalian species. On the other hand, the effect of age on testicular endocrine function is highly variable between and within species. Our studies have shown that the sharp decrease in serum testosterone in the aged male rat can be restored by chronic HCG stimulation of the testes; this suggests that the decrease in serum testosterone is caused by inadequate interstitial cell stimulation.

Table 2
SERUM LH AND FSH LEVELS IN MALES

Species	Age	LH (nmol)[a]	FSH (nmol)[a]	Ref.
Human	30—50 years	2.7 IU/1	3.7 IU/1	
	>50 years	8.9	6.8	8
	21—50 years	1.42 IU/1	1.95 IU/1	
	>70 years	3.04	7.27	15
Rat	3—4 months	0.59	7.33	
	21 months	0.18	5.53	124
	4—5 months	0.48	—	128
	24—28 months	0.25		
	5 months	0.44	—	129
	22—26 months	0.24		
	4—6 months	0.77	—	167
	23—30 months	0.18		
Mouse	12 months	0.50	53.3	54
	28 months	0.50	55.7	

[a] Calculated from published values on the basis of a molecular weight of 34,000 for rat LH and 30,000 for rat FSH, except in the studies on humans, for which adequate information on potency and structure of the pure hormones is not yet available.

The endocrine function of testicular interstitial tissue is primarily regulated by LH stimulation. Decreased blood testosterone concentrations have been reported in aged human males and male rats. If the feedback control system for LH secretion and testicular Leydig cells is functioning normally, this decreased testosterone should result in sufficient stimulation of pituitary LH secretion to restore testosterone secretion. (There are apparently significant sex differences in gonadotropin control systems in men and women; it is recognized that a large increase in gonadotropin secretion occurs in postmenopausal women, presumably as a consequence of reduced steroid hormone negative feedback caused by failure of follicular development and luteinization in the ovaries of these women.) Representative serum gonadotropin concentrations from aging males of several species are shown in Table 2. Significant age effects on serum gonadotropins have been reported for all these species except the mouse. The reproductive control system of the aging male mouse appears to be functionally normal, allowing it to maintain similar blood testosterone, LH and FSH concentrations, and similar pituitary responsiveness to LH-releasing hormone (LHRH) stimulation as in young adult male mice. Although serum LH concentrations in both aged men and rats are different from mature adult LH concentrations, they are changed in opposite directions. The decrease in testosterone secretion by aged men is accompanied by increased serum concentrations of FSH and LH.[8,15] However, the increased gonadotropin secretion is not sufficient to elevate serum testosterone to concentrations found in young men. Although several studies[112,114] have shown reduced testicular secretion of testosterone in response to HCG stimulation in aged compared to young men (presumably indicating decreased Leydig cell function), the aged testis has sufficient reserve capacity to increase blood testosterone to concentrations found in younger men.[160] These data suggest that the increase in LH secretion in aged men is not sufficient to stimulate testosterone secretion in quantities typical of young men, and implicate age-related alterations in the ability of the hypothalamus to secrete adequate LHRH in response to the decreased blood testosterone in aged men.

The decline in hypothalamic responsiveness to hormonal feedback is more evident in the aged male rat than in the human. The aged male rat has consistently been shown to have reduced serum gonadotropin concentrations.[124,151,167] These data indicate that the hypothalamic-pituitary gonadotropin control system does not respond to decreased testosterone concentrations. Although the aged male rat exhibits smaller increases in serum LH following a single LHRH injection, we have shown that multiple LHRH stimulations cause similar increases in serum LH in young and aged male rats.[128] These experiments indicate that age-related alterations in hypothalamic responsiveness may be a primary lesion in the reproductive control system of the aged male rat.

It is accepted that the hypothalamus synthesizes and secretes hormonal factors which are major regulators of anterior pituitary secretion.[78] Most evidence suggests that release of hypothalamic hormones into the hypothalamic-hypophyseal portal vessels involves the function of neurotransmitters of the central nervous system, particularly the catecholamines. Alterations in hypothalamic concentrations of dopamine and norepinephrine, particularly within the median eminence, are associated with the release of gonadotropin-releasing hormone and prolactin.[53,126,132,166]

A large body of experimental data indicates a negative feedback relationship between serum testosterone concentrations and hypothalamic gonadotropin-releasing hormone and pituitary gonadotropin release. We and many other investigators believe the hypothalamus is a primary site of age-related alterations in reproductive control systems.[12,43,124] Some experiments suggest decreased hypothalamic sensitivity to control input with increased age,[43,149,150] whereas others have hypothesized increased hypothalamic sensitivity to hormonal controls.[12]

Age-related alterations in hypothalamic gonadotropin-releasing hormone content could affect the responsiveness of the reproductive control system. Similar concentrations of biologically active gonadotropin-stimulating activities were found in hypothalamic extracts from young and aged intact and gonadectomized male and female rats.[129] These data suggest that changes in hypothalamic gonadotropin-releasing hormone content cannot be associated with decreased pituitary gonadotropin secretion in aged male rats.

Several laboratories have studied aging effects on hypothalamic neurotransmitters.[53,132,169] Most studies have either considered age effects on hypothalamic monamine content or measured neurotransmitter turnover as an index of activity in laboratory rats and mice. These studies show a consistent decrease in hypothalamic dopamine and norepinephrine content. In addition, decreased dopamine and norepinephrine turnover was found in the hypothalmus of aged rats.[169] On the other hand, although hypothalamic serotonin content was not altered in aged rats, the older male group had increased serotonin turnover. These rat data are substantiated by similar results with male mice.[54] The older mice had decreased median eminence dopamine content and as much as a 50% decrease in hypothalamic norepinephrine turnover. The changes in hypothalamic neurotransmitter function in aged male mice and rats are consistent with the hypothesis that alterations in hypothalamic neurotransmitter function are a major factor in the loss of testosterone secretion and fertility in these animals.

In summary, significant changes occur in the male reproductive control systems of most mammalian species studied. These changes often include decreased libido, decreased spermatogenesis, infertility, and decreased testosterone secretion. Although the decrease in testicular endocrine function is variable, most experiments indicate increased capacity for testosterone secretion among aged males. Some studies have shown decreased acute pituitary responsiveness to LHRH stimulation, presumably due to a degree of endocrine disuse atrophy; however, most experiments do not indicate significant alterations in pituitary gonadotropin secretory capacity. Age-related alterations of hypothalamic responsiveness to control input have been implicated in most species. In some instances, hypothalamic responsiveness appears to be the primary lesion in the reproductive control system of aging males; in other species it appears to be a contributing factor to these alterations.

Female

The most fundamental effect of aging on the mammalian female reproductive control system is the irreversible decline in oocytes which commences during neonatal life and continues through the aging of the reproductive system. The best known and most widely documented aging effect on female reproduction is the loss of ovarian function which occurs in women. Although the number of normal oocytes is exhausted at or shortly after the menopause in women,[97] other species experience reproductive failure when substantial numbers of oocytes remain in the ovaries.[177] In most instances, follicular development and ovulation can be stimulated in species that exhibit age-related loss of fertility; this suggests that the loss of oocytes is not the primary factor in the failure to reproduce.

The effect of age on reproductive function has been most extensively studied in the laboratory rodent, particularly the rat. The current understanding of age effects in the rodent suggests two phases of reproductive senescence.[54] The first phase is characterized by the loss of fertility in animals with regular ovarian cycles, begins before midage in the rat, and is believed to be potentially similar to the premenopausal decline in fertility in women. The second phase begins later in the rat's life span and is characterized by alterations in the animal's ovarian cycles.

The first change in vaginal cytological patterns in the rat is the development of constant estrous states. Later, increased numbers of aging female rats develop repetitive pseudopregnancies or may eventually enter a noncyclic, diestrous state.[12] A large number of studies have shown that the loss of ovarian function in the aged rat is not accompanied by the increase in gonadotropin secretion which is characteristic of the postmenopausal woman.[82]

A great deal of attention has recently been directed toward the identification of specific lesions occurring with age in the hypothalamic-pituitary-gonadal control system of the laboratory rodent. Most studies show decreased litter size prior to decreased ovulatory rates.[4] Age-related alterations affecting fertilization and development of the preimplanted egg have been proposed. The viability of oocytes from aged females has been studied by transplanting fertilized eggs from old donors to young recipients. Although an initial study of ova transplanted from aged to young female hamsters indicated decreased fertility compared to control transplants from young donors to young recipients, subsequent studies using somewhat different postovulatory transplant times have shown similar viability of aged compared to young donor ova transplanted to young recipient mice and rabbits.[68,97,178] In addition, these same studies show sharply decreased survival of eggs transplanted from young donors to aged recipients.

These data indicate that the decrease in fertility of aged mammalian females occurs much earlier than any recognized alteration in ovarian reproductive potential; they implicate alterations with age in the ability of the reproductive tract (presumably the uterus) to sustain normal gestation. Age alterations in uterine function have been implicated in the decrease in fertility characteristic of premenopausal women and midaged rodent species. Failure of the uterus to sustain pregnancy could involve either anatomical changes in reproductive tract tissues which affect their ability to sustain the conceptus, or age changes in endocrine stimulation of uterine function. Decreased endometrial decidual tissue development has been reported in aged hamsters and mice.[21,89] Since this change in decidualization could reflect alterations in either the amount of hormonal stimulation or tissue responsiveness, several investigators have considered the effect of age on ovarian steroid secretion.

Table 3
PROGESTAGEN LEVELS IN MAMMALIAN FEMALES

A. Serum Levels in Human and Rabbit Females

Species	Condition	Compound measured	Concentration (nmol)[a]	Ref.
Human	Premenopausal, follicular	17-OH progesterone	1.24	2
	Premenopausal, luteal		4.83	
	Postmenopausal		0.74	
Rabbit	Young, 5-day pregnancy	Progesterone	31.5	174
	Old, 5-day pregnancy		31.3	
	Young, 18-day pregnancy	Progesterone	51.1	174
	Old, 18-day pregnancy		57.0	

B. Progesterone Levels in Rat Serum at Various Stages of the Estrous Cycle

Stage	Progesterone concentration (nmol)[a]				Ref.
	3 months	12 months	18 months	24 months	
Proestrous	55	26	29	23	
Estrous	29	20	19	14	130
Diestrous	46	27	26	24	

C. Progesterone Levels in Rat Serum after Various Periods of Pregnancy

Day of pregnancy	Progesterone concentration (nmol)[a]			Ref.
	4 months	13 months	22 months	
1	16	13	10	
6	235	127	322	
11	202	140	290	
16	228	127	36	132
19	241	225	—	
22	26	91	—	

[a] Calculated from published values on the basis of a molecular weight of 308 for progesterone, and 324 for 17-OH progesterone.

Both direct and indirect estimates have been made on the effect of aging on luteal progesterone secretion (Table 3). Reports of reduced numbers of luteal cells in aging mice,[51,70,77] and increased implantation of embryos in aging hamsters receiving young ovarian implants (to increase their progesterone secretion)[22] and in mice treated with progesterone injections[69] suggest reduced luteal progesterone secretion. On the other hand, similar plasma progesterone levels have been reported during pregnancy in young and aged rabbits.[107] A recent study of the effect of increased age on progesterone secretion in female Long-Evans rats demonstrated that progesterone concentrations were consistently reduced in the aging rats (Table 3B), although serum progesterone concentrations showed similar patterns of change during proestrous, estrous, and diestrous stages of the ovarian cycle as in young mature rats. Determination of possible physiological effects of these reduced progesterone concentrations on the gonadotropin surge of proestrus, the development of the fertilized egg, or on the implantation mechanisms await additional experimentation.

Table 4
ESTROGEN LEVELS IN HUMAN FEMALES

Age (years)	Condition	Serum estrogen (pmol)[a] Estradiol	Estrone	Ref.
18—25	Intact	150	220	
51—65	Intact	75	186	184
	Ovariectomized	68	182	
Premenopausal	Follicular	154		
	Luteal	218		73
Postmenopausal		79		
		24	95	111
		49	—	1
		—	110	99

[a] Calculated from published values on the basis of a molecular weight of 266 for estradiol and 264 for estrone.

A study of aging effects on serum progesterone during pregnancy and pseudopregnancy in mated cycling rats and constant estrous rats is summarized in Table 3C.[130] Successful pregnancy was reduced to 50% in 11-month-old rats and 25% in the 13-month-old group, with no successful pregnancies occurring in older groups. Mean progesterone concentrations were not different between the various aged mated cycling or mated constant estrous aged groups through postcoital day 11. Serum progesterone was higher in the younger cycling rats which produced litters than in the other groups during the last half of gestation. These data suggest normal luteal tissue development and early function in the aged rat, and implicate inadequate placental luteotropic stimulation in the aged groups.

Another experiment in this study considered the effect of age on serum progesterone in early and late gestation in rats producing normal litters. Mean gestation length was 1.5 days longer in 13-month-old compared to 4-month-old rats. The only difference in progesterone levels was a sharper decline in late pregnancy in the young group which corresponded with the earlier parturition time. The increased gestation length in aged rats is substantiated by a recent report of similar observation in aged mice.[196]

The influence of progesterone on gestation could be influenced by age-related alterations in uterine responsiveness to the hormone. For instance, normal cytosol receptor function is essential for progesterone function. Since estradiol and progesterone cytosol receptor concentrations are influenced by steroid hormones, preovulatory deficits of these hormones in the aged rats could cause a deficit in steroid receptors and inhibit uterine responsiveness to the hormones. Additional experiments are needed to address this important point.

Very little information is currently available concerning effects of age on estrogen secretion in laboratory rodents; this process could be important in many of the changes occurring in reproduction in rodent species. Our preliminary data indicate reduced proestrous estrogen secretion in aged compared to young cycling rats, with an intermediate estrogen concentration found in aging constant estrous females.

Although there is considerably more data on estrogen and progesterone function in aging women than in rodents, most of these experiments have concerned changes in the menopausal years (Tables 3 and 4). As women approach menopause, failure of ovulation and corpus luteum formation becomes an increasingly common occurrence.[177] There is also evidence that the corpora lutea formed in these women may be anatomically and endocrinologically abnormal, resulting in shortened men-

Table 5
SERUM LH AND FSH LEVELS IN FEMALES

		LH		FSH	
Species	Age	Concentration (nmol)[a]	Ref.	Concentration (nmol)[a]	Ref.
Human	21—17 years	10 U/1		1.1	
	45—56 years	172 U/1	99	3.3	36
Rat	3 months	0.29		0.47	
	22 months	0.14	113	1.25	119
	4 months	1.39			
	26 months	0.64	123	—	—

[a] Concentrations calculated as in Table 2.

strual cycles or early abortion of the conceptus if pregnancy has occurred.[37,137] Mean values for pregnandiol in 24-hr urine,[104] luteal progesterone secretion,[168] and plasma 17-hydroxyprogesterone[1] have all been reported to be decreased in postmenopausal women. It is well-established that the ovarian secretion of estrogen, particularly estradiol, decreases in the menopausal woman.[73] It has recently been recognized that a major source of estrogens in the postmenopausal woman is the peripheral metabolism of androgens — primarily of ovarian origin — to estrogens.[142] Ovarian vein concentrations of estrogens in postmenopausal women are only about a third those of premenopausal women, while androgen synthesis is increased to about twice the level of premenopausal ovarian secretion.

Although there are major endocrinological alterations established as occurring with the menopause, many unanswered problems exist in our understanding of specific age-related lesions which may occur in the hypothalamic-pituitary-gonadal reproductive control system in aging women. An age-related change in the sensitivity of a hypothalamic-pituitary unit to steroid feedback has been proposed. However, the sharp increase in postmenopausal FSH and LH secretion and the induction of gonadotropin surges by steroid hormone treatment of postmenopausal women challenges this theory.[140] Another factor in the infertility of aging women is an age-related alteration in the responsiveness of oocytes. Although oocytes are exhausted in aging women shortly after menopause, a recent study demonstrated some anatomically normal primordial follicles in anovulatory menopausal women.[38] These findings suggest an age-related change in ovary or follicular sensitivity to gonadotropins in the menopausal years.[113]

Pituitary gonadotropin secretion is sharply increased in postmenopausal women (Table 5). Increased gonadotropin secretion in premenopausal women has been hypothesized as a factor which contributes to the loss of oocytes;[49] however, most studies have not shown increased gonadotropin secretion in women until after the climacteric.[36,105] The increase in gonadotropin secretion in postmenopausal women appears to occur as a direct consequence of reduced ovarian estradiol and progesterone secretion since restoration of these hormones reduced gonadotropin secretion.[140] FSH and LH concentrations increase and lose their typical cyclicity during the menstrual cycles of the early climacteric.[3,195]

Although aged female rodents lose their reproductive capacity long before they reach their maximal longevity, there is no evidence for increased gonadotropin secretion associated with this infertility (Table 5). The appearance of ovarian interstitial deficiency cells which can be restored with LH injection suggested reduced gonadotropin stimulation of the aged rat ovary.[12] This suggestion of inadequate gonadotropin secretion in aged female rats is supported by direct measurements of serum gonadotropins in

Table 6
LEVELS OF PROLACTIN IN RAT SERUM

Sex	Age (months)		Prolactin concentration (nmol)[a]		Ref.
	Young	Old	Young	Old	
Male	3	24	0.76	3.34	34
	4—6	22—30	0.69	2.10	151
Female	3	22	0.29	0.40	119
	4—6	23—30	0.21	13.8	167

[a] Calculated from published values on the basis of a molecular weight of 21,000 daltons.

aged groups. The aged female rat has been shown to maintain increased serum prolactin, but reduced LH concentrations (Tables 5 and 6).[90,167,187] The increase in serum LH following ovariectomy is smaller in aged compared to young female rats.[167] In addition, we have found reduced serum LH concentrations in proestrous aged rats compared to young rats; these data could reflect decreased pituitary capacity for gonadotropin secretion. Although there was decreased pituitary responsiveness to a single LHRH stimulus,[187] subsequent experiments showed that both aged and young female rats had similar serum LH concentrations following multiple LHRH stimulations.[128] This observation of a similarity in pituitary response to LHRH stimulation in young and aged rats is similar to reports of a lack of age differences in pituitary response to LHRH in women.[179,191] The increase in gonadotropin secretion following ovariectomy and LHRH stimulation indicates that the aged rat can sustain higher serum gonadotropin concentrations than those which normally occur during aging; this suggests that failure of normal hypothalamic stimulation of pituitary gonadotropin contributes to the loss of normal ovarian function and infertility.

Aging effects on the ability of hypothalamic neurons to synthesize LHRH could contribute to the decrease in gonadotropin secretion in female rats, but such differences have not been demonstrated in aged male or female rats.[129] These data suggest that age alterations in the ability of the rat hypothalamus to secrete LHRH (rather than aging effects on LHRH synthesis) contribute to the decrease in pituitary LH secretion. Many researchers have shown that the release of hypothalamic hormones, including LHRH, into the portal vessels in the median eminence can be influenced by alterations in hypothalmis neurotransmitters. In particular, hypothalamic dopamine and norepinephrine function has been associated with LHRH secretion.[61,163] The decrease in hypothalamic dopamine and norepinephrine content and turnover in aged rats suggests that loss of catecholamine function could contribute to the decrease in hypothalmic LHRH release and loss of fertility in these rats.

There is considerable indirect evidence supporting the hypothesis that decreased hypothalamic catecholamine function is a major contributor to the failure of aged rats to reproduce. There is a decreased responsiveness of the hypothalamic-pituitary unit to L-dopa injection in aged rats.[186] The decrease in control system responsiveness was found for both the stimulation of LH secretion and the inhibition of prolactin secretion. As mentioned previously, one of the first alterations in the ovarian cycle of the aging rat is the development of the constant estrous state. Electrical stimulation of the preoptic region of the hypothalamus induces the resumption of estrous cycles and ovulation in the aged constant estrous rat.[35,194] A large variety of treatments including

Table 7
EFFECTS OF AGE ON GROWTH HORMONE IN MAN

Property	Age range (years)	Sex	Change with age	Ref.
Blood levels				
Basal	9—92	Male, female	No change	23, 47, 162, 180
	16—76	Male	Increased	162
Decrease by glucose	22—81	Male	No change	47
Increase by arginine	17—90	Male	No change	23, 29
Increase during sleep	8—62	Male, female	Decreased	29, 55
Induction by insulin	20—84	Male, female	Decreased	134
Rate of secretion	9—62	Male, female	Decreased	55
GH-producing cells in pituitary	20—80	Male, female	No change	28
Binding of GH to liver membranes	20—79	Male, female	No change	30

progesterone, ACTH, stress, L-dopa, lergotrile, iproniazid, and epinephrine have been shown to be capable of reinitiating ovarian cycles in aging constant estrous rats. Although some of these treatments may reinitiate ovarian cycles by affecting neurotransmitter function, direct evidence of effects of these agents on hypothalamic monoamines is lacking. Progesterone, ACTH, stress, and epinephrine could all act by increasing progesterone concentration which in turn could stimulate gonadotropic secretion by the hypothalamic-pituitary unit.

In summary, more than a single mechanism seems to be involved with aging effects on the reproductive control system. Aging rats and menopausal women show decreased ovarian steroid secretion which results in decreased negative feedback and increased gonadotropin secretion in women, and decreased stimulation of the gonadotropin release mechanism in rats. Current information indicates uncertainty about hypothalamic involvement with decreased fertility in aging women. On the other hand, decreased sensitivity of hypothalamic gonadotropin control mechanisms to control input is without question a significant alteration in the aging laboratory rat and mouse.

GROWTH HORMONE AND SOMATOMEDIN

In contrast to the situation with the gonadotrophins, it appears that there is no well-established change with age in levels or secretion of growth hormone. Virtually all the studies of this hormone have been in humans (thus involving unavoidable difficulties in controlling and evaluating differences among individual clinical subjects); the data are summarized in Table 7. Although there are no consistent changes with age in basal levels of GH or induction of GH secretion by arginine, substantial age-related decreases in the elevation of GH during sleep or following insulin administration have been reported. However, as Muggeo et al.[134] pointed out, the decrease with age in the effect of insulin could be secondary to an impaired hypoglycemic response to insulin.

Some time ago, Root and Oski[159] reported that certain effects of GH were depressed in old patients. Recently, Florini and Roberts[57] demonstrated that circulating levels of somatomedins were significantly decreased when 26- to 28-month-old Fischer 344 rats were compared with 5- and 14- to 17-month-old animals. It is now clear that the somatomedins mediate many of the actions of GH;[13] these observations suggest that age-related decreases in anabolic processes may result from impaired secretion or potency of the somatomedins.

Table 8
THYROID HORMONE LEVELS IN HUMANS

Age (years)	Serum levels of thyroid hormones (nmol)[a] Thyroxine	Triiodothyronine	Ref.
20—64	98	1.9	
65—92	80	0.92	83
20—39	98	1.7	
40—59	91	1.5	173
69—79	94	1.2	
20—30	99	2.2	
70—80	78	1.8	17
25—35	123	—	
80—89	124	—	141

[a] Calculated from published data on the basis of a molecular weight of 800 for thyroxine, and 673 for triiodothyronine.

THYROID FUNCTION

The strong influences of thyroid hormone on total body metabolic processes have made studies of the relationship of age and thyroid function particularly attractive. Stimulation of metabolic rate by cold exposure in rats, or exposure of *Drosophila* to elevated temperature has been shown to accelerate pathological lesions and markedly shorten life span. There are similarities between hypothyroidism and the effects of aging on metabolism in humans. Aging is characterized by decreased metabolic rate and impairment of fat and protein metabolism. These correlates have led to the hypothesis that biological aging may be accompanied by hypothyroidism.

Aging is known to affect iodide dynamics in humans. Renal iodide clearance has been shown to decrease in aged humans.[62,188] Changes in renal iodide clearance are accompanied by increased plasma iodide concentration in women[76,188] and decreased thyroid iodide clearance rates.[62,76,188] The iodide accumulation rate is also decreased in aged human subjects.[92] However, it is felt that this decrease in uptake reflects decreased peripheral thyroid hormone degradation, leading to decreased TSH stimulation of iodide uptake rather than as a part of generalized thyroid deficiency in aging.

Another useful index of thyroid function is thyroid response to TSH stimulation. Although some studies show decreased functional pituitary TSH secretory reserve with aging,[109,164] other experiments do not.[16] These data indicate that considerable thyroid reserve is retained in the aged and any decrease in this parameter with aging is of limited magnitude.

The effect of aging on blood thyroid hormone levels has also been studied. Although some studies indicate the blood thyroxine[62] and protein-bound iodide concentration are not affected by age,[26,141] other experiments suggest a modest decline of about 20% in serum T_4 or PBI (Table 8). A more significant age effect on thyroid hormones concerns the clearance of T_4. The T_4 clearance rate is reduced so that by the 9th decade it is about half that of young adults (Table 9).[74,91,139,188] Since serum T_4 concentrations remain nearly constant, thyroid secretion rate is also sharply reduced in the aged.

The concentration of thyroid binding globulin is minimally affected by aging,[26,85] suggesting that changes in blood T_4 binding do not significantly contribute to the reduced T_4 clearance rate in the aged and that free hormone concentrations are similar in young and aged subjects.

Table 9
THYROXINE METABOLISM DURING HUMAN AGING[74]

Age (years)	Distribution vol (1)	Half-life (days)	Thyroxine degradation rate (μg T_4 1/day)
21	12.34	6.61	88.65
65	11.65	9.10	58.84
83	9.34	9.25	43.89

Another factor affecting the rate of metabolism of T_4 concerns its extrathyroidal conversion to triiodothyronine.[93] It is now recognized that many of the metabolic activities of thyroid hormones are associated with T_3 which is formed by this peripheral deiodination of T_4.[87] Several studies indicate decreased T_3 concentrations in the aged.[17,83,85] This decrease in T_4 deiodination probably contributes to the reduced metabolism of T_4. On the other hand, caloric deprivation, stress, and illness[133,143,181] have also been shown to decrease systemic T_4 to T_3 conversion. In summary, the decrease in T_4 secretion and metabolism and apparent reduction in conversion of T_4 to T_3 in the aged suggest functional hypothyroidism in the aged. On the other hand, aged tissues may require less thyroid hormone for maintenance of metabolic function. Resolution of these uncertainties will require additional experimentation.

Thyroidal T_4 secretion is normally regulated by pituitary TSH secretion. Pituitary TSH synthesis and secretion reflects the amount of hypothalamic thyrotropin releasing hormone (TRH) stimulation, and thyroid hormone feedback inhibition which pituitary thyrotrophs receive. Current studies indicate near normal basal concentrations of TSH in the blood of aged humans and rats.[14,17,39] Pituitary responsiveness to TRH has recently been used as an index of aging effects on TSH secretion. The current data are controversial. In human studies, all experiments show increased TSH secretion following TRH treatment. Some studies report decreased TSH responsiveness in elderly men but not in women.[14,173] Others found decreased responsiveness in aging women but not men,[92] while another reported increased TRH responsiveness in the elderly.[141] To these authors' knowledge nothing is known about the ability of the hypothalamus to respond to control input, such as decreased temperature, which regulates TRH secretion in the aged. It is assumed by many that hypothalamic neurotransmitters control TRH release. The recognition that hypothalamic neurotransmitter content and turnover decreases with age in laboratory rodents suggests that hypothalamic TRH responsiveness may be impaired in aged subjects.

In summary, functional hypothyroidism as a consequence of or a contribution to biological aging remains an attractive hypothesis. This hypothesis is supported by considerable clinical and biological data. Blood concentrations of T_4 and TSH are not appreciably affected by increased age. Likewise, the aged pituitary and thyroid retain significant functional secretory reserve capacity. A more significant age alteration in thyroidal function is the reduction in extrathyroidal conversion of T_4 to the more biologically potent T_3. In addition, almost nothing is known about age effects on thyroid hormone activity, such as the amount of thyroid hormone receptors or tissue response to hormone-receptor combination.

ADRENAL CORTEX

Decreased physiological reserve and impairment of homeostatatic controls are characteristic of biological aging in many tissues and control systems. Since adrenocortical secretions are important endocrine components in homeostasis, the effect of biological

Table 10
CHANGES IN GLUCOCORTICOID SECRETION AND METABOLISM IN AGING HUMAN SUBJECTS

Age	Cortisol[a] nmol/100 mℓ	Cortisol half-life (min)	Cortisol secretion rate mg/24 hr	Ref.
25—40 years	34	112		192
>80 years	40	169		
21—35 years			23.6	157
65—73 years			17.7	
20 years	50			24
70—90 years	43			

[a] Calculated from published data on the basis of a molecular weight of 361.

aging on adrenocortical function has generated considerable interest. One of the first biological phenomena recognized to be associated with adrenocortical function was that a large variety of physical and psychogenic stressors stimulated adrenocortical secretion and that increased adrenocortical secretions were involved in the ability of the person or animal to survive the stress. A higher rate of mortality is associated with stress in elderly patients.[24] It has been proposed that age-related decreases in adrenocortical function could be related to this increase in mortality.

However, changes in adrenal morphology with biological aging are not dramatic. Adrenal weights and cortical widths were similar in young and aging humans.[63,79] Although aged male beagle dogs have smaller adrenal weights, female beagle adrenal weights were increased with age.[41] Adrenals from several species show increased connective tissue with age.[24,95] There is also an increased amount of adrenocortical age pigment (consisting of lipochrome granules) with increased age.[146,176] Another microscopic feature of the aging adrenal is the formation of adrenocortical nodules.[44] The development of adrenocortical nodules is associated with several structural changes in adrenals. There occurs a proliferation of connective tissue, enlargement of sinusoidal capillaries, hemorrhage, and impairment of vascularity in nodule-containing adrenals. The incidence of nodules increased with age in humans and was associated with the development of hypertension.

Considerable attention has been given to the effect of aging on the adrenocortical control system. Our current understanding of this control system indicates that ACTH, the primary regulator of glucocorticoid secretion, is regulated by combined effects of negative feedback from glucocorticoids and a temporal stimulation of hypothalamic corticotropin-releasing hormone by neural factors influenced by activity-sleep patterns. Several studies have shown that the glucocorticoid secretion rate is reduced from 25 to 40% in aging humans (Table 10).[24,157] This reduction in secretory rate is accompanied by a reduction in glucocorticoid excretion and an increase in circulatory half-life resulting in nearly stable blood cortisol concentrations in aged humans.[24,192] Aged humans also showed temporal blood cortisol concentrations similar to young controls, indicating that the neural mechanisms controlling ACTH release were functionally intact. In a series of studies we have shown similar resting glucocorticoid concentrations in aging rats, cattle, and goats.[86,153,154] The results of these experiments, showing similar blood glucocorticoid concentrations associated with reduced adrenocortical glucocorticoid secretion rate in laboratory animals and humans, suggest that the ACTH control mechanisms of these species are not affected by increased age.

Several laboratories have studied the effect of aging on adrenocortical responsiveness to ACTH. Our work showed decreased adrenocortical responsiveness in terms of the magnitude of increased glucocorticoid concentration after ACTH or stress stimulation in aged rats, goats, and cattle.[86,153,154] On the other hand, most studies on humans show essentially normal adrenal responsiveness in the aged. Adrenal response to the insulin tolerance test,[31,58,71] the metyrapone test,[23] ACTH stimulation,[25] and dexamethasone[58] were normal in the elderly compared to younger controls. In addition, it was shown in the same study that elderly patients have similar increases in plasma cortisol concentrations as young controls during surgical stress.

Studies of adrenocortical function in aged rats suggest alterations in adrenocortical control mechanisms in the older subjects (Table 11). A study of adrenocortical responsiveness to chronic ACTH stimulation showed higher corticosterone concentrations after ACTH stimulation in young compared to aged rats (Table 11A).[87] Although chronic ACTH injections resulted in decreased adrenocortical stimulation after ether vapor stress in young rats, the responsiveness of the aged rats to ether stress was not reduced. These data suggest that the hypothalamic-pituitary control mechanism for ACTH release was responding differently to elevated serum corticosterone in young and aged rats. The sensitivity of young and aged rat hypothalamic-pituitary corticotropin control mechanisms to direct corticosteroid negative feedback was next studied by measuring stress responsiveness after dexamethosone inhibition of the control system (Table 11B).[150] Both chronic and acute dexamethasone treatments produced greater adrenocortical inhibition in young than in aged rats which again suggests increased sensitivity to glucocorticoid negative feedback in young groups. In another study, the responsiveness of the adrenocortical control system was tested during a restraint stress treatment regime.[149] Again, in these experiments, the adrenocortical control mechanisms of young rats were more responsive to restraint stress-induced increases in corticosterone secretion. These studies suggest a decreased sensitivity of the adrenocortical control system to glucocorticoid negative feedback in the aged rat. Direct measurements of the sensitivity of the adrenocortical control systems of aged humans have not been reported. However, one study suggests increased adrenal responsiveness to the metyrapone test on day 4 postoperative in elderly compared to young patients.[24] This report is similar to data from the rat and suggests that the adrenocorticotropin control system of the aged human may also be less sensitive to glucocorticoid negative feedback.

The effect of aging on tissue responsiveness to glucocorticoid hormones has received some attention. One study reported threefold greater increases in glucose-6-phosphatose and fructose-1,6-diphosphatose activity following dexamethazone injection in 1-month-old compared to 15-month-old-rats.[161] However, others have found an increase in the time required for enzyme induction in aged rats with no age effect on the maximal tissue response to the hormones.[5,144] These studies suggest aging effects on the kinetics of cellular response, but minimal effects on the overall response of a tissue to adrenocortical hormones.

Comparatively little attention has been given to the effect of age on aldosterone control systems. The adrenocortical secretory rate, the metabolic clearance rate, and the circulatory level of aldosterone have all been shown to be decreased in aged humans.[56] In addition, plasma renin activity was found to be decreased in aged subjects.[189] These reports suggest significant age effects on aldosterone control mechanisms which warrant additional experimental study.

One of the initial observations concerning the effect of age on adrenocortical function was the decline in urinary 17-ketosteroid secretion.[75] A progressive decline in adrenal androgen secretion has been identified by several investigators.[126,185] Although the measured decline in adrenal androgen secretion is dramatic, its physiological importance is unclear.

Table 11
CORTICOSTERONE LEVELS IN AGING RATS; EFFECTS OF ACTH AND STRESS TREATMENTS

A. Effects of 2 Weeks of Daily ACTH Treatment on Adrenocorticol Response to Acute ACTH and Ether Stress

		Serum corticosterone (nmol/mℓ)				
		After ether stress		After ACTH stimulation		
Sex	Treatment	Young (3—5 months)	Aged (22—26 months)	Young (3—5 months)	Aged (22—26 months)	Ref.
Male	Control	1710	1620	2030	1810	87
	After 2 wks, 10 μ ACTH/day	880	1220	2890	1920	
Female	Control	2850	2400	2780	2710	87
	After 2 wks, 10 μ ACTH/day	1500	2690	3150	2970	

B. Corticosterone Following 14 Days of Dexamethasone Suppression

		Serum corticosterone (nmol/mℓ)		
Sex	Treatment	Young (4—6 months)	Aged (22—32 months)	Ref.
Male	Control	1670	1510	150
	Dexamethasone, 1 μg/100 g	790	880	
	Dexamethasone, 5 μg/100 g	180	560	
Female	Control	2390	2540	150
	Dexamethasone, 1 μg/100 g	1260	1620	
	Dexamethasone, 5 μg/100 g	360	680	

In summary, there is considerable evidence for functional changes in the adrenal glands of aged animals. Although some species show decreased reserve secretory capacity, this has not been shown to be characteristic of aged humans. All species which have been studied show normal resting blood glucocorticoid concentrations with increased age. Finally, there is evidence for decreased sensitivity of the adrenocortical control system to negative feedback inhibition of ACTH secretion in aged mammals.

PANCREAS

Diabetes mellitus is generally considered to be the most common metabolic disease in human populations. Decreased glucose tolerance has been well-documented in aging human populations.[10,11,125] There has been considerable debate concerning the incidence of diabetes mellitus in our society. The National Commission on Diabetes estimated that 16.7% of all persons reaching age 65 have diagnosed diabetes. By age 85, this study indicated that the incidence of diagnosed diabetes had increased to 26% of the population.[193] On the other hand, others have estimated much higher incidences of abnormal glucose tolerance in aged subjects.[175] These discrepancies indicate that different groups have applied different criteria in their estimations of the incidence of this disease; there has been considerable controversy over what criteria should be applied.

One approach to diagnosing diabetes in the aged is to use criteria similar to those applied to younger age groups; this usually leads to identification of more than 50% of those over age 70 as diabetics.[175] Others have suggested that only persons with elevated fasting glucose be considered diabetics.[171] The National Commission on Diabetes has recommended an approach which allows proportional decreases in glucose tolerance in normal aging subjects.[147]

Although identification of decreased glucose tolerance with aging is well-established, factors associated with the increased blood glucose after carbohydrate loading are unclear. One factor which has received consideration is the ability of the pancreas to respond to control input during aging. The experimental data related to insulin secretion following pancreatic stimulation are inconsistent. Several studies report decreased insulin secretion following pancreatic challenge.[46,52,193] One study measured plasma concentrations of insulin, growth hormone, and glucagon following i.v. administration of glucose or arginine.[46] This study showed a higher fasting glucose concentration in aged men even though their fasting concentrations of insulin, growth hormone, and glucose were unchanged. These workers interpreted the increase in fasting glucose concentration with age as indicating a reduced pancreatic secretion of insulin. Another study showed a slower secretory response by the pancreas following glucose treatment in aged compared to young human subjects which could contribute to higher glucose concentrations in the older group.[96] On the other hand (Table 12), others have not found reduced insulin response to pancreatic stimulation in the aged,[32,106] and some investigators have found increased blood insulin concentrations in aged subjects after a glucose load.[190]

Measurement of insulin concentrations in the blood of the elderly can be complicated by increased pancreatic secretion of immunoreactive compounds with altered biochemical structure and reduced biological activity. Although these immunoreactive compounds have not been structurally identified, they are frequently referred to as proinsulin. Aged subjects have been shown to have higher blood concentrations of proinsulin than mature adults.[45] Most studies of insulin secretion or blood insulin concentration in the aged have assumed that all the insulin was of similar biological activity. It seems probable that in at least some cases increased secretion of proinsulin contributes to the discrepancies between measured serum insulin concentrations and biological activity of insulin characterized by decreased glucose tolerance in the aged.

Table 12
INSULIN LEVELS AND SECRETION IN HUMANS

Age (years)	Serum insulin levels (pM)[a] at specified time after administration of glucose load 0 (basal)	30 min	60 min	120 min	Ref.
20—39	49	—	245	159	
40—59	72	—	342	189	94
60 +	107	—	445	199	
23	67	400	387	207	
55	60	534	634	354	19

[a] Calculated from reported data on the basis of a molecular weight of 6000 and a potency of 25 units/mg; thus, 100 pmol is equivalent to 15 μU/mℓ or 0.6 ng/mℓ.

It has also been shown that insulin secretion is normally enhanced by GI hormones which are stimulated by food in the gut.[116] This GI hormone stimulation is of major functional significance. Activation of this endocrine system results in greater insulin release and lower blood glucose concentration when glucose is administered via the gut compared to i.v. infusion.[118] It is possible that the responsiveness of this endocrine system could be affected by aging and contribute to the decreased pancreatic responsiveness to control input in the aged.

Age alterations in pancreatic structure could also contribute to beta cell insensitivity in the aged. Pancreatic structural changes in the aged include fewer beta cells and pancreatic vascular degeneration.[27] These structural changes in the pancreas could contribute to reduced beta cell responsiveness to glucose stimulation in the elderly.

Obesity is another important factor which complicates interpretation of the data concerned with pancreatic function in the aged. Increased fat deposits are characteristic of increased age. Even if obvious obesity is eliminated from data collected in aged subjects, the elderly show progressive loss of muscle tissue and increased fat deposition.[59,138] Increased obesity is recognized to result in increased tissue resistance to insulin activity.[100] It is likely that relative or overt obesity in the aged results in increased insulin requirements to maintain normal carbohydrate metabolism. The increased insulin secretion would contribute to the normal or often increased levels of immunoreactive insulin measured in aged subjects with decreased glucose tolerance.

The increased capillary basement membrane thickness, which is a recognized complication in diabetics, could also contribute to decreased tissue responsiveness to insulin in the aged.[102,172] The relationship of this increase in basement membrane thickness to aging is of interest. Increased basement membrane thickness has been demonstrated in subjects with genetic predisposition for diabetes.[172] At least one study of diabetes has shown increased basement membrane thickness with aging in both control and diabetic subjects.[102]

In summary, current evidence suggests that several components of the insulin regulatory system may be affected by aging. There are structural alterations in the pancreas with increased age. Although measured serum insulin concentrations are not consistently affected by aging, there is evidence that beta cell responsiveness is decreased, and the aged pancreas may be secreting increased amounts of proinsulin, a compound with reduced biological activity. Finally, there is substantial evidence for increased tissue resistance to insulin activity in the aged.

PARATHYROIDS AND MINERAL METABOLISM

One of the most consistent physiological changes occurring with aging is the progressive decrease in bone mineralization. The decrease in bone density generally occurs at about the age at which significant reduction in reproductive function occurs. These changes are particularly consistent in postmenopausal women. Although the hypothesis of decreased gonadal hormone directly contributing to the loss of bone mineral is attractive, the data are not conclusive and several other age-related alterations in factors which regulate mineral metabolism may contribute to bone loss.

One factor which contributes to the alteration in mineral metabolism during aging is intestinal calcium absorption. A progressive decrease in intestinal calcium absorption has been measured in aging humans and animals.[9] Thus calcium absorption is insufficient to maintain serum calcium concentrations; this deficiency has been postulated to contribute to increased bone catabolism with aging.[158]

In men, serum calcium concentrations decrease progressively after 20 years of age.[158] On the other hand, serum parathyroid hormone (PTH) concentration was increased in men from age 20 to 50, then was progressively decreased through 90 years of age.[60] The lack of a clear inverse relationship between blood concentrations of calcium and measured serum parathyroid hormone suggests significant (but yet unidentified) alterations in the parathyroid hormone regulatory system in aging men.

The patterns of serum calcium and PTH of aging women do not parallel those of men (Table 13).[158] Calcium concentrations increased moderately from 20 to 59 years of age, followed by a progressive decrease. Serum PTH decreased from 20 to 49 years of age and then increased in older women. Although the inverse relationship between serum calcium and PTH concentrations in women suggests intact parathyroid control function, experimentally increased serum calcium did not lower PTH concentration in aged osteoporatic women.[155]

A major factor related to the amount of bone mass in humans is the individual's sex. Bone mass is greater at all ages in men compared to women.[65,66,121,123] Although both sexes lose bone mass with age, the loss occurs earlier and is of greater magnitude in women. Bone loss is accelerated by the loss of ovarian function at menopause or after ovariectomy.[6,40,120,122] The initial bone loss in postmenopausal women can be reduced by estrogen therapy.[7,80,122,145] In some instances, treatment with estrogen has been reported to result in increased bone mass after ovariectomy.[110] Other studies have shown that estrogen therapies can reduce fractures and height reduction in osteoporatic women.[84] To be effective, these treatments have required substantial estrogen dosages which are sufficient to induce uterine endometrial withdrawal bleeding.

The exact interaction between estrogen, calcium, and PTH regulation remains unclear. In addition, the aforementioned beneficial effects of estrogen therapy may be transitory. One study showed that postmenopausal estrogen therapy increased bone density for the first 5 to 10 years of treatment.[42] After this interval, the differences in mineralization between those receiving estrogen and controls was progressively reduced until after 15 to 20 years of estrogen therapy; no difference was found in bone mass between estrogen-treated and control groups. Additionally, another study has shown that the benefits of estrogen therapy in overtly osteoporatic women was reduced after only 2 to 3 years of therapy.[156] These studies suggest that age-related demineralization of bone in women involves more than the loss of estrogen.

The rate of bone catabolism exceeds that of bone synthesis in osteoporesis.[98] Increased sensitivity to PTH with reduced estrogen availability has been postulated to contribute to bone demineralization and osteoporesis in women.[64] Estrogens are thought to suppress hyperparathyroidism by parathyroid adenomas presumably by antagonizing the actions of PTH on bone. Although hyperparathyroidism occurs in all

Table 13
PARATHYROID HORMONE AND CALCIUM LEVELS IN HUMANS

A. Parathyroid Hormone in Serum (pmol)[a]

Sex	Age (years) 20—39	40—49	60—69	80+	Postmenopausal	Ref.
Male	43	42	23	26	211	60

B. Parathyroid Hormone Levels ($\mu\ell$ eq/mℓ)

Sex	Age (years) 20—30	30—40	50—60	70—80	80—90	Ref.
Male	5.8	9.5	16.5	11.4	6.5	158
Female	11.8	8.6	11.3	13.3	17.7	158

[a] Calculated from published data on the basis of a molecular weight of 9000 daltons.

adult age groups, its greatest incidence occurs between 40 and 60 years of age.[81,135,148] A recent review of hyperparathyroidism indicates that this disease can be associated with multiple causes and can induce pathologies in several physiological systems.[158]

Another factor which can influence mineral metabolism with aging is thyrocalcitonin. Thyrocalcitonin has been shown to reduce serum calcium concentrations by reducing bone salt resorption. The effectiveness of thyrocalcitonin is reduced in aging rats over a wide range of hormone treatments.[88] In addition, reduced thyrocalcitonin secretion after hypercalcemia was found in aging rats and sheep. Although the potential usefulness of thyrocalcitonin to combat age-related demineralization and osteoporesis is attractive, minimal long-term studies of the effectiveness of the hormone have not been completed.

In summary, bone demineralization, including osteoporesis, is increased with aging. Several factors including excessive parathyroid hormone secretion, changes in parathyroid hormone activities, decreased thyrocalcitonin, reduced dietary intake or intestinal absorption of calcium, or differences in renal calcium absorption are involved with the decrease in bone mineralization. In senile osteoporesis the rate of bone mineral turnover is altered in that the amount or bone resorption is increased while bone formation continues within normal limits.

REFERENCES

1. **Abraham, G. E., Lobotsky, J., and Lloyd, C. W.,** Metabolism of testosterone and androstenedione in normal and ovariectomized women, *J. Clin. Invest.,* 48, 696, 1969.
2. **Abraham, G. E., Swerdloff, R. S., and Tulchinsky, D.,** Radioimmunoassay of plasma 17-hydroxy progesterone, *J. Clin. Endocrinol.,* 33, 42, 1971.
3. **Adamopoulos, D. A., Loraine, J. A., and Dove, G. A.,** Endocrinological studies in women approaching the menopause, *J. Obstet. Gynaecol. Br. Commonw.,* 78, 62, 1971.
4. **Adams, C. E.,** Aging and reproduction in the female mammal with particular reference to the rabbit, *J. Reprod. Fertil. Suppl.,* 12, 1, 1970.
5. **Adelman, R. C., Freeman, C., and Cohen, B. S.,** Enzyme adaptation as a biochemical probe of development and aging, *Adv. Enzyme Regul.,* 10, 365, 1972.
6. **Aitken, J. M., et al.,** Osteoporosis after oophorectomy for non-malignant disease in premenopausal women, *Br. Med. J.,* 2, 325, 1973.
7. **Aitken, J. M., Hart, D. M., and Lindsay, R.,** Oestrogen replacement therapy for prevention of osteoporosis after oophorectomy, *Br. Med. J.,* 3, 515, 1973.
8. **Albeaux-Fernet, M., Bohler, C. C. S., and Karpas, A. E.,** Testicular function in the aging male, in *Geriatric Endocrinology,* Greenblatt, R. B., Ed., Raven Press, New York, 1978, 201.
9. **Alevizaki, C. C., Ikkos, D. B., and Singhelakis, P.,** Progressive decrease of true intestinal calcium absorption with age in normal man, *J. Nucl. Med.,* 14, 760, 1973.
10. **Andres, R.,** Effect of age in interpretation of glucose and tolbutamide tolerance tests, in *Diabetes Mellitus: Diagnosis and Treatment,* Vol. 3, Fajans, S. S. and Sussman, K. E., Eds., American Diabetes Association, New York, 1971b, 115.
11. **Andres, R. and Tobin, J. D.,** Aging and the disposition of glucose: explorations in aging, *Adv. Exp. Med. Biol.,* 61, 239, 1974.
12. **Aschheim, P.,** Aging in the hypothalamic-hypophyseal-ovarian axis in the rat, in *Hypothalamus, Pituitary, and Aging,* Everitt, A. V. and Burgess, J. A., Eds., Charles C Thomas, Springfield, Ill., 1976, 376.
13. **Asch, R. H. and Greenblatt, R. B.,** The aging ovary: morphologic and endocrine correlations, in *Geriatric Endocrinology,* Greenblatt, R. B., Ed., Raven Press, New York, 1978, 141.
14. **Azizi, F., Vagenakis, A. G., Portnay, G. I., Rapoport, B., Ingbar, S. H., and Braverman, L. E.,** Pituitary-thyroid responsiveness to intramuscular thyrotropin-releasing hormone based on analyses of serum throxine, triiodothyronine, and thyrotropin concentrations, *N. Engl. J. Med.,* 292, 273, 1975.
15. **Baker, H. W. G., Burger, H. G., Kekretser, D. M., Hudson, B., O'Connor, S., Wang, C., Mirovics, A., Court, J., Dunlop, M., and Rennie, G. C.,** Changes in the pituitary-testicular system with age, *Clin. Endocrinol. (Oxford),* 5, 349, 1976.
16. **Baker, S. P., Gaffney, G. W., Shock, N. W., and Landowne, M.,** Physiological responses of five middle-aged and elderly men to repeated administration of thyroid-stimulating hormone, *J. Gerontol.,* 14, 37, 1959.
17. **Bermudex, F., Surks, M. I., and Oppenheimer, J. H.,** High incidence of decreased serum triiodothyronine concentration in patients with nonthyroidal disease, *J. Clin. Endocrinol. Metab.,* 41, 27, 1975.
18. **Bishop, M. W. H.,** Aging and reproduction in the male, *J. Reprod. Fertil. Suppl.,* 12, 65, 1970.
19. **Björntorp, P., Berchtold, P., and Tibblin, G.,** Insulin secretion in relation to adipose tissue in men, *Diabetes,* 20, 65, 1971.
20. **Blaha, G. C.,** Effect of age of the donor and recipient on the development of transferred golden hamster ova, *Anat. Rec.,* 150, 413, 1964.
21. **Blaha, G. C.,** Effects of age, treatment, and method of induction on deciduomata in the golden hamster, *Fertil. Steril.,* 18, 477, 1967.
22. **Blaha, G. C.,** The influence of ovarian grafts from young donors on the development of transferred ova in the aged golden hamster, *Fertil. Steril.,* 21, 268, 1970.
23. **Blichert-Toft, M.,** Secretion of corticotrophin and somatotrophin by the senescent adenophypophysis in man, thesis, *Acta Endocrinol. Suppl.,* 195, 1975.
24. **Blichert-Toft, M.,** The adrenal glands in old age, in *Geriatric Endocrinology,* Greenblatt, R. B., Ed., Raven Press, New York, 1978, 81.
25. **Blichert-Toft, M., Blichert-Toft, B., and Jensen, H. K.,** Pituitary-adrenocortical stimulation in the aged as reflected in levels of plasma cortisol and compound S., *Acta Chir. Scand.,* 136, 665, 1970.
26. **Braverman, L. E., Dawber, N. A., and Ingbar, S. H.,** Observations concerning the binding of thyroid hormones in sera of normal subjects of varying ages, *J. Clin. Invest.,* 45, 1273, 1966.
27. **Burgess, J. A.,** Diabetes mellitus and aging, in *Hypothalamus, Pituitary and Aging,* Everitt, A. V. and Burgess, J. A., Eds., Charles C Thomas, Springfield, Ill., 1976, 497.

28. **Calderon, L., Ryan, N., and Kovacs, K.,** Human pituitary growth hormone cells in old age, *Gerontology,* 24, 441, 1978.
29. **Carlson, H. E., Gillin, J. C., Gorden, P., and Snyder, F.,** Absence of sleep-related growth hormone peaks in aged normal subjects and in acromegaly, *J. Clin. Endocrinol. Metab.,* 34, 1102, 1972.
30. **Carr, D. and Friesen, H. G.,** Growth hormone and insulin binding to human liver, *J. Clin. Endocrinol. Metab.,* 42, 484, 1976.
31. **Cartlidge, N. E. F., Black, M. M., Hall, M. R. P., and Hall, P.,** Pituitary function in the elderly, *Gerontol. Clin.,* 12, 65, 1970.
32. **Chlouverakis, C., Jarrett, R. J., and Keen, H.,** Glucose tolerance, age, and circulating insulin, *Lancet,* 1, 806, 1967.
33. **Choufoer, J. C., Van Rhijn, M., and Querido, A.,** Endemic goitre in Western New Guinea. II. Clinical picture, incidence, and pathogenesis of endemic cretinism, *J. Clin. Endocrinol.,* 25, 385, 1967.
34. **Clemens, J. A. and Bennett, D. R.,** Do aging changes in the preoptic area contribute to the loss of cyclic endocrine function?, *J. Gerontol.,* 32, 19, 1977.
35. **Clemens, J. A. and Meites, J.,** Neuroendocrine status of old constant estrous rats, *Neuroendocrinology,* 7, 249, 1971.
36. **Coble, Y. D., Kohler, P. O., Cargille, C. M., and Ross, G. T.,** Production rates and metabolic clearance rates of human follicle-stimulating hormone in premenopausal and postmenopausal women, *J. Clin. Invest.,* 48, 359, 1969.
37. **Collett, M. E., Wertenberger, G. E., and Fiske, V. M.,** The effect of age upon the pattern of the menstrual cycle, *Fertil. Steril.,* 5, 437, 1954.
38. **Costoff, A. and Mahesh, V. B.,** Primordial follicles with normal oocytes in the ovaries of postmenopausal women, *J. Am. Geriatr. Soc.,* 23, 193, 1975.
39. **Cuttelod, S., Lemarchand-Beraud, T., Magnenat, P., Perret, C., Poli, S., and Venotti, A.,** Effect of age and role of kidneys and liver on thyrotropin turnover in man, *Metabolism,* 23, 101, 1974.
40. **Dalén, N., Lamke, B., and Wallgren, A.,** Bone-mineral losses in oophorectomized women, *J. Bone J. Surg.,* 56A, 1235, 1974.
41. **Das, L. N. and Magilton, J. H.,** Age changes in the relationship among endocrine glands of the beagle, *Exp. Gerontol.,* 6, 297, 1971.
42. **Davis, M. E. and Lanzl, L. H.,** Estrogens and the aging process: the detection, prevention, and retardation of osteoporosis, *JAMA,* 196, 219, 1966.
43. **Dilman, V. M.,** The hypothalamic control of aging and age-associated pathology: the elevation mechanism of aging, in *Hypothalamus, Pituitary and Aging,* Everitt, A. V. and Burgess, J. A., Eds., Charles C Thomas, Springfield, Ill., 1976, 634.
44. **Dobbie, J. W.,** Adrenocortical nodular hyperplasia: the aging adrenal, *J. Pathol.,* 99, 1, 1969.
45. **Duckworth, W. C. and Kitabchi, A. E.,** Effect of age, obesity, and degree of carbohydrate intolerance on proinsulin response to oral glucose, *Diabetes,* 21, (Suppl. 1), 356, 1972b.
46. **Dudl, R. J. and Ensinck, J. W.,** The role of insulin, glucagon, and growth hormone in carbohydrate homeostasis during aging, *Diabetes,* 21, Suppl. 1, 357, 1972.
47. **Dudl, R. J., Ensinck, J. W., Palmer, H. E., and Williams, R. H.,** Effect of age on growth hormone secretion in man, *J. Clin. Endocrinol. Metab.,* 37, 11, 1973.
48. **Eleftheriou, B. E. and Lucas, L. A.,** Age-related changes in testes, seminal vesicles, and plasma testosterone levels in male mice, *Gerontologia,* 20, 231, 1974.
49. **Everitt, A. V.,** The female climacteric, in *Hypothalamus, Pituitary and Aging,* Everitt, A. V. and Burgess, J. A., Eds., Charles C Thomas, Springfield, Ill., 1976, 419.
50. **Everitt, A. V. and Burgess, J. A., Eds.,** *Hypothalamus, Pituitary and Aging,* Charles C Thomas, Springfield, Ill., 1976.
51. **Fekete, E.,** A comparative study of the ovaries of virgin mice of the DBA and C57 black strains, *Cancer Res.,* 6, 263, 1946.
52. **Felig, P.,** Pathophysiology of diabetes mellitus, *Med. Clin. N. Am.,* 55, 821, 1971.
53. **Finch, C. E.,** Catecholamine metabolism in the brains of aging male mice, *Brain Res.,* 52, 261, 1973.
54. **Finch, C. E.,** Reproductive senescence in rodents: factors in the decline of fertility and loss of regular estrous cycles, in *The Aging Reproductive System,* Schneider, E. L., Ed., Raven Press, New York, 1978, 193.
55. **Finkelstein, J. W., Roffwarg, H. P., Boyar, R. M., Kream, J., and Hellman, L.,** Age-related change in the twenty-four-hour spontaneous secretion of growth hormone, *J. Clin. Endocrinol. Metab.,* 35, 665, 1972.
56. **Flood, C., Gherondache, C., Pincus, G., Tait, J. F., Tait, S. A. S., and Willoughby, S.,** The metabolism and secretion of aldosterone in elderly subjects, *J. Clin. Invest.,* 46, 960, 1967.
57. **Florini, J. R. and Roberts, J. R.,** Effect of rat age on blood levels of somatomedin-like growth factors, *J. Gerontol.,* 1979, in press.

58. **Friedman, M., Green, M. F., and Sharland, D. E.,** Assessment of hypothalamic-pituitary-adrenal function in the geriatric age group, *J. Gerontol.,* 24, 292, 1969.
59. **Fryer, J. H.,** Studies of body composition in men aged 60 and over, in *Biological Aspects of Aging,* Shock, N. W., Ed., Columbia University Press, New York, 1962, 59.
60. **Fujita, T., Orimo, H., Okano, K., Yoshikawa, M., Shimo, R., Inove, T., and Itami, Y.,** Radioimmunoassay of serum parathyroid hormone in postmenopausal osteoporosis, *Endocrinol. Jpn.,* 19, 571, 1972.
61. **Fuxe, K. and Hokfelt, T.,** Catecholamines in the hypothalamus and pituitary gland, in *Frontiers in Neuroendocrinology,* Ganong, W. F. and Martini, L., Eds., Oxford University Press, Oxford, 1969, 47.
62. **Gaffney, G. W., Gregerman, R. I., and Shock, N. W.,** Relationship of age to the thyroidal accumulation, renal excretion, and distribution of radioiodide in euthyroid man, *J. Clin. Endocrinol. Metab.,* 22, 784, 1962.
63. **Galloway, N. O., Foley, C. F., and Lagerbloom, P.,** Uncertainties in geriatric data. II. Organ size, *J. Am. Geriatr. Soc.,* 13, 20, 1965.
64. **Gallagher, J. C. and Nordin, B. E. C.,** Treatment with estrogens of primary hyperparathyroidism in postmenopausal women, *Lancet,* 1, 503, 1972.
65. **Garn, S. M., Nagy, J. M., and Sandusky, S. T.,** Differential sexual dimorphism in bone diameters of subjects of European and African ancestry, *Am. J. Phys. Anthropol.,* 37, 127, 1972.
66. **Garn, S. M., Poznanski, A. K., and Nagy, J. M.,** Bone measurement in the differential diagnosis of osteopenia and osteoporosis, *Radiology,* 100, 509, 1971.
67. **Ghanadian, R., Lewis, J. G., and Chisholm, G. D.,** Serum testosterone and dihydrotestosterone changes with age in rat, *Steroids,* 25, 753, 1975.
68. **Gosden, R. G.,** Survival of transferred C57BL mouse embryos: effects of age of donor and recipient, *Fertil. Steril.,* 25, 348, 1974.
69. **Gosden, R. G.,** Ovarian support of pregnancy in aging inbred mice, *J. Reprod. Fertil.,* 42, 423, 1975.
70. **Green, J. A.,** Some effects of advancing age on the histology and reactivity of the mouse ovary, *Anat. Rec.,* 129, 333, 1957.
71. **Green, M. F. and Friedman, M.,** Hypothalamic-pituitary-adrenal function in the elderly, *Gerontol. Clin.,* 10, 334, 1968.
72. **Greenblatt, R. B., Ed.,** *Geriatric Endocrinology,* Raven Press, New York, 1978.
73. **Greenblatt, R. B., Colle, M. L., and Mahesh, V. B.,** Ovarian and adrenal steroid production in the postmenopausal woman, *Obstet. Gynecol.,* 47, 383, 1976.
74. **Gregerman, R. I., Gaffney, G. W., and Shock, N. W.,** Thyroxine turnover in euthyroid man with special reference to changes with age, *J. Clin. Invest.,* 41, 2065, 1962.
75. **Hamilton, H. B. and Hamilton, J. B.,** Aging in apparently normal men, *J. Clin. Endocrinol.,* 8, 433, 1948.
76. **Hansen, J. M., Skovsted, L., and Siersbaek-Neilsen, K.,** Age-dependent changes in iodine metabolism and thyroid function, *Acta Endocrinol. (Copenhagen),* 79, 60, 1975.
77. **Harman, S. M. and Talbert, G. B.,** The effect of maternal age on ovulation, corpora lutea of pregnancy, and implantation failure in mice, *J. Reprod. Fertil.,* 23, 33, 1970.
78. **Harris, G. W.,** Unsolved problems in the portal vessel-chemotransmitter hypothesis, in *Hypophysiotropic Hormones of the Hypothalamus: Assay and Chemistry,* Meites, J., Ed., Williams & Wilkins, Baltimore, 1970, 1.
79. **Haugen, O. A.,** The adrenal glands of elderly men in relation to abnormal prostatic growth, *Acta Pathol. Microbiol. Scand.,* 81, 831, 1973.
80. **Heaney, R. P. and Recker, R. R.,** Estrogen effects on bone remodeling at menopause, *Clin. Res.,* 23, 535A, 1975.
81. **Hecht, A., Gershberg, H., and St. Paul, H.,** Primary hyperparathyroidism, *JAMA,* 233, 519, 1975.
82. **Heller, C. G. and Heller, E. J.,** Gonadotropic hormone: urine assays of normally cycling, menopausal, castrated, and estrin-treated human females, *J. Clin. Invest.,* 18, 171, 1939.
83. **Hermann, J., Rusche, H. J., Kroll, H. J., Hilger, P., and Kruskemper, H. L.,** Free triiodothyronine (T_3) and thyroxine (T_4) serum levels in old age, *Horm. Metab. Res.,* 6, 239, 1974.
84. **Hernberg, C. A.,** Treatment of postmenopausal osteoporosis with estrogens and androgens, *Acta Endocrinol.,* 34, 51, 1960.
85. **Hesch, R. D., Gatz, J., Pope, J., Schmidt, E., and von zur Huhlen, A.,** Total and free triiodothyronine and thyroid-binding globulin concentration in elderly human persons, *Eur. J. Clin. Invest.,* 6, 139, 1976.
86. **Hess, G. D. and Riegle, G. D.,** Adrenocortical responsiveness to stress and ACTH in aging rats, *J. Gerontol.,* 25, 354, 1970.
87. **Hess, G. D. and Riegle, G. D.,** Effects of chronic ACTH stimulation on adrenocortical function in young and aged rats, *Am. J. Physiol.,* 222, 1458, 1972.

88. **Hirsch, P. F. and Munson, P. L.,** Thyrocalcitonin, *Physiol. Rev.*, 49, 548, 1969.
89. **Holinka, C. H. and Finch, C. E.,** Age-related changes in the decidual responses of the C57BL/6J mouse uterus, *Biol. Reprod.*, 16, 385, 1977.
90. **Huang, H. H., Marshall, S., and Meites, J.,** Capacity of old vs. young female rats to secrete LH, FSH, and prolactin, *Biol. Reprod.*, 14, 538, 1976.
91. **Inada, M., Koshiyame, K., Torizuka, K. A., Kagi, H., and Miyake, T.,** Clinical studies for the metabolism of ^{131}I-labeled L-thyroxine, *J. Clin. Endocrinol. Metab.*, 24, 775, 1964.
92. **Ingbar, S. H.,** The influence of aging on the human thyroid economy, in *Geriatric Endocrinology,* Greenblatt, R. B., Ed., Raven Press, New York, 1978, 13.
93. **Ingbar, S. H. and Woeber, K. A.,** The thyroid gland, in *Textbook of Endocrinology,* 4th ed., Williams, R. H., Ed., W. B. Saunders, Philadelphia, 1968, 232.
94. **Jarrett, R. L., Chlouverakis, C., and Keen, H.,** Glucose tolerance, age, and circulating insulin, *Lancet,* 1, 806, 1967.
95. **Jayne, E. P.,** Cytology of the adrenal gland of the rat at different ages, *Anat. Rec.*, 115, 459, 1953.
96. **Joffe, B. I., Vinik, A. I., and Jackson, W. P. U.,** Insulin reserve in elderly subjects, *Lancet,* 1, 1292, 1969.
97. **Jones, E. C.,** The aging ovary and its influence on reproductive capacity, *J. Reprod. Fertil. Suppl.*, 12, 17, 1970.
98. **Jowsey, J.,** Quantitative microradiography: a new approach in the evaluation of metabolic bone disease, *Am. J. Med.*, 40, 485, 1966.
99. **Judd, H. L., Lucas, W. E., and Yen, S. S. C.,** Serum 17-estradiol and estrone levels in postmenopausal women with and without endometrial cancer, *J. Clin. Endocrinol. Metab.*, 43, 272, 1976.
100. **Karam, J. H., Grodsky, G. M., and Forsham, P. M.,** Excessive insulin response to glucose in obese subjects as measured by immunochemical assay, *Diabetes,* 12, 197, 1963.
101. **Kent, J. R. and Acone, A. B.,** Plasma testosterone levels and aging in males, in *Androgens in Normal and Pathological Conditions,* Vermeulen, A. and Exley, D., Eds., Excerpta Medica Foundation, Amsterdam, 1966, 31.
102. **Kilo, C., Vogler, N., and Williamson, J. R.,** Muscle capillary basement membrane changes related to aging and to diabetes mellitus, *Diabetes,* 21, 881, 1972.
103. **Kinsey, A. C., Pomeroy, W. B., and Martin, C. E.,** *Sexual Behavior in the Human Male,* W. B. Saunders, Philadelphia, 1948.
104. **Klopper, A. I. and Wilson, G. R.,** A method for the assay of oestriol in pregnancy urine, *Obstet. Gynaecol. Br. Commonw.*, 69, 533, 1962.
105. **Kohler, P. O., Ross, G. T., and Odell, W. D.,** Metabolic clearance and production rates of human luteinizing hromone in pre- and postmenopausal women, *J. Clin. Invest.*, 47, 38, 1968.
106. **Langs, H. M., Andres, R., Pozefsky, T., and Gregerman, R. I.,** Responses in serum insulin concentration to the cortisone glucose tolerance test (CGTT): the importance of age, *Diabetes,* 15, 539, 1966.
107. **Larson, L. L., Spilman, C. H., Dunn, H. O., and Foote, R. H.,** Reproductive efficiency in aged female rabbits given supplemental progesterone and oestradiol, *J. Reprod. Fertil.*, 33, 31, 1973.
108. **Leathem, J. H. and Albrecht, E. D.,** Effect of age on testis Δ^5-3β-hydroxysteroid dehydrogenase in the rat, *Proc. Soc. Exp. Biol. Med.*, 145, 1212, 1974.
109. **Lederer, J. and Bataille, J. P.,** Senescence et fonction thyroidienne, *Ann. Endocrinol. (Paris),* 30, 598, 1969.
110. **Lindsay, R., Aitken, J. M., Anderson, J. B., Hart, D. M., MacDonald, E. B., and Clarke, A. C.,** Long-term prevention of postmenopausal osteoporosis by oestrogen: evidence for an increased bone mass after delayed onset of oestrogen treatment, *Lancet,* 1, 1038, 1976.
111. **Longcope, C.,** Metabolic clearance and and blood production rates of estrogens in postmenopausal women, *Am. J. Obstet. Gynecol.*, 11, 778, 1971.
112. **Longcope, C.,** The effect of human chorionic gonadotrophin on plasma steroid levels in young and old men, *Steroids,* 21, 583, 1973.
113. **Longcope, C.,** Steroid production in pre- and postmenopausal women, in *The Menopausal Syndrome,* Greenblatt, R. B., Ed., Medcom Press, New York, 1974.
114. **MacLeod, J. and Gold, R. Z.,** The male factor in fertility and infertility. VII. Semen quality in relation to age and sexual activity, *Fertil. Steril.*, 4, 194, 1953.
115. **Martin, C. E.,** Frequency of male sexual activity in relation to measures of physiologic function and body composition, in *Proc. 10th Int. Congr. Gerontol., Vol. 1, Plenary Sessions, Symposia,* The Congress, Jerusalem, 1975, 183.
116. **Mayhew, D. A., Wright, P. H., and Ashmore, J.,** Regulation of insulin secretion, *Pharmacol. Rev.*, 21, 185, 1969.
117. **McCullagh, S. F.,** The Huon Peninsula endemic. IV. Endemic goitre and congenital defect, *Med. J. Aust.*, 1, 884, 1963.

118. **McIntyre, N., Holdsworth, C. D., and Turner, D. S.,** Intestinal factors in the control of insulin secretion, *J. Clin. Endocrinol. Metab.,* 25, 1317, 1965.
119. **McPherson, J. C., Costoff, A., and Mahesh, V. B.,** Effects of aging on the hypothalamic-hypophyseal-gonadal axis in female rats, *Fertil. Steril.,* 28, 1365, 1977.
120. **Meema, H. E., Bunker, M. L., and Meema, S.,** Loss of compact bone due to menopause, *Am. J. Obstet. Gynaecol.,* 26, 333, 1965.
121. **Meema, H. E. and Meema, S.,** Measurable roentgenologic changes in some peripheral bones in senile osteoporosis, *J. Am. Geriatr. Soc.,* 11, 1170, 1963.
122. **Meema, H. E. and Meema, S.,** Prevention of postmenopausal osteoporosis by hormone treatment of the menopause, *Can. Med. Assoc. J.,* 99, 248, 1968.
123. **Meema, S., Bunker, M. L., and Meema, H. E.,** Preventive effect of estrogen on postmenopausal bone loss, *Arch. Int. Med.,* 135, 1436, 1975.
124. **Meites, J., Huang, H. H., and Simpkins, J. W.,** Recent studies on neuroendocrine control of reproductive senescence in rats, in *The Aging Reproductive System,* Schneider, E. L., Ed., Raven Press, New York, 1978, 213.
125. **Metz, R., Surmaczynska, B., Berger, S., and Sobel, G.,** Glucose tolerance, plasma insulin, and free fatty acids in elderly subjects, *Ann. Intern. Med.,* 64, 1042, 1966.
126. **Migeon, C. J., Keller, A. R., Lawrence, B., and Shepard, T. H.,** Dehydroepiandrosterone and androsterone levels in human plasma. I. Effect of age and sex; day-to-day and diurnal variations, *J. Clin. Endocrinol.,* 17, 1051, 1957.
127. **Miller, A. E. and Riegle, G. D.,** Serum testosterone and testicular response to HCG in young and aged male rats, *J. Gerontol.,* 33, 197, 1978.
128. **Miller, A. E. and Riegle, G. D.,** Serum LH levels following multiple LHRH injections in aging rats, *Proc. Soc. Exp. Biol. Med.,* 157, 494, 1978.
129. **Miller, A. E. and Riegle, G. D.,** Hypothalamic LH-releasing activity in young and aged intact and gonadectomized rats, *Exp. Aging Res.,* 4, 145, 1978.
130. **Miller, A. E. and Riegle, G. D.,** Temporal changes in serum progesterone in aged female rats, *Endocrinology,* 106, 1579, 1980.
131. **Miller, A. E. and Riegle, G. D.,** Serum progesterone during pregnancy and pseudopregnancy and gestation length in the aging rat, *Biol. Reprod.,* 22, 751, 1980.
132. **Miller, A. E., Shaar, C. J., and Riegle, G. D.,** Aging effects on hypothalamic dopamine and norepinephrine content in the male rat, *Exp. Aging Res.,* 2, 475, 1976.
133. **Moshang, T., Parks, J. S., Baker, L., Vaidya, V., Utiger, R. D., Bongiovanni, A. M., and Snyder, P. J.,** Low serum triiodothyronine in patients with anorexia nervosa, *J. Clin. Endocrinol. Metabl.,* 40, 470, 1975.
134. **Muggeo, M., Fedele, D., Tiengo, A., Molinari, M., and Crepaldi, G.,** Human growth hormone and cortisol response to insulin stimulation in aging, *J. Gerontol.,* 30, 545, 1975.
135. **Muller, H.,** Sex, age, and hyperparathyroidism, *Lancet,* 1, 449, 1969.
136. **Newman, G. and Nichols, C. R.,** Sexual activities and attitudes in older persons, *JAMA,* 173, 33, 1960.
137. **Novak, E. R.,** Ovulation after fifty, *Obstet. Gynecol.,* 36, 903, 1970.
138. **Novak, L. P.,** Aging, total body potassium, fat-free mass, and cell mass in males and females between ages 18 and 85 years, *J. Gerontol.,* 27, 438, 1972.
139. **Oddie, T. H., Meade, J. H., and Fisher, D. L.,** An analysis of published data on thyroxine turnover in human subjects, *J. Clin. Endocrinol. Metabl.,* 26, 425, 1966.
140. **Odell, W. D. and Swerdloff, R. S.,** Progesterone-induced luteinizing and follicle-stimulating hormone surge in postmenopausal women: a simulated ovulatory peak, *Proc. Natl. Acad. Sci. U.S.A.,* 61, 529, 1968.
141. **Ohara, H., Kobayaski, T., Shiraishi, M., and Wada, T.,** Thyroid function of the aged as viewed from the pituitary-thyroid system, *Endocrinol. Jpn.,* 21, 377, 1974.
142. **Poortman, J., Thijssen, J. H. H., and Schwarz, F.,** Androgen production and conversion to estrogens in normal postmenopausal women and in selected breast cancer patients, *J. Clin. Endocrinol. Metab.,* 37, 101, 1973.
143. **Portnay, G. I., O'Brien, J. T., Rudolph, M., Vagenakis, A. G., Azizi, F., Arky, R. A., Ingbar, S. H., and Braverman, L. E.,** The effects of starvation on the concentration and binding of thyroxin- and triiodothyronine in serum and on the response to TRH, *J. Clin. Endocrinol. Metab.,* 39, 191, 1974.
144. **Rahman, Y. E. and Peraino, C.,** Effects of age on patterns of enzyme adaptation in male and female rats, *Exp. Gerontol.,* 8, 93, 1973.
145. **Recker, R. R., Saville, P. D., and Heaney, R. P.,** Effect of estrogens and calcium carbonate on bone loss in postmenopausal women, *Ann. Int. Med.,* 87, 649, 1977.
146. **Reichel, W.,** Lipofuscin pigment accumulation and distribution in five rat organs as a function of age, *J. Gerontol.,* 23, 145, 1968.

147. Report of the Workgroup on Definition and Diagnosis of Diabetes Mellitus, in Report of the National Commission on Diabetes to the Congress of the United States, Vol. 3 (Part 1), Department of Health, Education and Welfare, Washington, D.C., 1976, 45.
148. **Riddick, F. A.,** Hyperparathyroidism in the aged, *Geriatrics,* 22, 94, 1967.
149. **Riegle, G. D.,** Chronic stress effects on adrenocortical responsiveness in young and aged rats, *Neuroendocrinology,* 11, 1, 1973.
150. **Riegle, G. D. and Hess, G. D.,** Chronic and acute dexamethasone suppression of stress activation of the adrenal cortex in young and aged rats, *Neuroendocrinology,* 9, 175, 1972.
151. **Riegle, G. D. and Meites, J.,** Effects of aging on LH and prolactin after LHRH, L-DOPA, methyl dopa, and stress in the male rat, *Proc. Soc. Exp. Biol. Med.,* 151, 507, 1976.
152. **Riegle, G. D. and Miller, A. E.,** Aging effects on the hypothalamic-hypophyseal-gonadal system in the rat, in *The Aging Reproductive System,* Schneider, E. L., Ed., Raven Press, New York, 1978, 159.
153. **Riegle, G. D. and Nellor, J. E.,** Changes in pituitary-adrenal function during aging in cattle, *J. Gerontol.,* 22, 83, 1967.
154. **Riegle, G. D., Prezekop, F., and Nellor, J. E.,** Changes in adrenocortical responsiveness to ACTH infusion in aging goats, *J. Gerontol.,* 23, 187, 1968.
155. **Riggs, B. L., Arnaud, C. D., Jowsey, J., Goldsmith, R. S., and Kelly, P. J.,** Parathyroid function in primary osteoporosis, *J. Clin. Invest.,* 52, 181, 1973.
156. **Riggs, B. L., Jowsey, J., Goldsmith, R. S., Kelly, P. J., Hoffman, D. L., and Arnaud, C. D.,** Short- and long-term effects of estrogen and synthetic anabolic hormone in postmenopausal osteoporosis, *J. Clin. Invest.,* 51, 1659, 1972.
157. **Romanoff, L. P., Morris, C. W., Welch, P., Rodriguez, R. M., and Pincus, G.,** The metabolism of cortisol-4-C^{14} in young and elderly men, *J. Clin. Endocrinol.,* 21, 1413, 1961.
158. **Roof, B. S. and Gordan, G. S.,** Hyperparathyroid disease in the aged, in *Geriatric Endocrinology,* Greenblatt, R. B., Ed., Raven Press, New York, 1978, 33.
159. **Root, A. W. and Oski, F. A.,** Effects of human growth hormone in elderly males, *J. Gerontol.,* 24, 98, 1969.
160. **Rubens, R., Dhont, M., and Vermeulen, A.,** Further studies on Leydig cell function in old age, *J. Clin. Endocrinol. Metab.,* 39, 40, 1974.
161. **Rugh, R. and Wohlfromm, M.,** The reproductive performance of the laboratory mouse: maternal age, litter size, and sex ratio, *Proc. Soc. Exp. Biol. Med.,* 136, 685, 1967.
162. **Sandberg, H., Yoshimine, N., Maeda, S., Symons, D., and Zavodnick, J.,** Effect of an oral glucose load on serum immunoreactive insulin, free fatty acid, growth hormone, and blood sugar level in young and elderly subjects, *J. Am. Geriatr. Soc.,* 21, 433, 1973.
163. **Sawyer, C. H., Hilliard, J., Kanematsu, S., Scaramuzzi, R., and Blake, C. A.,** Effects of intraventricular infusion of norepinephrine and dopamine on LH release and ovulation in the rabbit, *Neuroendocrinology,* 15, 328, 1974.
164. **Scazigga, B., Lemarchand-Beraud, T., and Vanotti, A.,** in *Problems de Geriatrie,* Sandoz, Paris, 1968, 15.
165. **Schneider, E. L., Ed.,** *The Aging Reproductive System,* Raven Press, New York, 1978.
166. **Shaar, C. J. and Clemens, J. A.,** The role of catecholamines in the release of anterior pituitary prolactin in vitro, *Endocrinology,* 95, 1202, 1974.
167. **Shaar, C. J., Euker, J. S., Riegle, G. D., and Meites, J.,** Effects of castration and gonadal steroids on serum luteinizing hormone and prolactin in old and young rats, *J. Endocrinol.,* 66, 45, 1975.
168. **Sherman, B. M., West, J. H., and Korenman, S. G.,** The menopausal transition: analysis of LH, FSH, estradiol, and progesterone concentration during menstrual cycles of older women, *J. Clin. Endocrinol. Metab.,* 42, 629, 1976.
169. **Simpkins, J. W., Mueller, G. P., Huang, H. H., and Meites, J.,** Evidence for depressed catecholamine and enhanced serotonin metabolism in aging male rats: possible relation to gonadotropin secretion, *Endocrinology,* 100, 1672, 1977.
170. **Singhal, R. L.,** Effect of age on the induction of glucose-6-phosphatase and fructose-1, 6-diphosphatase in rat liver, *J. Gerontol.,* 22, 77, 1967.
171. **Siperstein, M. D.,** The glucose tolerance test, *Adv. Int. Med.,* 20, 297, 323.
172. **Siperstein, M. D., Unger, R. H., and Madison, L. L.,** Studies of capillary basement membranes in normal subjects, diabetic, and prediabetic patients, *J. Clin. Invest.,* 47, 1973, 1968.
173. **Snyder, P. J. and Utiger, R. D.,** Response to thyrotropin-releasing hormone (TRH) in normal man, *J. Clin. Endocrinol. Metab.,* 34, 380, 1972.
174. **Spilman, C. H., Larson, L. L., Concannon, P. W., and Foote, R. H.,** Ovarian function during pregnancy in young and aged rabbits: temporal relationship between fetal death and corpus luteum regression, *Biol. Reprod.,* 7, 223, 1972.
175. **Streeten, D. H. P., Gerstein, M. M., Warmor, B. M., and Doisy, R. J.,** Reduced glucose tolerance in elderly human subjects, *Diabetes,* 14, 579, 1965.

176. **Szabo, R., Dzsinich, D., Okros, I., and Stark, E.,** The ultrastructure of the aged rat zona fasciculata under various stressing procedures, *Exp. Gerontol.*, 5, 335, 1970.
177. **Talbert, G. B.,** Effect of aging of the ovaries and female gametes on reproductive capacity, in *The Aging Reproductive System,* Schneider, E. L., Ed., Raven Press, New York, 1978, 59.
178. **Talbert, G. B. and Krohn, P. L.,** Effect of maternal age on viability of ova and uterine support of pregnancy in mice, *J. Reprod. Fertil.*, 11, 399, 1966.
179. **Tsai, C. C. and Yen, S. S. C.,** Acute effects of intravenous infusion of 17β-estradiol on gonadotrophin release in pre- and postmenopausal women, *J. Clin. Endocrinol. Metab.*, 32, 766, 1971.
180. **Utiger, R. D.,** Extraction and radioimmunoassay of growth hormone in human serum, *J. Clin. Endocrinol. Metab.*, 24, 60, 1964.
181. **Vagenakis, A. G., Burger, A., Portnay, G. I., Rudolph, M., O'Brien, J. T., Azizi, F., Arky, R., Nicod, P., Ingbar, S. H., and Braverman, L. E.,** Diversion of peripheral thyroxine metabolism from activating to inactivating pathways during complete fasting, *J. Clin. Endocrinol. Metab.*, 41, 191, 1975.
182. **Van Wyk, J. J. and Underwood, L. W.,** Relation between growth hormone and somatomedin, *Annu. Rev. Med.*, 26, 427, 1975.
183. **Vermeulen, A.,** Leydig cell function in old age, in *Hypothalamus, Pituitary and Aging,* Everitt, A. V. and Burgess, J. A., Eds., Charles C Thomas, Springfield, Ill., 1976, 458.
184. **Vermeulen, A.,** The hormonal activity of the postmenopausal ovary, *J. Clin. Endocrinol. Metab.*, 42, 247, 1976.
185. **Vihko, R.,** Gas chromatographic-mass spectrometric studies on solvolyzable steroids in human peripheral plasma, *Acta Endocrinol. (Copenhagen) Suppl.*, 109, 1966.
186. **Watkins, B. E., McKay, D. W., Meites, J., and Riegle, G. D.,** L-DOPA effects on serum LH and prolactin in old and young female rats, *Neuroendocrinology,* 19, 331, 1976.
187. **Watkins, B. E., Meites, J., and Riegle, G. D.,** Age-related changes in pituitary responsiveness to LHRH in the female rat, *Endocrinology,* 97, 543, 1975.
188. **Wayne, E. J., Koutras, D. A., and Alexander, W. D.,** *Clinical Aspects of Iodine Metabolism,* Blackwell, Oxford, 1964.
189. **Weidmann, P., Byttennere-Bursztein, S., Maxwell, M. H., and Lima, J.,** Effect of aging on plasma renin and aldosterone in normal man, *Kidney Int.*, 8, 325, 1975.
190. **Welborn, T. A., Stenhouse, N. S., and Hohnstone, C. G.,** Factors determining serum insulin response in a population sample, *Diabetologia,* 5, 263, 1969.
191. **Wentz, A. C., Jones, G. S., and Rocco, L.,** Gonadotropin responses following luteinizing hormone releasing hormone administration in normal subjects, *Obstet. Gynecol.*, 45, 239, 1975.
192. **West, C. D., Brown, H., Simons, E. L., Carter, D. B., Kumagai, L. F., and Englert, E.,** Adrenocortical function and cortisol metabolism in old age, *J. Clin. Endocrinol.*, 21, 1197, 1961.
193. **Williams, R. H.,** The pancreas, in *Textbook of Endocrinology,* W. B. Saunders, Philadelphia, 1968.
194. **Wilson, C. A.,** Hypothalamic amines and the release of gonadotrophins and other anterior pituitary hormones, *Adv. Drug Res.*, 8, 119, 1974.
195. **Yahia, C., Taymor, M. L., and Buytendorp, A.,** Day to day variation in LH excretion in carcinoma of the endometrium and normal menopause, *Am. J. Obstet. Gynecol.*, 88, 730, 1964.
196. **Finch, C. E.,** personal communication, 1979.

CHANGES IN HORMONE RECEPTORS DURING ADULTHOOD AND SENESCENCE

George S. Roth

THE ROLE OF HORMONE RECEPTORS IN HORMONE ACTION

Although hormones are extraordinarily diverse with respect to size, molecular type, and physiological responses elicited, essentially all of these molecules begin their actions in the same general way: by attachment to specific cellular receptors. Receptors are protein molecules located either intracellularly or on the plasma membrane. Some membrane receptors, such as those for catecholamines, glucagon, and ACTH, are functionally linked to the enzyme adenylate cyclase and mediate responses dependent on production of cyclic AMP.[1] For others, such as the insulin receptor, a clear mechanism of action has not yet been established.[1] Some intracellular hormone receptors, such as those for steroids, shuttle from the cytoplasm to the nucleus when complexed with hormone and act directly on the genome.[2,3] In all of these cases important biological effects ultimately ensure.

Receptors also may exert a certain degree of control over the responses which they mediate. In many cases the degree of biological response is dependent upon the amount of complexes which form between receptors and hormones.[4,5] Even more important, it has been shown that during many altered physiological states, including diseases, development, and biological cycles, changes in hormone receptor levels occur which appear to be closely related to changes in biological responsiveness.[4,5] For example, during development in the rat, hepatic glucocorticoid receptor concentrations increase concommitantly with the ability to induce tyrosine aminotransferase.[6] Also, during the diurnal light and dark cycle, rat pineal β-adrenergic receptor levels fluctuate up and down in parallel with the ability to induce N-acetyltransferase.[7,8] Thus, the receptor-binding step in many hormone actions seem to pay a key role both in initiating and regulating physiological responsiveness.

AGE-RELATED HORMONE RECEPTOR CHANGES AND THEIR ROLE IN ALTERED RESPONSIVENESS

All of the molecular events in hormone actions subsequent to receptor binding are candidates for alteration with increasing age. However, because of the close relationship of hormone receptors to responsiveness in numerous situations changes in receptors are likely sites for altered biological responses to hormones during aging. Numerous examples of such altered hormonal responsiveness over the life span have been reviewed in the literature.[4,5] In some cases such responsiveness is not significantly altered during senescence but may change during maturation. In a few situations, responsiveness may actually increase with increasing age. However, in the majority of cases ability to respond to particular hormones decreases during the senescence phase of the life span.

Many studies on hormone receptors during the aging process have now been published. These can be divided into various groups on the basis of several criteria, including intracellular vs. extracellular receptors, hormone classes, tissue and/or cell types, and animal species. For the purposes of this review, such investigations are classified according to hormones. Three have been selected arbitrarily: (1) steroid receptors, (2) polypeptide receptors, and (3) nonpolypeptide, nonsteroid receptors. The first group initially act intracellularly, while the second and third groups act initially at the cell

Table 1
CHANGES WITH AGE IN STEROID HORMONE RECEPTORS

Receptor	Tissue or cell	Species	Change	Concomitant change in biological response	Ref.
Cortico-steroid	Splenic lympho-cytes	Rat	D	Inhibition of uridine uptake	9
	Cerebral cortex	Rat	D		10
	Cerebral cortex	Mouse	N		11
	Cortical neurons	Rat	D		12
	Skeletal muscle	Rat	D		10
	Adipose tissue	Rat	D		10
	Adipocytes	Rat	D	Inhibition of glucose oxida-tion	13
	Liver	Human	D		14
	Liver	Rat	N, DE		10, 15
	Liver	Mouse	N		16
	Thymus	Rat	DE		15
	Lung fibroblasts (WI-38)	Human	D	Prolongation of in vitro life span	17
	Hypothalamus	Mouse	N		11
	Pituitary	Mouse	N		11
Androgen	Liver	Rat	D	Induction of α2u globulin	18
	Ventral prostate	Rat	D	Maintenance of cell content	19, 20
	Lateral prostate	Rat	D		21
	Dorsal prostate	Rat	N		21
	Anterior prostate	Rat	N		21
	Prostate	Dog	N		22
	Testes	Rat	D		23
	Seminal vesicles	Rat	N, I		21, 24
	Hypothalamus	Rat	D		23
	Pituitary	Rat	D		23
	Cerebral cortex	Rat	DE		23
Estrogen	Uterus	Rat	D	Induction of phosphofruc-tokinase	25, 26
	Uterus	Mouse	D		27
	Brain	Rat	D	Induction of acetylcholines-terase	28, 29
	Seminal vesicles	Rat	I		24

Note: D = decrease during senescence; N = no change; DE = decrease during early adulthood; and I = increase during senescence.

membrane (with the exception of thyroid hormones which act intracellularly). Studies on these receptors during aging are catalogued in Tables 1, 2, and 3. It should be noted that in almost all of these studies the changes which occur are in receptor concentrations, whereas binding affinities are not altered significantly with age.

SIGNIFICANCE OF RECEPTOR STUDIES TO AGING RESEARCH

Although a few conflicting reports are listed in the tables, it is clear that changes in certain hormone receptor concentrations constitute a fairly common manifestation of the aging process. It is also clear that about 70% of the concentration changes reported thus far are reductions, either during senescence or earlier in the adult life span. This is in contrast to the situation for cellular enzymes in general where no consistent pattern as to increases, decreases, or lack of changes with age has emerged[48] (see also "Enzyme Levels in Animals of Various Ages"). Furthermore, receptor losses in most

Table 2
CHANGES WITH AGE IN POLYPEPTIDE HORMONE RECEPTORS

Receptor	Tissue or cell	Species	Change	Concomitant change in biological response	Ref.
Insulin	Skin fibroblasts	Human	D, I	Stimulation of glucose	30, 31
	Liver	Rat	DE		32
	Liver	Mouse	N		33
	Heart	Mouse	N		33
Glucagon	Adipocyte	Rat	DE	Stimulation of lipolysis	34
Gonado-tropin	Teses	Rat	D		35
Growth hormone	Liver	Mouse	N		33
Prolactin	Prostate	Rat	DE		36
	Seminal vesicles	Rat	DE		36
Epidermal growth factor	Lung fibroblasts (WI-38)	Human	I		37
Low density lipoprotein	Lung fibroblasts (WI-38)	Human	D		38
	Skin fibroblasts	Human	N		39

Note: D = decrease during senescence; N = no change; DE = decrease during early adulthood; and I = increase during senescence.

Table 3
CHANGES WITH AGE IN NONPOLYPEPTIDE, NONSTEROID HORMONE RECEPTORS

Receptor	Tissue or cell	Species	Change	Concomitant change in biological response	Ref.
β-Adrenergic	Lymphocytes	Human	D		40
	Adipocytes	Rat	D	Lypolysis	41
	Cerebellum	Rat	D		42
	Corpus striatum	Rat	D		42
	Erythrocyte	Rat	DE	Stimulation of adenylate cyclase	43
	Pineal	Rat	DE		42
	Cerebral cortex	Rat	N		43
Dopamine	Corpus striatum	Rat	D		44
		Rabbit	D	Stimulation of adenylate cyclase	45
Acetylcholine	Cerebral cortex	Rat	D		46
	Cerebellar cortex	Rat	D		46
Thyroid	Cerebral hemisphere	Rat	DE		47

Note: D = decrease during senescence; N = no change; and DE = decrease during early adulthood.

cases are at least 50 to 70% over the life span, whereas enzyme activities in general rarely change more than 25%.

Age changes in receptors are consistent with the idea proposed by many that the manifestations of aging should not be reflected uniformly in the expression of all genes, but most strikingly for certain key regulatory genes.[49,50] As such, hormone receptor systems offer important models for studying the control of genetic information transfer during aging. More important, however, is the fact that examination of altered hormone action may help to bridge the gap between more superficial measurements of life span and vigor and highly refined molecular biological studies.

REFERENCES

1. **Cuatrecasas, P.**, Membrane receptors, *Annu. Rev. Biochem.*, 43, 169, 1974.
2. **King, R. J. B. and Mainwaring, W. I. P.**, *Steroid Cell Interactions*, University Park Press, Baltimore, 1974.
3. **O'Malley, B. W. and Means, A. R., Eds.**, *Receptors for Reproductive Hormones*, Plenum Press, New York, 1973.
4. **Roth, G. S.**, in Hormonal receptor and responsiveness changes during aging: genetic modulation, *Genetic Effects on Aging*, Bergsma, D. and Harrison, D. H., Eds., Alan R. Liss, New York, 1978, 365.
5. **Roth, G. S.**, Hormone action during aging: alterations and mechanisms, *Mech. Ageing Dev.*, 9, 499, 1979.
6. **Singer, S. and Litwack, G.**, Effects of age and sex on ^{3}H-cortisol uptake, binding, and metabolism in liver and on enzyme induction capacity, *Endocrinology*, 88, 1448, 1971.
7. **Kebabian, J. W., Zatz, M., Romero, J. A., and Axelrod, J.**, Rapid changes in rat pineal B-adrenergic receptor: alterations in 1-(^{3}H) alprenolol binding and adenylate cyclose, *Proc. Natl. Acad. Sci. U.S.A.*, 72, 3735, 1975.
8. **Romero, J. A. and Axelrod, J.**, Regulation of sensitivity to beta adrenergic stimulation in induction of pineal N-acetyltransferase, *Proc. Natl. Acad. Sci. U.S.A.*, 72, 1661, 1975.
9. **Roth, G. S.**, Reduced glucocorticoid responsiveness and receptor concentration in splenic leukocytes of senescent rats, *Biochim. Biophys. Acta*, 399, 145, 1975.
10. **Roth, G. S.**, Age-related changes in specific glucocorticoid binding by steroid responsive tissues of rats, *Endocrinology*, 94, 82, 1974.
11. **Nelson, J. F., Holinka, C. F., Latham, K. R., Allen, J. K., and Finch, C. E.**, Corticosterone binding in cytosols from brain regions of mature and senescent male C57BL/6J mice, *Brain Res.*, 115, 345, 1976.
12. **Roth G. S.**, Reduced glucocorticoid binding site concentration in corticol neuronal perikarya from senescent rats, *Brain Res.*, 107, 345, 1976.
13. **Roth, G. S. and Livingston, J. N.**, Reductions in glucocorticord inhibition of glucose oxidation and presumptive glucocorticord receptor content in rat adipocytes during aging, *Endocrinology*, 99, 831, 1976.
14. **Singer, S., Ito, H., and Litwack, G.**, ^{3}H-cortisol binding by young and old human liver cytosol proteins *in vitro*, *Int. J. Biochem.*, 4, 569, 1973.
15. **Petrovic, J. S. and Markovic, R. Z.**, Changes in cortisol binding to soluble receptor proteins in rat liver and thymus during development and aging, *Dev. Biol.*, 45, 176, 1975.
16. **Latham, K. R. and Finch, C. E.**, Hepatic glucocorticoid binders in mature and senescent C57 BL/65 male mice, *Endocrinology*, 98, 1480, 1976.
17. **Rosner, B. A. and Cristofalo, V. J.**, *Fed. Proc.*, 37, 888, 1978.
18. **Roy, A. K., Milin, B. S., and McMinn, D. M.**, *Biochem. Biophys. Acta*, 354, 213, 1974.
19. **Shain, S. A. and Boesel, R. W.**, *Mech. Ageing Dev.*, 6, 219, 1977.
20. **Shain, S. A., Boesel, R. W., and Axelrod, L. R.**, *Arch. Biochem. Biophys.*, 167, 247, 1973.
21. **Robinette, C. L. and Mawhinney, M. G.**, *Fed. Proc.*, 36, 344, 1977.
22. **Shain, S. A. and Boesel, R. W.**, Androgen receptors of the aging canine prostate, *Proc. 59th Annu. Meet. Endocr. Soc.*, p. 332, 1977.
23. **Chouknyiska, R. and Vassileva-Popova, J. G.**, *C. R. Acad. Bulg. Sci.*, 30, 133, 1977.
24. **Robinette, C. L. and Mawhinney, M. G.**, Effects of aging on the estrogen receptor in rat seminal vesticles, *Fed. Proc.*, 37, 283, 1978.
25. **Holinka, C. F., Nelson, J. F., and Finch, C. E.**, *Gerontologist*, 15, 30, 1975.
26. **Singhal, R. L., Valadares, H. R. E., and Ling, G. M.**, *Am. J. Physiol.*, 217, 793, 1969.
27. **Nelson, J. F., Holinka, C. F., and Finch, C. E.**, *Abstr. 29th Annu. Meet. Gerontol. Soc.*, 34, 86, 1976.

28. **Kanungo, M. S., Patnaik, S. E., and Koul, O.,** *Nature,* 253, 366, 1975.
29. **Moudgil, V. K. and Kanungo, M. S.,** *Biochim. Biophys. Acta,* 329, 211, 1973.
30. **Ito, H., Orimo, H., and Shimada, H.,** Reduced insulin action in vitro and the binding of ^{125}I-insulin to cultured human skin fibroblasts with aging, *Abstr. 5th Intl. Congr. Endocrinol.,* p. 261, 1976.
31. **Rosenbloom, A. and Goldstein, S.,** Insulin binding to cultured human fibroblasts increase with normal and precocious aging, *Science,* 193, 412, 1976.
32. **Freeman, C., Karoly, K., and Adelman, R. C.,** *Biochem. Biophys. Res. Comm.,* 54, 1573, 1973.
33. **Sorrentino, R. M. and Florini, J. R.,** Variations among individual mice in binding of growth hormones and insulin to membranes from animals of different ages, *Exp. Aging Res.,* 2, 191, 1976.
34. **Livingston, J. N., Cuatrecasas, P., and Lockwood, D. H.,** *J. Lipid Res.,* 15, 26, 1974.
35. **Vassileva-Popova, J.,** Developmental changes in gonadol binding of gonadotrophins, *Proc. 5th Asia Oceania Congr. Endocrinol.,* p. 242, 1974.
36. **Barkey, R. J., Shani, J., Amit, T., and Barzilai, D.,** *J. Endocrinol.,* 74, 163, 1977.
37. **Ladda, R.,** personal communication, 1978.
38. **Gallup, P.,** personal communication, 1979.
39. **Bierman, E.,** personal communication, 1979.
40. **Schocken, D. D. and Roth, G. S.,** Reduced beta adrenergic receptor concentrations in aging man, *Nature,* 267, 856, 1977.
41. **Guidicelli, Y. and Pequery, R.,** β-adrenergic receptors and catecholamine sensitive adenylate cyclase in rat fat cell membranes: influence of growth, cell size, and aging, *Eur. J. Biochem.,* 90, 413, 1978.
42. **Greenberg, L. H., Dix, R. K., and Weiss, B.,** Age-related changes in ^{3}H-dihydroalprenolol binding in rat brain, in *Pharmcological Intervention of the Aging Process,* Cristofalo, V. J., Roberts, J., and Adelman, R. C., Eds., Plenum, New York, in press.
43. **Bylund, D. B., Tellez-Inon, M. T., and Hollenberg, M. D.,** Age-related parallel decline in beta adrenergic receptors, adenyl cyclase, and phosphodiesterase activity in rat erythrocyte membranes, *Life Sci.,* 21, 403, 1977.
44. **Joseph, J. A., Berger, R. E., Engel, B. T., and Roth, G. S.,** Age-related changes in the nigrostriation: a behavioral and biochemical analysis, *J. Gerontol.,* 33, 643, 1978.
45. **Makman, M. H., Ahn, H. S., Thal, L. J., Sharpless, N. S., Dvorkin, B., Horowitz, S. G., and Rosenfeld, M.,** Aging and monoamine receptors in brain, *Fed. Proc.,* 308, 1922, 1979.
46. **James, T. C. and Kanungo, M. S.,** Alteration in atropine sites of the brain as a function of age, *Biochem. Biophys. Res. Comm.,* 72, 170, 1976.
47. **Timiras, P. S. and Bignami, A.,** in *Special Review of Experimental Aging Research: Progress in Biology,* Elias, M. F., Eleftheriou, B. E., and Elias, P. K., Eds., Bar Harbor, Maine, 1976, 351.
48. **Finch, C. E.,** Enzyme activities, gene function, and aging in mammals, *Exp. Gerontol.,* 7, 53, 1972.
49. **Cutler, R. G.,** Nature of aging and life maintenance processes, *Interdisciplinary Topics in Gerontology,* Vol. 9, S. Karger, Basel, 1976, 83.
50. **Martin, G. M.,** Genetic syndromes in man with potential relevance to the pathobiology of aging in *Genetic Effects of Aging,* Bergsma, D. and Harrison, D. H., Eds., Alan R. Liss, New York, 1978, 5.

ENZYME ADAPTATION DURING AGING

Mark F. Obenrader, James L. Sartin, and Richard C. Adelman

The ability to initiate adaptive changes in the activity of a large number of enzymes is impaired during aging and evident in various tissues of different species in response to a broad spectrum of stimuli. The expression of such age-related adaptive alterations in enzyme induction has been categorized into four general patterns of response[1] (Figure 1):

Type 1 — Induction initiation time is altered (increased or decreased), but magnitude of the response is not influenced during aging.

Type 2 — Magnitude of response is altered (increased or decreased) without changes in temporal pattern of induction.

Type 3 — Both the temporal pattern and magnitude of response is modified during aging.

Type 4 — Enzyme adaptive responsiveness is not altered during aging.

Where enzyme inductions are assessed at only one time point, the response cannot be characterized according to the above scheme. These data are tabulated in Table 1, and the age effect on the magnitude of the adaptive responses are indicated by arrows (↑, increase; ↓, decrease).

The data presented here represent a summary of the age-related adaptive responses in enzyme induction. Where possible, an attempt has been made to indicate the pattern (type) of age-related response. Since patterns of enzyme adaptation are susceptible to considerable variation related to difference in species and strain, sex, and conditions of environmental maintenance, additional information also has been included. It should be noted that enzyme induction studies reflecting developmental rather than senescent changes have not been considered.

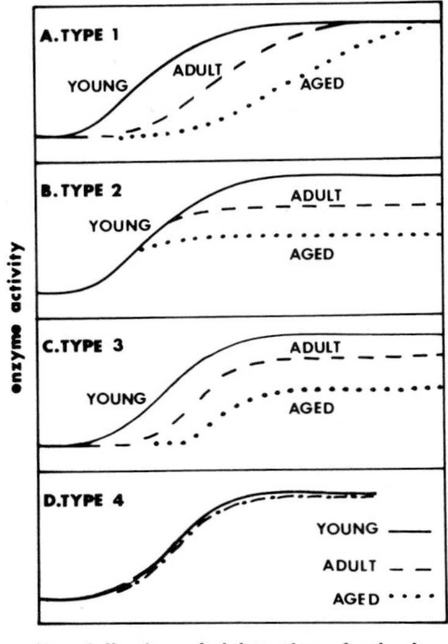

FIGURE 1. Patterns of age-dependent enzyme adaptation. (From Adelman, R. C., in *Enzyme Induction*, Parke, D.V., Ed., Plenum Press, New York, 1975. With permission.)

Table 1
ENZYME INDUCTION DURING AGING

Enzyme	Species (stock or strain)	Sex	Ages (months)	Tissue	Inducer	Adaptive response[a]	Ref.
Adenylate cyclase	Rat (Wistar)	Male, female	3, 12, 24	Liver	Epinephrine	↑[b]	2
					Fluoride	↑[b]	1
					Glucagon	↑[b]	
	Rat (Wistar)	Male	2, 6, 12, 24	Fat cells	ACTH	↓[b]	3
					Epinephrine	↓[b]	
					Fluoride	↓[b]	
	Rat (Wistar CF)	Male	1, 8, 30	Fat cells	Epinephrine	↓[b]	4
					Norepinephrine	↓[b]	
	Rat (Charles River CD-F)	Male	4, 12, 24, 30	Brain (corpus striatum)	Dopamine	↓[b]	5
Alkaline phosphatase	Mouse (C57B1/6J)	Female (ovarectomized)	6, 11, 21	Uterus	Estradiol	↓[b]	6
Aminopyrine N-demythylase	Rat (Wistar)	Female	1.3, 3.3, 9.9, 19.8	Liver	Phenobarbital	↓[b]	7
Aniline hydroxylase	Rat (Wistar)	Female	1.3, 3.3, 9.9, 19.8	Liver	Phenobarbital	↓[b]	7
Catalase	*Drosophila*	Male	0.25, 1.75	Whole fly	3-amino-1,2,4-triazole	Type III	8
Cytochrome P450 reductase	Rat (Wistar)	Male	3, 12, 27	Liver	Polychlorinated biphenyls	Type IV	9
Deoxythymidylate synthetase	Rat (Sprague-Dawley)	Male	2, 12	Salivary gland	Isoproterenol	Type III	10
DNA polymerase B	Rat (Wistar)	Female	4, 19	Liver	Bleomycin	No change[b]	11
Fatty acid synthetase	Mouse (C57B1/6J)	Male	1, 8, 10, 18	Liver	Shift to fatless diet	↓[b]	12
Fructose-1,6-di-phosphatase	Rat	Male	2, 12, 24	Liver	Hydrocortisone	↓[b]	13
				kidney	Hydrocortisone	↓[b]	
				Spleen	Hydrocortisone	↑[b]	14
	Rat (Wistar)	Male	1, 3, 6, 9, 12, 15	Liver	Dexamethasone	↓[b]	

Glucokinase	Rat (Sprague-Dawley)	Male, female	2, 14, 24	Liver	Glucose	Type I	15, 16
	Rat (Sprague-Dawley)	Male	2, 18, 24	Liver	ACTH	Type IV	17
					Cortisol	Type IV	
					Insulin	Type IV	
					Glucagon	Type IV	
Glucose-6-phosphatase	Rat (Wistar)	Male	1, 3, 6, 9, 12, 15	Liver	Dexamethasone	↓[b]	14
	Rat	Male	2, 12, 24	Liver	Hydrocortisone	↓[b]	13
				Kidney	Hydrocortisone	↓[b]	
				Spleen	Hydrocortisone	↑[b]	
	Rat (Sprague-Dawley)	Male, female	1, 12	Liver	High casein diet	Type II	18
Glutamine synthetase	Rat	Female	2, 18	Liver	Cortisone	Type II	19
α-Glycerol phosphate dehydrogenase	Rat (Wistar)	Female	12, 28	Liver	3,3,5-Triiodothyronine	Type IV	20, 21
Hexabarbitol hydroxylase	Rat (Wistar)	Female	1.3, 3.3, 9.9, 19.8	Liver	Phenobarbitol	↓[b]	7
NADPH: cytochrome *c* reductase	Rat (Wistar)	Female	1.3, 3.3, 9.9, 19.8	Liver	Phenobarbitol	↓[b]	7
	Rat (Sprague-Dawley)	Male	2, 14, 24	Liver	Phenobarbitol	Type I	16
	Rat (Wistar)	Male	3, 12, 27	Liver	Polychlorinated biphenyls	Type IV	9
NADPH: neotetrazolium reductase	Rat (Wistar)	Female	1.3, 3.3, 9.9, 19.8	Liver	Phenobarbitol	↓[b]	7
NADPH: oxidase	Rat (Wistar)	Female	1.3, 3.3, 9.9, 19.8	Liver	Phenobarbitol	↓[b]	7
P-nitrobenzoic acid nitroreductase	Rat (Wistar)	Female	1.3, 3.3, 9.9, 19.8	Liver	Phenobarbitol	↓[b]	7
Ornithine aminotransferase	Rat (Sprague-Dawley)	Male, female	1, 12	Liver	High casein diet	Type II	18
Ornithine decarboxylase	Rat (Wistar)	Male	3, 23	Liver	Dexamethasone	No change[b]	22
Phosphofructokinase	Rat (Wistar)	Male	1, 2, 3, 6, 12	Prostate	Testosterone	↓[b]	23
				Seminal vesicle	Testosterone	↓[b]	

Table 1 (continued)
ENZYME INDUCTION DURING AGING

Enzyme	Species (stock or strain)	Sex	Ages (months)	Tissue	Inducer	Adaptive response[a]	Ref.
6-Phospgluconate and glucose-6-phosphate dehydrogenases	Mouse (C56B1/6J)	Male	1, 8, 10, 18	Liver	Shift to fatless	↓[b]	12
Prolyl hydroxylase	Human	—	Passages 38, 55	Fibroblasts (WI-38)	Ascorbate	↓[b]	24
Serine dehydratase	Rat (Sprague-Dawley)	Male, female	1, 12	Liver	High casein diet	Type I	18
Thymidine kinase	Rat (Spraque-Dawley)	Male	2, 12	Salivary gland	Isoproterenol	Type III	10
Tryptophan pyrrolase	Rabbit (N ew Zealand)	Female	2, 4—10	Liver	Fasting	Type III	25
	Rat (Fischer 344)	Male	1, 6, 12	Liver	Tryptophan	↓[b]	26
Tyrosine aminotransferase	Mouse (C56B1/6J)	Male	16, 28	Liver	Cold	Type I	27
					Corticosterone	Type IV	
					Insulin	Type IV	
	Rat (Sprague-Dawley)	Male	2, 18, 24	Liver	ACTH	Type I	28
	Rat (Sprague-Dawley)	Male	2, 18, 24	Liver	Insulin	Type IV	17
					Cortisol	Type IV	
					Glucagon	Type IV	

[a] ↓ = decrease; ↑ = increase.
[b] Measurement of magnitude of response only, no time course. Old values compared to young values.

REFERENCES

1. **Adelman, R. C.,** in *Enzyme Induction,* Parke, D. V., Ed., Plenum Press, New York, 1975, 301.
2. **Kalish, M. I., Katz, M. S., Pineyro, M. A., and Gregerman, R. I.,** *Biochim. Biophys. Acta,* 483, 452, 1977.
3. **Cooper, B. and Gregerman, R. I.,** *J. Clin. Invest.,* 57, 161, 1977.
4. **Giudicelli, Y. and Pecquery, R.,** *Eur. J. Biochem.,* 90, 413, 1978.
5. **Puri, S. K. and Volicer, L.,** *Mech. Ageing Dev.,* 6, 53, 1977.
6. **Holinka, C. F., Hetland, M. D., and Finch, C. E.,** *Biol. Reprod.,* 17, 262, 1977.
7. **Kato, R. and Takanaka, A.,** *J. Biochem.,* 63, 406, 1968.
8. **Nicolosi, R. J., Baird, M. B., Massie, H. R., and Samis, H. V.,** *Exp. Gerontol.,* 8, 101, 1973.
9. **Birnbaum, L. S. and Baird, M. B.,** *Exp. Gerontol.,* 13, 469, 1978.
10. **Roth, G. S., Karoly, K., Britton, V. J., and Adelman, R. C.,** *Exp. Gerontol.,* 9, 1, 1974.
11. **Ove, P. and Coetzee, M. L.,** *Mech. Ageing Dev.,* 8, 363, 1978.
12. **Eisenbach, L., Shimron, F., and Yagil, G.,** *Exp. Gerontol.,* 11, 63, 1976.
13. **Frolkis, V. B., Bezrukov, V. V., and Muradian, Kh. K.,** *Exp. Gerontol.,* 14, 65, 1979.
14. **Singhal, R. L.,** *J. Gerontol.,* 22, 77, 1967.
15. **Adelman, R. C.,** *J. Biol. Chem.,* 245, 1032, 1970.
16. **Adelman, R. C.,** *Exp. Gerontol.,* 6, 75, 1971.
17. **Adelman, R. C. and Freeman, C.,** *Endocrinology,* 90, 1551, 1972.
18. **Rahman, Y. E. and Peraino, C.,** *Exp. Gerontol.,* 8, 93, 1973.
19. **Rao, S. S. and Kanungo, M. S.,** *Mech. Ageing Dev.,* 1, 61, 1972.
20. **Bulos, B., Shukla, S., and Sacktor, B.,** *Mech. Ageing Dev.,* 1, 227, 1972.
21. **Bulos, B., Sacktor, B., Grossman, I. W., and Altman, N.,** *J. Gerontol.,* 26, 13, 1971.
22. **Ferioli, M. E., Ceruti, G., and Comoll, R.,** *Exp. Gerontol.,* 11, 153, 1976.
23. **Singhal, R. L.,** *J. Gerontol.,* 22, 343, 1967.
24. **Chen, K. H., Evans, C. A., and Gallop, P. M.,** *Biochem. Biophys. Res. Commun.,* 74, 1631, 1977.
25. **Wu, S. Y. and Rosenthal, H. L.,** *Proc. Soc. Exp. Biol. Med.,* 122, 414, 1966.
26. **Haining, J. L. and Correll, W. W.,** *J. Gerontol.,* 24, 143, 1969.
27. **Finch, C. E., Foster, J. R., and Mirsky, A. E.,** *J. Gen. Physiol.,* 54, 690, 1969.
28. **Adelman, R. C.,** *Nature,* 228, 1095, 1970.

Theories of Aging

BIOLOGICAL THEORIES OF AGING

N. W. Shock

INTRODUCTION

Aging is, in general, associated with a gradual decline in the performance of most organ systems[1,2] with a loss in reserve capacities. Ultimately, the losses in any organ system may become so large that the animal is no longer capable of meeting the environmental demands for continued existence and death ensues.

In some organ systems such as the kidney, the progressive loss of functional capacity with age[3] can be ascribed to the loss of functioning cells.[4] Other postmitotic nondividing cells also show progressive loss with advancing age,[5] e.g., nerve cells[6,7] and muscle cells. Thus one of the basic problems of gerontology has been to explain why cells die as an animal ages.

A number of cellular theories have been proposed to explain the death of cells in the animal. Many of these theories are based on data derived from cultivating isolated cells in tissue culture. Hayflick[9,10] made a major contribution to our understanding of cellular aging by discovering that most cellular systems are able to undergo only 40 to 50 doublings, thus showing that cell systems have finite life spans and are not immortal.

CELLULAR THEORIES

There is at present no single theory which can adequately explain all of the phenomena of aging. Rather, there are a number of theories which focus on specific aspects of aging. Biological theories of aging may be genetic, nongenetic, or physiological.[11] The fundamental assumption of genetic theories of aging is that the life span of any animal species is determined by a program which resides in the genes of the species and ultimately in the information contained in the DNA molecules through a variety of steps to the ultimate formation of proteins which are critical for the continued function of specific cells in the animal. Thus, aging may result from damage to the DNA or errors in the transmission of information essential to the formation of final products.[12]

Nongenetic theories place emphasis on the changes that may occur with the passage of time in cellular proteins after they have been formed. These changes may represent chemical or structural changes induced by environmental factors. Both genetic and nongenetic theories emphasize changes that occur at the cellular and tissue levels.

Since there are some tissues where cell loss with aging is very small or nonexistent[13] and many tissues can regenerate under conditions of stress, it is doubtful whether all of the phenomena of aging can be explained by cellular phenomena alone. Survival of an individual organism depends on the effectiveness with which performance of different cells and organ systems are integrated to meet the stresses of living.[14,15] Thus, the ultimate key to the phenomena of aging in intact animals may lie in the mechanisms of communication between cells, tissues, and organs. Hence, physiological theories of aging place major emphasis on the effects of aging on regulatory mechanisms.

Genetic Theories

The average age of death varies markedly among different species of animals. Therefore, on the average the may fly lives only one day; the housefly, 30 days; the rat, 3 years; the dog, 12 years; the horse, 25 years; and the human, 70 years.[16] It is, therefore, presumed that there is some genetic program which sets the maximum life span for each species. Even within a single species, genetically determined differences in life span occur as indicated from selective inbreeding experiments with flies in which strains of flies with different life spans were produced.[17] Since the inbred strains had shorter life spans than the original wild strain, it has been concluded that factors related to long life are associated with many different genes so that a large gene pool is advantageous for longevity.

Support for theories of preprogrammed, genetically determined aging has also been provided by studies which indicate that when maintained in tissue cultures, at least some cells of the body are capable of undergoing a limited number of divisions (approximately 40 to 50) after which they age and die.[8] Furthermore, the number of cell divisions that can be effected by cells in culture diminishes progressively with the age of the donor.[18,19]

Humans with long-lived parents and grandparents live, on the average, about 6 years longer than those with parents and grandparents who died before the age of 50.[20] From the evidence available, it seems clear that: (1) there is a genetic program which sets the upper limits of life span in a species, (2) there is some familial characteristic that influences differences in life span among individuals of a given species, and (3) the expression of the basic genetic program can be altered by environmental factors.

DNA Readout — Codon Restriction

It is now recognized that all genetic information depends on the precise molecular structure of different parts of the very large DNA molecules.[21] It is also known that only a small part of the total information coded in the DNA molecule is utilized by a cell at any given time. Thus, during development different "messages" operate in a sequential manner and different proteins are formed. This general theory of gene activation and repression has been extended to explain cellular aging.[22,23] Strehler[24] has developed in great detail the codon restriction theory of aging which basically suggests that as a result of differentiation, cells lose their ability to translate genetic information. Central to the theory is the observation that aging is accompanied by changes in the types of tRNA synthetases present in the cell.

It is also possible that with advancing age, messages previously read and utilized by the cell are no longer accessible. von Hahn[25] has shown that histones are more tightly bound to chromatin in cells from old animals than in young. His interpretation of these results is that with aging, critical areas of information coded in specific parts of the DNA molecules are no longer available.

DNA Damage — Somatic Mutation

Any alterations in the molecular structure of the DNA molecules could alter the "message" and thus result in slight differences in the structure of proteins formed, such as enzymes which would interfere with their physiological functions. Furthermore, alterations in the structure of the DNA molecules would result in mutations when the cell divides; consequently, maintenance of the structural integrity of the DNA molecules is essential for continued existence of a cell line.

In view of the relatively low incidence of spontaneous mutations, it is extremely doubtful that aging is the result of changes in the structure of the DNA molecule. Since one of the primary effects of exposure to radiation is damage to DNA with subsequent induction of mutations, it was often stated that "radiation accelerates aging". It is true that exposure to nonlethal doses of radiation significantly reduces the length of life in experimental animals as well as humans, and the degree of life shortening is directly related to the dose level.[26]

However, subsequent research has shown that the primary lesions of aging and radiation are not identical.[27] In the first place, the effects of radiation occur primarily in dividing cell lines such as the bone marrow stem cells involved in the production of red blood cells, as well as leucocytes and epithelial cells of the gut. Effects are seen after cell division when mutations occur. In contrast, age effects are primarily centered in cell lines that no longer divide in the adult animal, e.g., nerve and muscle cells. It is no longer believed that radiation accelerates the biological effects of aging.

Curtis[28] postulated that aging was basically the result of spontaneous mutations which occur in somatic cells. Although it was not possible to identify structural changes in the DNA molecule itself, experiments were conducted with rats and mice which showed that the incidence of abnormal chromosomes increased: (1) remarkably after exposure to radiation and (2) progressively with age in nonradiated animals. It was also shown that abnormal chromosomes accumulated more rapidly in short-lived species (rat, mouse) than in long-live species (dog).

The ''hit'' theory of aging, proposed by Szilard,[29] is a variation of the somatic mutation theory. According to this theory, ''hits'' occur at random over the lifetime of the animal which inactivate a gene or part of a DNA molecule. When some critical number of hits have occurred, the cell or animal dies.

At the present time, the somatic mutation theory of aging is not regarded as very probable. In the first place, calculations of the rate at which somatic mutations are apt to occur in the absence of exposure to ionizing radiation is much too low to account for overall age changes in an animal.[30] Furthermore, recent studies have shown that most cells contain mechanisms for the repair of damaged DNA molecules,[31,32] although there is no substantial evidence that the effectiveness of the DNA repair mechanism declines in senescent animals.[33] It is apparently more effective in long- rather than short-lived species.[31]

Species differences in the ability of animals to tolerate DNA damage rather than to repair it could also be a reason for their different life spans. The presence of multiple copies of the same message coded within the DNA molecule would thus offer protection when one copy was damaged. Medvedev[34] has cited data which show that the number of repetitions of genes for the major rRNA is 5 to 10 in bacteria, 100 to 130 in *Drosophila* and 250 to 600 in vertebrates. Thus there is a rough correlation between the number of repetitions of a gene and life span of species. However, Cutler[35] could find no clear correlation between the percentage of reiterated DNA and longevity or between the amount of ribosomal gene redundancy and life span among different mammalian species. However, when he examined the genes involved in transcribing mRNA in the brain of mice, cows, and humans, he found that the average redundancy was greater in humans than in cows, and greater in cows than in mice.

Error Theories

Although the basic information necessary for the formation of all of the many different proteins involved in cell function resides in the coded messages within the DNA molecule, many steps are involved in the formation of specific proteins. These processes involve the formation of a number of RNAs. It was Medvedev[36] who first recognized that errors in the transmission of information through the RNAs could have important implications for cellular aging. This theory, known as the error theory, has been further developed and amplified.[37,38] According to this theory, aging and death of a cell are the result of errors which may occur at any step in the sequence of information transfer, resulting in the formation of a protein or enzyme which is not an exact copy and is, therefore, unable to carry out its function properly. The ''error'' may be simply the incorporation of the wrong amino acid in the protein or a slight error in the normal amino acid sequence. Because of the relatively short half-life of RNA molecules, they are being formed continuously during the lifetime of the cell in order to provide replacement of enzyme molecules. The possibility of inducing errors is thus a continuing hazard to the cell.

Orgel[38] has argued that the ability of a cell to produce functional proteins, such as enzymes, depends not only on the accuracy of the genetic information as coded in the DNA molecules, but also on the competence of the protein synthetic apparatus, i.e., the enzymes involved in transcription and translation of the information from the DNA to the final protein product. According to his theory, aging is the result of errors in enzymes involved in translation and transcription rather than in the formation of RNAs. Orgel claimed that although the initial frequency of errors in a cell may be low, in the absence of cell division (as in an adult animal) there will be with the passage of time an exponential increase in the frequency of errors in the proteins synthesized which leads to an "error catastrophy" and the death of the cell. Orgel[39] pointed out that inaccurate protein synthesis and inaccurate DNA synthesis are coupled phenomena so that it is extremely difficult to separate their effects. In attempting to explain cellular aging, the error hypothesis must include both types of errors.

Evidence supporting the error hypothesis is largely based on experiments with fruit flies in which "errors" in specific enzymes were experimentally produced by feeding the flies analogues of certain amino acids.[40] Flies with experimentally induced errors had shorter life spans than normals.

A critical test of the error hypothesis is the identification of abnormal enzymes or proteins in cells and tissues of senescent animals. Direct evidence that old cells contain higher levels of proteins with incorrect amino acids is rather scarce because detecting these errors is technically very difficult. Nevertheless, it has been shown that with advancing age, tissues and cells contain defective enzymes which could have been produced by mistranslation. Thus, Holliday and Tarrant[41] showed that the proportion of the heat labile fractions of the enzymes glucose-6-phosphate dehydrogenase and 6-phosphogluconate dehydrogenase extracted from young and old fibroblasts increased markedly with age. They also found that the heat labile fraction of enzyme found in old cells had an altered substrate specificity indicating the possible presence of errors. By using immunologic techniques it has also been possible to show an age-associated increase in the proportion of inactive lactic dehydrogenase in human fibroblasts, isocitrate lyase in the nematode, and aldolase in mice livers.[42] Structural differences in aldolase separated from old and young mouse muscle have been reported by Gershon and Gershon.[43]

Although there is experimental evidence that errors do occur at the cellular level with aging, it is doubtful that the error theory can account for all of the phenomena of aging. Furthermore, the general theory is relatively nonspecific since errors can occur at so many different points between the information source (DNA) and the final protein product. Although errors may be detected, the experiments seldom permit the identification of the point at which the error occurred. It is also difficult to distinguish error effects from possible somatic mutations. The error theory, although not yet proved, is a viable one deserving further research.

Nongenetic Theories

These theories focus on the changes that take place with the passage of time in structural and functional elements of cells, including molecules, after they have been formed. It is assumed that these changes impair their effectiveness.

Wear and Tear Theory

This theory is based on the assumption that living organisms behave like machines.[44] That is, with repeated use, parts wear out, defects occur, and the machinery finally fails to function. However, the man-machine analogy is not a very good one. Unlike machines which cannot repair themselves, living organisms have developed many mechanisms which permit self-repair.

The primary evidence for wear and tear theories stems from the observations that life span of poikilothermic animals is shortened by increasing the environmental temperature and lengthened by lowering it. This phenomenon has been reported for fruit flies,[45,46] rotifers,[47] and *campanularia*.[48] Since the rates of all chemical reactions increase with rising temperatures, it was assumed that the increased ''rate of living'' shortened life span by increasing ''wear and tear''.

It has long been known that among different animal species life span is inversely related to basal oxygen consumption.[49,50] Short-lived species such as the rat and mouse have much higher rates of basal oxygen consumption per unit of body weight than do longer-lived species such as the elephant and man.

More recently Sacher[51-53] has derived multiple regression equations to predict life span on the basis of brain and body weight, resting or basal oxygen consumption, and body temperature. The multiple regression equation was derived from data on a sample of 85 mammalian species ranging from mice to elephants. The original four-parameter equation could be transformed to a two-parameter equation, based on substituting two independently defined functions of basal metabolism and the ratio of brain to body weight. Sacher concluded that species longevity increases as two major determiners of the entropy production of the species decreases. Although these results demonstrate a clear inverse relationship between basal metabolic rate and life span over a broad spectrum of mammalian species, it is still to be demonstrated that a similar relationship holds for individual animals of differing life span within the same species. It is also hazardous to infer causality from such studies.

Deprivation Theories

Deprivation theories assume that impaired cellular function and cell death are the result of inadequate delivery of essential nutrients or oxygen. These theories are based primarily on the increasing prevalence of atherosclerosis with advancing age in humans and the well-known deleterious effects of vascular degeneration on cellular and tissue functions. However, when the blood supply to a tissue is impaired by vascular disease, all of the cells in the area supplied degenerate and die. This is in sharp contrast to the chance distribution of cells which disappear from a tissue or organ with advancing age. Studies on humans have failed to show a significant decrement in blood concentrations of oxygen or essential nutrients with advancing age. Carpenter and Loyhd[54] have speculated that with advancing age, changes occur in cell membranes which limit the diffusion of oxygen and nutrients from the blood to the inside of living cells. However, there is little experimental data to indicate that this is the case. It is, therefore, extremely doubtful that senescence can be ascribed to cellular deprivation.

Accumulation Theories

Impaired cellular function with advancing age has also been ascribed to the accumulation of deleterious substances in aging animals. Carrel and Ebeling[55] reported that serum taken from old chickens inhibited the growth of cells in tissue culture. This observation led to the presumption that some substance deleterious to cellular growth accumulated in the blood as the chicken aged. Despite numerous attempts, however, no such substance has been isolated and chemically identified.

The most positive evidence for the accumulation theory comes from the identification of highly insoluble lipofuscin particles which accumulate in cells of various tissues such as neurones, muscle fibers of the heart, the adrenal cortex, and the testicle with advancing age.[56] It has been argued that the presence of these insoluble particles interferes with normal cellular metabolism and ultimately results in cell death. However, no direct evidence for impaired physiological function in cells with high levels of age pigment has been obtained.

Free Radical Theories

Free radicals are chemical compounds which contain an unpaired electron in an outer orbital. This unpaired electron makes free radicals highly reactive; they are produced as transient intermediates in the course of normal metabolism as well as from spontaneous random reactions. Much of the cellular damage caused by ionizing radiation is thought to occur from the formation of free radicals derived from the ionization of water. The presence of antioxidants, such as vitamin E, inhibits the formation of free radicals in cells. On the basis of these known facts, Harman[57] has proposed that aging and cell death stem from the damaging effects of free radicals. To test this hypothesis, Harman added a number of antioxidants, e.g., 2-mercaptoethylamine and butylated hydroxytoluene, to the diet of mice. Some of the antioxidants increased the average life span of the mice while others, such as Vitamin E, did not. In no case was the maximum life span increased. Furthermore, no record of the food intake of the animals was taken. Thus, if the added antioxidant was distasteful to the mouse so that he ate less, the increase in average life span might have been due to restriction in food intake which is known to increase life span in mice.[58] In view of the contradictory evidence available and limitations in experimental design, the free radical theory of aging must be regarded as still unproved.

Cross-Linking Theories

With the passage of time, many macromolecules of biological importance develop cross-linkages or bonds either between component parts of the same molecule or between molecules themselves. The formation of these cross-links alters the physical and chemical properties of the molecules involved so that they no longer function in a normal manner. Since these cross-links are apt to be very stable they accumulate with the passage of time. The cross-linking theory first proposed by Bjorksten[59] holds that the accumulation of cross-linked molecules is a primary cause of aging.

The primary experimental evidence for this theory derives from experiments on the extracellular protein collagen.[60] It is well-established that with aging cross-links develop between the two intertwined strands of the collagen molecule and between adjacent strands. Formation of these cross-links results in the well-known loss of elasticity with advancing age in many tissues of the body such as the skin and blood vessels. Kohn[61] has hypothesized that these changes in collagen may have far reaching effects on many organ systems and be the common factor that induces the physiological decrements that occur with aging.

From these observed facts with respect to the extracellular protein collagen, it has been assumed that similar cross-links are formed in intracellular proteins (enzymes) as well as in the DNA molecule itself.[62] Although cross-linking between different parts of the DNA molecule has been observed in vitro, no evidence has yet appeared indicating that these changes also occur in vivo. Until evidence that cross-linking occurs in intracellular proteins and nuclear constituents in vivo, the theory must be regarded as speculation.

In summary, it must be said that although there are a number of theories of cellular aging, none have been firmly established on the basis of clear-cut experimental evidence. Each theory focuses on specific aspects of aging, but none is capable of explaining all of the known facts. Among those which seem to be more probable than others are codon expression and error and cross-linking theories, but a great deal of experimental work remains to be done.

BIOLOGICAL THEORIES OF AGING

Physiological theories of aging attempt to explain aging and the life span of various species of animals either on the basis of a failure in the performance of a single organ system or, more reasonably, in terms of impairment in physiological control mechanisms.[14] Physiological theories of aging which deal with aging of the total animal will be briefly summarized in terms of broad generalities.

Single Organ Theories

Almost every organ system has at one time or another been regarded as the key to aging.

Cardiovascular System

Since cardiovascular disease is the primary cause of death among elderly people, deterioration in the performance of the heart and blood vessels has been regarded as the primary cause of aging. According to this hypothesis, aging results from the reduction in blood supply to critical organs, such as the brain and heart, which is based on the development of atherosclerosis. However, atherosclerosis is a disease process which also occurs in the young and many cause death at any age. Furthermore, aging occurs in many lower animal species where no blood vessels are present, e.g., fruit flies, rotifers, and nemotodes. Hence the hypothesis that aging is basically caused by a reduction in blood supply does not have general biological significance, even though it is an important cause of death among humans.

Thyroid

Since the thyroid gland is the primary regulator of metabolic rate in mammals, it too has been assigned a key role in aging since it was believed that metabolic rate, even at the cellular level, diminishes progressively with age. However, more detailed studies have shown that the age-related fall in basal metabolism is a reflection of tissue loss.[63] The oxygen consumption of individual cells does not change significantly with age. Other experiments have shown that the response of the thyroid gland to exogenous administration of thyroid-stimulating hormone is not influenced by the age of the subject.[64] Hence the theory that aging is due to failure of the thyroid gland must be rejected as untenable.

Gonads

Failure of both male and female sex glands to secrete adequate amounts of sex hormones has been a popular theory of aging in the past. There is, however, no experimental evidence to support this theory. The administration of testosterone and androgens to men and estrogens to women[65] to combat the effects of aging has had a long and stormy history. Although the administration of these hormones often relieves some of the aggravating symptoms that sometimes occur at the menopause, the effects are temporary and long-term administration has potential hazards,[66] especially that of stimulating cancer. There is no evidence that the sex glands play a key role in aging.

Immune System — Autoimmunity

The immune system protects the body not only against invading microorganisms, but also against atypical mutant cells which may form in the body. The production of antibodies reaches a peak in adolescence and then declines.[67]

One assumption is that the basic impairment in the immune system is a loss in the ability to recognize slight deviations in molecular structure and cellular characteristics so that cells which have undergone mutation and would ordinarily be destroyed by the immune system are no longer recognized, and are permitted to grow and develop to the detriment of the animal. Similarly, impairment of cell recognition ability might result in the development of antibodies which inactivate normal cells in various tissues.

It may also be hypothesized that even though recognition occurs, the immune system of the senescent animal is unable to produce an adequate supply of antibodies or phagocytic cells. Heidrick and Makinodan[68] have shown that in senescent mice the reduced production of antibodies and phagocytic cells is due to a fall in the rate of cell division in the stem cells. Thus the impairment in performance of the immune system has a cellular basis.

The autoimmune theory of aging[69,70] proposes that aging results from the production of antibodies which react with normal cells of the body and destroy them. This hypothesis gains its greatest support from the age-related increase of autoimmune antibodies bound in the blood,[70] and the similarity between the symptoms of many of the so-called autoimmune diseases and the phenomena of aging.[71]

Although evidence for the key role of the immune system in aging is still sketchy, the general hypothesis is an attractive one since it integrates some of the cellular theories, such as somatic mutations and error theories, with age changes in the responses of the total animal; it can be experimentally tested and deserves further investigation.

Physiological Control Mechanisms

It is now becoming apparent that the overall performance of an animal is closely related to the effectiveness of a variety of control mechanisms which regulate the interplay between different organs and tissues.[14,15] Frolkis[72] has advanced the hypothesis that aging and death of an animal is the result of failure of adaptive mechanisms. Since adaptation to environmental stresses involves the appropriate functioning of control mechanisms, the adaptation hypothesis can be considered as a special case of the broader theory of control mechanism failure or the breakdown of homeostasis.

In the mammal, primary control mechanisms to produce adaptive responses operate through the endocrine or nervous systems. Although relatively few studies on the specific effects of aging on control mechanisms have been carried out, there are a number of examples that indicate that this would be a fruitful approach.[14]

Endocrine Controls

Since the pituitary gland plays a control role in the modulation of activity of the adrenal gland, the thyroid, and the gonads, aging has been ascribed to failure of this gland to carry out its appropriate functions.[73] The extensive literature on the relation between aging and the pituitary gland has been recently summarized by Everitt and Burgess.[74] Many studies point to the importance of the pituitary in maintaining a variety of regulatory functions. In some instances, the age impairment in function is located in the target organ. For example, the response of the kidney to a standard amount of pituitary antidiuretic hormone is significantly less in the aged subject than in the young.[75]

With advancing age, the rate at which excess glucose is removed from the blood is significantly reduced.[76] The removal of the excess glucose is regulated primarily by the release of insulin from the pancreas. Extensive experiments have shown that the age deficit is due to the reduced sensitivity of the beta cells of the pancreas to a slight rise in blood glucose level.[77]

It is clear that endocrine control mechanisms play an important role in aging as seen in the intact animal.

Nervous System Controls

The nervous system also plays an important role in regulating many activities. Performances which require coordinated movements mediated through the nervous system show greater decrements with age than do component parts of the total performance. For example, maximum breathing capacity which requires coordinated muscular movements shows a significantly greater age decrement than does vital capacity.[78] Similarly, the age decrement in a coordinated exercise such as crank turning shows a greater age decrement than the static strength of the muscles involved in cranking.[79] Under normal circumstances, a rise in blood pressure results in a fall in heart rate. The response is mediated through the nervous system. When blood pressure was experimentally increased by 50 mm Hg in old and young rats by the continuous infusion of phenylephrine, the lowering of the heart rate was significantly less in the old than in the young animals.[80]

There is both clinical and experimental evidence to show that with advancing age the regulation of body temperature is less effective. Young subjects can maintain body temperature when the environmental temperature is either increased or decreased, whereas old subjects show a significant change.[81] Old subjects are also much more susceptible to heat stroke and hypothermia than are young.

The ability to perform muscular work requires the integrated activity of the nervous, cardiovascular, respiratory, and muscular systems. Many studies have shown that perhaps the greatest decrements with age lie in the area of exercise and maximum work performance.[82] Although age decrements are found in each of the organ systems involved, they are less than the decrements in total performance. It is clear that the coordination and integration of the responses of different organ systems plays an important role in aging.

SUMMARY

There are at present a number of theories of aging. However, even at the cellular level no single theory is able to account for all of the phenomena of aging. It is now clear that some of the theories are more probable than others. There is little doubt that each animal species has some genetic program which places a limit on its maximum life span, even though the mechanisms by which this genetic code operates is still not known. The cellular theories which seem most fruitful to pursue seem to be the codon-restriction hypothesis, the error theory, and the cross-linking theory.

In addition to cellular theories, it is also necessary to develop theories which will take into account interactions between cells as well as control mechanisms which regulate responses that require the integrated performance of different organ systems. At present the autoimmune hypothesis is one that holds great promise for the future. In addition, theories which focus their attention on regulatory mechanisms will do much to clarify the processes of aging as reflected in the performance and behavior of the total animal. It is extremely doubtful that a single theory can explain all of the aspects of aging. Aging is a highly complex phenomenon which will no doubt require different explanatory principles for different aspects of the process.

REFERENCES

1. **Shock, N. W.,** The physiology of aging, *Sci. Am.,* 206(1), 100, 1962.
2. **Shock, N. W.,** The biological basis of aging, in *Frontiers of Medicine,* Meade, G. M., Ed., Plenum Press, New York, 1977, 167.
3. **Davies, D. F. and Shock, N. W.,** Age changes in glomerular filtration rate, effective renal plasma flow, and tubular excretory capacity in adult males, *J. Clin. Invest.,* 29, 496, 1950.
4. **Arataki, M.,** The postnatal growth of the kidney, with special reference to the number and size of the glomeruli (albino rat), *Am. J. Anat.,* 36, 399, 1926.
5. **Shock, N. W.,** Age changes in physiological functions in the total animal: the role of tissue loss, in *The Biology of Aging,* Strehler, B. L., Ed., AIBS Publication No. 6, Washington, D.C., 1960, 258.
6. **Corsellis, J. A. N.,** Neuronal loss in the aging brain, *Proc. 10th Int. Congr. Gerontol.,* 1, 109, 1975.
7. **Brody, H. and Vijayashankar, N.,** Cell loss with aging, in *The Aging Brain and Senile Dementia,* Nandy, K. and Sherwin, I., Eds., Plenum Press, New York, 1977, 15.
8. **Andrew, W., Shock, N. W., Barrows, C. H., Jr., et al.,** Correlation of age changes in histological and chemical characteristics in some tissues of the rat, *J. Gerontol.,* 14, 405, 1959.
9. **Hayflick, L.,** The cellular basis for biological aging, in *Handbook of the Biology of Aging,* Finch, C. E. and Hayflick, L., Eds., Van Nostrand Reinhold, New York, 1977, 159.
10. **Hayflick, L.,** The cell biology of aging, *J. Invest. Dermatol.,* 73, 8, 1979.
11. **Shock, N. W.,** Biological theories of aging, in *Handbook of the Psychology of Aging,* Birren, J. E. and Schaie, K. W., Eds., Van Nostrand Reinhold, New York, 1977, 103.
12. **Shock, N. W.,** Physiological theories of aging, in *Theoretical Aspects of Aging,* Rockstein, M., Ed., Academic Press, New York, 1974, 119.
13. **Beutow, D. E.,** Cellular content and cellular proliferation changes in the tissues and organs of the aging mammal, in *Cellular and Molecular Renewal in the Mammalian Body,* Cameron, I. L. and Thrasher, J. D., Eds., Academic Press, New York, 1971, 87.
14. **Shock, N. W.,** Systems integration in *Handbook of the Biology of Aging,* Finch, C. E. and Hayflick, L., Eds., Van Nostrand Reinhold, New York, 1977, chap. 25.
15. **Shock, N. W.,** Systems physiology and aging: introduction, *Fed. Proc.,* 38, 161, 1979.
16. **Comfort, A.,** *The Biology of Senescence,* 3rd ed., Elsevier, New York, 1979.
17. **Maynard-Smith, J.,** Review lectures on senescence: the causes of aging, *Proc. R. Soc. Biol. Sci.,* 157, 115, 1962.
18. **Goldstein, S.,** Human genetic disorders that feature premature onset and accelerated progression of biological aging, in *The Genetics of Aging,* Schneider, E. L., Ed., Plenum Press, New York, chap. 7.
19. **Martin, G. M., Sprague, C. A., and Epstein, C. J.,** Replicative life span of cultivated human cells; effect of donor's age, tissue, and genotype, *Lab. Invest,* 23, 86, 1970.
20. **Dublin, L. I.,** *Length of Life: A Stůdy of the Life Table,* Ronald Press, New York, 1949, 379.
21. **Watson, J. D.,** *The Double Helix,* New American Library, New York, 1969, 143.
22. **Kunungo, M. S.,** A model for aging, *J. Theor. Biol.,* 53, 253, 1975.
23. **Strehler, B. L.,** Implications of aging research for society, *Fed. Proc.,* 34, 5, 1975.
24. **Strehler, B. L.,** *Time, Cells and Aging,* 2nd ed., Academic Press, New York, 1977.
25. **von Hahn, H. P.,** Failures of regulation mechanisms as causes of cellular aging, in *Advances in Gerontological Research,* Vol. 3, Strehler, B. L., Ed., Academic Press, New York, 1971, 1.
26. **Sacher, G. A.,** Life table modification and life prolongation, in *Handbook of the Biology of Aging,* Finch, C. E. and Hayflick, L., Eds., Van Nostrand Reinhold, New York, 1977, chap. 24.
27. **Walburg, H. W., Jr.,** Radiation-induced life-shortening and premature aging, *Adv. Radiat. Biol.,* 5, 145, 1975.
28. **Curtis, H. J.,** *Biological Mechanisms of Aging,* Charles C Thomas, Springfield, Ill., 1966, 133.
29. **Szilard, L.,** On the nature of the aging process, *Proc. Natl. Acad. Sci. U.S.A.,* 45, 30, 1959.
30. **Maynard-Smith, J.,** Theories of aging, in *Topics in the Biology of Aging,* Krohn, P. L., Ed., Interscience, New York, 1966, 1.
31. **Hart, R. W. and Setlow, R. B.,** Correlation between deoxyribonucleic acid excision repair and life span in a number of mammalian species, *Proc. Natl. Acad. Sci. U.S.A.,* 71, 2169, 1974.
32. **Wheeler, K. T. and Lett, J. T.,** On the possibility that DNA repair is related to age in nondividing cells, *Proc. Natl. Acad. Sci. U.S.A.,* 71, 1892, 1974.
33. **Tice, R. R.,** Aging and DNA repair capability, in *The Genetics of Aging,* Schneider, E. L., Ed., Plenum Press, New York, 1978, 53.
34. **Medvedev, Z. A.,** Repetition of molecular-genetic information as a possible factor in evolutionary changes in life span, *Exp. Gerontol.,* 7, 517, 1972.

35. **Cutler, R. G.,** Redundancy of information content in the genome of mammalian species as a protective mechanism determining aging rate, *Mech. Ageing Dev.*, 2, 381, 1974.
36. **Medvedev, Z. A.,** The molecular processes of aging, *Sowjetwiss Naturwiss, Beitr.*, 12, 1273, 1961.
37. **Medvedev, Z. A.,** The nucleic acids in development and aging, in *Advances in Gerontological Research,* Vol. 1, Strehler, B. L., Ed., Academic Press, New York, 1964, 181.
38. **Orgel, L. E.,** The maintenance of the accuracy of protein synthesis and its relevance to aging, *Proc. Natl. Acad. Sci. U.S.A.*, 49, 517, 1963.
39. **Orgel, L. E.,** Aging of clones of mammalian cells, *Nature (London)*, 243, 441, 1973.
40. **Harrison, B. J. and Holliday, R.,** Senescence and the fidelity of protein synthesis in *Drosophila, Nature (London)*, 213, 990, 1967.
41. **Holliday, R. and Tarrant, G. M.,** Altered enzymes in aging human fibroblasts, *Nature (London)*, 238, 26, 1972.
42. **Lamb, M. J.,** *Biology of Aging,* John Wiley & Sons, New York, 1977.
43. **Gershon, H. and Gershon, D.,** Altered enzyme molecules in senescent organisms: mouse muscle aldolase, *Mech. Ageing Dev.*, 2, 33, 1973.
44. **Sacher, G. A.,** Abnutzungstheorie, in *Perspectives in Experimental Gerontology,* Shock, N. W., Ed., Charles C Thomas, Springfield, Ill., 1966, chap. 26.
45. **Loeb, J. and Northrup, J. H.,** On the influence of food and temperature on the duration of life, *J. Biol. Chem.*, 32, 103, 1917.
46. **Strehler, B. L.,** Further studies on the thermally induced aging of *Drosophila melanogaster, J. Gerontol.*, 17, 347, 1962.
47. **Fanestil, D. D. and Barrows, C. H., Jr.,** Aging in the rotifer, *J. Gerontol.*, 20, 462, 1965.
48. **Brock, M. A. and Strehler, B. L.,** Studies on the comparative physiology of aging. IV. Age and mortality of some marine *Cnidaria* in laboratory, *J. Gerontol.*, 18, 23, 1963.
49. **Pearl, R.,** *The Rate of Living,* Knopf, New York, 1928.
50. **Sohol, R. S.,** Metabolic rate and life span, in *Interdisciplinary Topics in Gerontology,* Vol. 9, Cutler, R. G., Ed., S. Karger, Basel, 1976, 25.
51. **Sacher, G. A.,** Evaluation of the entropy and information terms governing mammalian longevity, in *Interdisciplinary Topics in Gerontology,* Vol. 9, Cutler, R. G., Ed., S. Karger, Basel, 1976, 69.
52. **Sacher, G. A.,** Longevity, aging, and death: an evolutionary perspective, *Gerontologist,* 18, 112, 1978.
53. **Sacher, G. A.,** Evolution of longevity and survival characteristics in mammals, in *The Genetics of Aging,* Schneider, E. L., Ed., Plenum Press, New York, 1978, 151.
54. **Carpenter, D. G. and Loynd, J. A.,** An integrated theory of aging, *J. Am. Geriatr. Soc.*, 16, 1307, 1968.
55. **Carrel, A. and Ebeling, A. H.,** Antagonistic growth principles of serum and their relation to old age, *J. Exp. Med.*, 38, 419, 1923.
56. **Strehler, B. L.,** On the histochemistry and ultrastructure of age pigment, in *Advances in Gerontological Research,* Vol. 1, Strehler, B. L., Ed., Academic Press, New York, 1964, 343.
57. **Harman, D.,** Free radical theory of aging: effect of free radical reaction inhibitors on the mortality rate of male LAF mice, *J. Gerontol.*, 23, 476, 1968.
58. **McCay, C. M.,** Chemical aspects of aging and the effect of diet upon aging, in *Cowdry's Problems of Aging,* 3rd ed., Lansing, A. I., Ed., Williams & Wilkins, Baltimore, 1952, 139.
59. **Bjorksten, J.,** The crosslinkage theory of aging, *J. Am. Geriatr. Soc.*, 16, 408, 1968.
60. **Verzâr, F.,** *Lectures on Experimental Gerontology,* Charles C Thomas, Springfield, Ill., 1963, 128.
61. **Kohn, R. R.,** *Principles of Mammalian Aging,* Prentice-Hall, Englewood Cliffs, N.J., 1978, 240.
62. **Bjorksten, J.,** Crosslinkage and the aging process, in *Theoretical Aspects of Aging,* Rockstein, M., Ed., Academic Press, New York, 1974, 43.
63. **Shock, N. W.,** Metabolism and age, *J. Chronic Dis.*, 2, 687, 1955.
64. **Baker, S. P., Gaffney, G. W., Shock, N. W., and Landowne, M.,** Physiological responses of five middle-aged and elderly men to repeated administration of thryoid-stimulating hormone (thyrotropin: TSH), *J. Gerontol.*, 14, 37, 1959.
65. **McGrady, P. M., Jr.,** *The Youth Doctors,* Coward McCann, New York, 1968, 352.
66. **Ryan, K. J. and Gibson, D. C., Eds.,** Menopause and Aging, Department of Health, Education and Welfare Publ. (NIH) No. 73-319, U.S. Government Printing Office, Washington, D.C., 1973, 125.
67. **Makinodan, T. and Yunis, E., Eds.,** *Immunology and Aging,* Plenum Press, New York, 1977, 208.
68. **Heidrick, M. L. and Makinodan, T.,** Nature of cellular deficiencies in age-related decline of the immune system, *Gerontologia,* 18, 305, 1972.
69. **Blumenthal, H. T. and Berns, A. W.,** Autoimmunity and aging, in *Advances in Gerontological Research,* Vol. 1, Strehler, B. L., Ed., Academic Press, New York, 1964, 289.
70. **Walford, R. L.,** *The Immunologic Theory of Aging,* Williams & Wilkins, Baltimore, 1969, 248.
71. **Burnet, F. M.,** *Immunology, Aging and Cancer,* W. H. Freeman & Company, San Francisco, 1976, 162.

72. **Frolkis, V. V.,** Regulatory process in the mechanisms of aging, *Exp. Gerontol.,* 3, 113, 1968.
73. **Dilman, V. M.,** The hypothalamic control of aging and age-associated pathology: the elevation mechanism of aging, in *Hypothalamus, Pituitary and Aging,* Everitt, A. V. and Burgess, J. A., Eds., Charles C. Thomas, Springfield, Ill., 1976, chap. 32.
74. **Everitt, A. V. and Burgess, J. A., Eds.,** *Hypothalamus, Pituitary and Aging,* Charles C Thomas, Springfield, Ill., 1976, 797.
75. **Miller, J. H. and Shock, N. W.,** Age differences in the renal tubular response to antidiuretic hormone, *J. Gerontol.,* 8, 446, 1953.
76. **Silverstone, F. A., Brandfonbrener, M., Shock, N. W., and Yiengst, M. J., et al.,** Age differences in the intravenous glucose tolerance test and the response to insulin, *J. Clin. Invest.,* 36, 504, 1957.
77. **Andres, R., Swerdloff, R., and Tobin, J. D.,** The effects of age on plasma insulin response to hyperglycemia: studies in man with a servo-control technique, in *Proc. 8th Int. Congr. Gerontol.,* Vol. 1, Federation of American Societies for Experimental Biology, Bethesda, Md., 1969, 36.
78. **Norris, A. H., Shock, N. W., Landowne, M., et al.,** Pulmonary function studies: age differences in lung volumes and bellows function, *J. Gerontol.,* 11, 379, 1956.
79. **Shock, N. W. and Norris, A. H.,** Neuromuscular coordination as a factor in age changes in muscular exercise, in *Medicine and Sport, Vol. 4,* Physical Activity and Aging, Brunner, D. and Jokl, E., Eds., S. Karger, Basel, 1970.
80. **Rothbaum, D. A., Shaw, D. J., Angell, C. S., and Shock, N. W.,** Age differences in the baroreceptor response of rats, *J. Gerontol.,* 29, 488, 1974.
81. **Krag, C. L. and Kountz, W. B.,** Stability of body temperature in the aged. I. Effect of the exposure of the body to cold, *J. Gerontol.,* 5, 227, 1950; II. Effect of exposure of the body to heat, *J. Gerontol.,* 7, 61, 1952.
82. **Norris, A. H. and Shock, N. W.,** Exercise in the adult years, in *Science and Medicine of Exercise and Sport,* 2nd ed., Johnson, W. R. and Buskirk, E. R., Eds., Harper & Row, New York, 1974, chap. 26.

Index

INDEX

A

Adenosine triphosphatase (ATPase)
 in human arteries, 168
 myofibrillar, see Myofibrillar ATPase
 myosin, see Myosin ATPase
 Na^+K^+, see Na^+K^+-ATPase
 in rat heart, 165, 166
 in rat liver, 180
 in rat muscle, 185
Adenosine triphosphate (ATP)
 ratio to ADP
  in rat heart muscle slices, 139
  in rat muscle, 143

B

C

D

E

F

G

H

I

K

L

M

N

O

P

Q

R

S

T

U

V

W

X

Z